Current Aspects of the Neurosciences

Volume 3

Current Aspects
of the Neurosciences

Volume 3

Edited by
Neville N. Osborne

Nuffield Laboratory of Ophthalmology
University of Oxford, UK

M
MACMILLAN
PRESS
Scientific & Medical

First published 1991

Published by
THE MACMILLAN PRESS LTD
Houndmills, Basingstoke, Hampshire RG21 2XS
and London
Companies and representatives
throughout the world

Filmset by Wearside Tradespools, Fulwell, Sunderland

Printed in Great Britain by WBC Print Ltd, Bridgend, Mid Glam.

British Library Cataloguing in Publication Data
Current aspects of the neurosciences.
Vol. 3
1. Man. Nervous system. Diseases
I. Osborne, Neville N. (Neville Nahash), *1942–*
616.8
ISSN 0956–4632
ISBN 0–333–54833–7

Contents

Preface

Most of the chapters in this volume of *Current Aspects of the Neurosciences* deal with molecular neurobiology and/or receptor analysis. This is consistent with the original aims of the series, which is to highlight new and fast-moving areas in neuroresearch.

The variety of approaches used to understand receptor function is illustrated. To study the localization of receptors, it is possible to use immunohistochemistry and autoradiography as well as *in situ* hybridization procedures. Binding studies and second-messenger analysis can also be used to provide detailed information about the pharmacology and characterization of receptor subtypes, while molecular biology application provides a means of elucidating receptor structures as well as supplying unambiguous data regarding subtypes of receptors as separate entities. Chapters dealing with all of these aspects are provided in this volume, thus giving the reader a balanced view of present-day research in this area.

The use of pharmacological agents to treat various forms of disease is of major importance and continues to be a major research area. This can effectively be done, however, if procedures are available to measure transmitter release/turnover in the *in situ* state. Chapter 2 has a direct bearing here, because it deals with the most recent of procedures available for providing a means of studying the turnover rate of the transmitter serotonin in the *in situ* state. Only with such methodology will it be possible ultimately to determine the effective clinical use of a drug.

Oxford, May 1990   N.N.O.

1

Molecular Neuroanatomy of Neurotransmitter Receptors: The Use of *in situ* Hybridization Histochemistry for the Study of Their Anatomical and Cellular Localization

M. T. VILARÓ, M. I. MARTINEZ-MIR, M. SARASA,
M. POMPEIANO, J. M. PALACIOS and G. MENGOD*

Preclinical Research, Sandoz Pharma Ltd, CH 4002 Basel, Switzerland
* To whom correspondence should be addressed

Contents

Current Aspects of the Neurosciences, Vol. 3. Edited by N. N. Osborne. © The Macmillan Press Ltd 1991

1.   Introduction

The concept of neurotransmitter receptor is now nearly a hundred years old. It was proposed initially by Ehrlich and Langley, to explain the mechanism of action of some drugs. The extreme selectivity of some cellular components to recognize members of a given chemical family led these investigators to propose that a 'receptive substance' or 'receptor' existed (Parascandola, 1980). It was not until the 1930s, with the work of A. J. Clark, that the first quantitative expression of drug–receptor interactions was provided (Brimble-combe, 1974). Since then, the receptor concept has developed and those 'receptive substances' are today known to be actual molecules. Initially, receptors were defined operationally in preparations of isolated organs by the differential response of those organs to series of drugs belonging to different chemical classes. It was through using this kind of preparation that the difference between muscarinic and nicotinic and between alpha and beta adrenergic receptors was found and the existence of these subtypes was proposed. With the introduction of radiolabelled molecules at the beginning of the 1970s, it was possible directly to label the receptor molecules in cell-free preparations, particularly in membranes. Little by little, the receptors were assuming a molecular aspect and, to quote E. J. Ariëns (1979), evolved 'from fiction to fact'. Thanks to the development of more and more selective compounds, it was possible to isolate the first receptor proteins. All this work has culminated in the last few years in the isolation and molecular cloning of the genes or cDNAs coding for many of these neurotransmitter receptors. The goal of the present review is to examine the impact that this progress in our understanding of the molecular nature of the receptors has had on our knowledge of neurotransmitter receptor localization.

2.   Classes of Neurotransmitter Receptor

Cloning of the genes that code for several neurotransmitter receptors has revealed the existence of two large superfamilies of receptors (Hall, 1987; Stevens, 1987). The characteristics of these two classes of receptors are summarized in Table 1.

One of these superfamilies, the so-called class I neurotransmitter receptors (Barnard *et al.*, 1987), includes a variety of receptors which constitute ion channels. The prototype of these ligand-gated ion channels is the nicotinic acetylcholine receptor (nAChR). Other members of the group are $GABA_A$, kainate (a glutamate receptor) and glycine receptors. These ligand-gated ion channels consist of several different subunits, which combine to form the ion channel. A common characteristic of all the subunits cloned so far is the occurrence of four hydrophobic amino acid stretches which are long enough to span the membrane, thus representing putative transmembrane helices. High degrees of sequence homology exist between the different subunits of a

Table 1 Characteristics of the two classes of neurotransmitter receptor (NTR)

Class I NTR	*Class II NTR*
Oligomeric glycoproteins (about 5 subunits)	Monomeric glycoproteins
4 transmembrane helices per subunit	7 transmembrane helices
Ligand-gated ion channels	Coupled to guanine nucleotide regulatory proteins
Cloned members 　Nicotinic cholinergic 　　muscle: $\alpha 1, \beta 1, \gamma, \delta, \epsilon$ 　　neuronal: $\alpha 2, \alpha 3, \alpha 4, \alpha 5, \beta 2, \beta 3, \beta 4$ 　GABA$_A$: $\alpha 1, \alpha 2, \alpha 3, \alpha 4, \beta 1, \beta 2, \beta 3,$ 　　$\gamma 2, \delta$ 　Glycine: 48 kD subunit 　Kainate: GluRK1	Cloned members 　Adrenergic: $\alpha_{1A}, \alpha_{1B}, \alpha_{2A}, \alpha_{2B}, \beta_1, \beta_2,$ 　　β_3 　Muscarinic cholinergic: *m1, m2, m3,* 　　*m4, m5* 　Serotonin: 5-HT$_{1A}$, 5-HT$_{1C}$, 5-HT$_2$ 　Dopamine: D2 (long and short forms) 　Angiotensin (*mas* oncogene) 　Tachykinins: SPR (substance P) 　　　　　　　(NK$_1$) 　　　　　　SKR (neurokinin A or 　　　　　　　substance K) (NK$_2$) 　　　　　　NKR (neurokinin B or 　　　　　　　neuromedin K) (NK$_3$)
Expected members 　Serotonin 5-HT$_3$ 　Other glutamate receptors (NMDA, 　　AMPA)	Expected members 　Adrenergic: α_{2C} 　Serotonin: 5-HT$_{1B}$, 5-HT$_{1D}$, 5-HT$_4$ 　Dopamine: D1 　Histamine: H$_1$, H$_2$, H$_3$ 　GABA$_B$ 　Neuropeptides: opiate receptors, 　　　　　　　CCK, somatostatin, 　　　　　　　NPY, neurotensin, 　　　　　　　etc.

given receptor and also between subunits of different receptors. However, it should be mentioned that the recently cloned kainate receptor (Gregor *et al.*, 1989; Hollmann *et al.*, 1989; Wada *et al.*, 1989), a member of the glutamate receptor family, does not show significant overall homology with any of the multiple subunits cloned for nAChRs, GABA$_A$ or glycine receptors.

The other superfamily of neurotransmitter receptors (class II) comprises receptors which are coupled to GTP binding proteins (G-proteins) which are, in turn, coupled to enzymes catalysing the synthesis of intracellular second messengers (Dohlman *et al.*, 1987). The first member of this family to be cloned was the β_2-adrenergic receptor, and subsequently a variety of other receptors have been cloned and shown to belong to this family—namely α-adrenergic, muscarinic cholinergic (MChR), several subtypes of serotonin (5-HT) receptors, dopamine D2, angiotensin and tachykinin receptors. All these receptors are monomeric glycoproteins whose hydropathicity profiles reveal the presence of seven hydrophobic domains (Hall, 1987). This kind of profile has also been described for bacteriorhodopsin and rhodopsin (Ovchinnikov, 1982). Electron diffraction studies indicate that bacteriorhodopsin contains seven α-helical rods spanning the membrane (Henderson and Unwin, 1975). Thus, on the basis of similar hydropathicity profiles and a certain amino acid sequence homology, the existence of seven putative transmembrane domains has also been proposed for rhodopsin and the G-protein-coupled family of neurotransmitter receptors. The amino terminal region of the receptor molecules is situated on the extracellular side of the membrane, whereas the carboxy terminus is on the cytoplasmic side. A longer third cytoplasmic loop connecting transmembrane segments V and VI is also a common characteristic of all the receptors belonging to this superfamily. The highest degrees of sequence homology between the members of a given receptor family (e.g. MChRs), as well as between members of different families, are found in the transmembrane regions, which have been proposed to constitute the ligand binding domain. In contrast, little or no homology is observed at the amino and carboxy terminal regions, which may, respectively, be involved in glycosylation and phosphorylation of the receptor proteins. Similarly, the third cytoplasmic loop is unique to each receptor subtype and it has been shown to be important for the coupling of the receptors to G proteins (O'Dowd *et al.*, 1989). The first members of this family that were cloned (i.e. β-adrenergic, MChRs, 5-HT$_{1A}$) were devoid of introns in their coding regions (O'Dowd *et al.*, 1989). Thus, it was thought that this could be a common characteristic of the members of this superfamily of receptors. However, recent studies have shown that this is not the case for the rat and human dopamine D2 receptors (Dal Toso *et al.*, 1989; Giros *et al.*, 1989; Grandy *et al.*, 1989; Monsma *et al.*, 1989; Selbie *et al.*, 1989; Chio *et al.*, 1990), and for the mouse 5-HT$_{1C}$ and rat 5-HT$_2$ receptors (Lübbert *et al.*, 1990).

In view of the results obtained in the multiple cloning studies reported so far, it becomes apparent that most of the subtype diversity observed within neurotransmitter receptor families emerges from the existence of various distinct genes which code for different receptor subtypes (Schofield *et al.*, 1990). However, other mechanisms can also contribute to the generation of diversity. Thus, for class I neurotransmitter receptors, their multisubunit structure offers the possibility of multiple combinations of the existing gene products to form functional receptors with specific properties. This has been shown to be the case for muscle nicotinic receptors, in which the adult form results from the substitution of an embryonic γ subunit with the adult ε subunit (Mishina *et al.*, 1986). Whether or not this is a widespread mechanism actually occurring in other systems is difficult to establish at present. Another means of generating heterogeneity within a given family of receptors is by alternative splicing of exons contained in a gene. In this case, receptors belonging to both classes seem to use this source of variability: the glycine receptor (see Schofield *et al.*, 1990) and the nicotinic receptor (Goldman *et al.*, 1987) from class I, and the dopamine D2 receptor (Dal Toso *et al.*, 1989;

Giros *et al.*, 1989; Grandy *et al.*, 1989; Monsma *et al.*, 1989; Selbie *et al.*, 1989; Chio *et al.*, 1990) from class II.

3. *Visualization of Neurotransmitter Receptors in Brain: Contribution of* in situ *Hybridization Histochemistry*

Receptor Autoradiography and Immunohistochemistry

The brain is an organ of great anatomical, cellular and connective complexity. Therefore, the understanding of many aspects of brain function requires the use of techniques affording a high degree of anatomical and cellular resolution. This is the case in the study of neurotransmitter receptor distribution. Historically, the first technique to be used for the visualization of the distribution of neurotransmitter receptors at the light microscopic level was receptor autoradiography or radioligand binding autoradiography (Kuhar *et al.*, 1986). The development of ligands with high affinity for a given receptor, and which can be radioactively labelled to high specific activities, has provided a wealth of information on the distribution and pharmacological characteristics of many of these receptors. With the combination of receptor autoradiography and computer-assisted image analysis systems, it is now possible to quantitate receptor densities on discrete brain areas, with a high degree of anatomical precision. This technique has been extensively used both in experimental animals and in human post-mortem tissues, allowing in the latter case the study of alterations in the distribution and densities of receptors caused by neurological diseases or drug treatment (Palacios *et al.*, 1986).

However, receptor autoradiography has a number of limitations, the most important one probably being the limited level of cellular resolution. This is related to the use of radioactively labelled ligands and photographic emulsions, since a certain degree of radiation scattering is inevitable. As a consequence, it is not possible in most cases to define the cell type which contains the receptor or to determine the pre- or postsynaptic location of the receptors. In some cases this problem can be solved in part by the combination of receptor autoradiography with selective cellular lesions. If receptor changes are observed in the lesioned animals, it is possible to draw conclusions about the localization of the receptors to particular cell populations. With the development of irreversible ligands for some neurotransmitter receptors, electron microscopy has been applied to the autoradiographic localization of these receptors (Hamel and Beaudet, 1984), but the level of resolution is still too low to assign silver grains to particular subcellular structures.

Another limitation of receptor autoradiography is the often limited specificity of the ligands used, particularly when different subtypes of receptors for a single neurotransmitter exist. Several of the available ligands are not selective enough to distinguish clearly one subtype from the others, making it difficult to determine the anatomical localization of the different subtypes.

The purification of the receptor molecules for some neurotransmitters has made possible the development of both polyclonal and monoclonal antibodies against some of these receptors. These antibodies have been used for the immunohistochemical visualization of receptors. Higher levels of cellular resolution are achieved with this technique, since several problems inherent to receptor autoradiography—namely ligand diffusion and radiation scatter—are not encountered with the use of antibodies (Richards *et al.*, 1987). However, when enzymatic reactions are used to visualize the primary antibody, a certain diffusion of the reaction products may occur. Electron microscopy has also been applied to the immunocytochemical localization of the receptors, and it has been possible to assign them to pre- and/or postsynaptic membranes (Richards *et al.*, 1987). Thus, a more detailed cellular and subcellular localization of neurotransmitter receptors can be achieved with immunohistochemical techniques. Monoclonal antibodies have also the theoretical advantage of being more selective than some receptor ligands. Despite the above-mentioned advantages of the immunohistochem-ical approach, it has an important drawback: accurate quantification, which has become relatively straightforward with receptor autoradiography, is at present difficult to achieve with the use of antibodies.

In situ Hybridization Histochemistry (ISHH)

Following the cloning and sequencing of the gene or cDNA coding for a neurotransmitter receptor, the possibility immediately arises of obtaining or synthesizing molecular probes that allow the detection and visualization of the mRNA coding for that receptor. Thus, a third technique can now be applied to the study of receptor distribution—i.e. *in situ* hybridization histochemistry (ISHH). This approach is certainly an invaluable tool in the study of the distribution of the different subtypes of receptors for a given neurotransmitter, since very often there are no specific ligands or antibodies available which can distinguish between the various subtypes.

Methodological Considerations

In order to detect the mRNA of interest, three different kinds of probes can be used: complementary DNA (cDNA), RNA and oligonucleotide.

cDNA and RNA probes can only be produced if one has access to the cloned cDNA or gene coding for the neurotransmitter receptor. cDNA probes are usually obtained by restriction enzyme digestion and subcloning of chosen regions of the gene and subsequent labelling by nick-translation or random-priming methods. The labelling of RNA probes involves subcloning of the desired fragment of the gene or cDNA into a plasmid transcription system. Single-stranded RNA probes complementary to the mRNA of interest can be then obtained upon transcription by the appropriate RNA polymerase in the presence of radioactively labelled ribonucleotides. (For further details of and considerations relating to these kinds of probes, see Coghlan *et al.*, 1985; Angerer *et al.*, 1987; Tecott *et al.*, 1987; Watson *et al.*, 1987.)

Oligonucleotide probes are single-stranded, synthetic DNA fragments which are designed to hybridize with the mRNA of interest. In our laboratory we favour the use of this type of probe for many reasons: they are fast and easy to obtain, providing access to a DNA synthesizer is available, and do not require long cloning and subcloning steps. Obviously, however, their design requires that the receptor mRNA sequence be published or available from the investigators who actually cloned the receptor gene or cDNA. The end-labelling and purification of oligonucleotide probes is also a relatively easy and fast procedure which yields probes with high specific activities. Perhaps the greatest advantage of using oligonucleotide probes is the possibility of obtaining probes highly specific for the mRNA of interest. This is especially important when multiple subtypes of receptors exist for a given neurotransmitter, since synthetic oligonucleotides can be designed to hybridize with regions of the mRNA which share very little or no identity among the different subtypes. In this way, probes which will recognize only one of the mRNA subtypes can be obtained and used to map the expression of the various subtypes. Moreover, in the case of some neurotransmitter receptor genes which may generate two receptor protein isoforms via alternative splicing, oligonucleotide probes can be designed in such a way that they recognize exclusively either the mRNA species lacking the spliceable sequences or the species containing them. This allows spatial and/or developmental patterns of expression of the different splice variants to be studied.

Another advantage of oligonucleotide probes is that they allow a number of precise control experiments to be performed in order to assess the specificity of the hybridization signal obtained. It is important to ascertain the specificity of the oligonucleotide probe itself by performing Northern analysis with RNA extracted from different regions of the brain. The RNA detected should be of a size corresponding to that originally described, if this information is available, and with a regional distribution in agreement with the pattern observed in ISHH experiments. For each mRNA analysed, at least two oligonucleotides complementary to different regions of the mRNA should be synthesized and used separately as hybridization probes in consecutive tissue sections. The hybridization pattern obtained must be the same for both probes, after similar exposure times. Competition or cohybridization studies should be carried out: specific hybridization signals are not observed when an excess of unlabelled oligonucleotide is included in the hybridization solution, the remaining signal giving an idea of the background levels. No alteration of the specific signal should be observed when the unlabelled oligonucleotide added in excess is complementary to a different region of the mRNA or to an equivalent region of a related mRNA—e.g. a different receptor subtype belonging to the same family. Different patterns of hybridization in serial sections with probes for related but different mRNAs—i.e. different subtypes of the same family—further supports the specificity of the signal. The thermal stability of the hybrids should be studied during, for example, the washing steps. A sharp decrease in the intensity of the hybridization signal should be observed at a temperature consistent with the theoretical T_m of the hybrids (the temperature at which 50% of the hybrids dissociate) (see Watson *et al.*, 1987; Lewis *et al.*, 1988).

If specific antibodies or selective ligands exist for a given receptor, further confirmation of the specificity of the hybridization signal can be obtained by performing immunohistochemistry or receptor autoradiography on sections consecutive to those used for ISHH. However, it should be borne in mind that ISHH permits the visualization of the perikarya which synthesize the neurotransmitter receptor, whereas both receptor autoradiography and immunohistochemistry uncover the final localization of the receptor polypeptides themselves, which can also be localized in the soma but which are generally transported to dendrites or axons and, therefore, distant from the cell bodies. This is an important fact to take into account when ISSH is used together with receptor autoradiography or immunohistochemistry to map the expression of neurotransmitter receptors in brain. Receptors found in a given nucleus may be synthesized by cells intrinsic to this nucleus, resulting in an overlap of the signal patterns obtained with ISHH and receptor autoradiography or immunohistochemistry. But it is often the case that receptors visualized in one nucleus are synthesized by afferents to this nucleus which may have the cell bodies located in distant brain areas. Then, the patterns of signal will be complementary rather than overlapping, an example being the primary sensory neurons in spinal ganglion that synthesize $GABA_A$ receptor isoforms; the receptors are then transported to afferent terminals in the spinal cord (Persohn *et al.*, 1990).

Limitations of *in situ* Hybridization Histochemistry

Despite its multiple advantages, ISHH is not devoid of limitations. The use of radioactive isotopes makes ISHH a hazardous and expensive methodology. A number of non-radioactive detection methods, which take advantage of enzymatic reactions or antibodies in order to detect the hybridized probe, have been applied to ISHH (Singer *et al.*, 1987). Although this approach obviates radiation hazards, the sensitivity of these non-isotopic methods is lower than that of conventional isotopic procedures. In the case of highly abundant mRNAs, this reduced sensitivity may not represent a problem. However, when dealing with transcripts of low or very low abundance (which seems to be the case for neurotransmitter receptors when compared with, for example, neuropeptides), the sensitivity of the method can be crucial in detecting those transcripts. Nevertheless, the combination of isotopic and non-isotopic probes in the same tissue section could provide a valuable approach to the study of the colocalization of various neurotransmitter receptor mRNAs to the same cell population.

Another limitation of ISHH is related to the fact that it gives an idea of the abundance of transcripts for a neurotransmitter receptor but not of the actual number of receptor molecules themselves. Translation rates may vary for the different mRNAs, as well as turnover rates for the different receptor proteins, and, therefore, a low number of transcripts could result in a high number of receptor proteins, and vice versa. For this reason, ISHH studies should be complemented, whenever possible, with receptor autoradiography or immunohistochemistry.

Finally, an exact quantification of transcripts in terms of, for example, 'number of mRNA molecules per cell' is still difficult to achieve at present. However, relative quantitative estimates can be obtained by microdensitometrical measurements of the autoradiograms.

4. *Class I Neurotransmitter Receptors:* In situ *Hybridization Histochemistry Studies*

As mentioned above, one of the characteristics of the receptors of class I is that they are made up by the combination of several subunits into a ligand-activated channel. These receptors appear to be extraordinarily diverse, owing to at least two different mechanisms: multiplicity of isoforms of the different subunits (see Table 1) and variety in the combination of chains. An additional complication arises from the absence of reliable information on the specific subunits being recognized by the available ligands, and even antibodies. Studies on nAChRs and $GABA_A$ receptors illustrate the problems arising from the great diversity of subunits detected in these two groups.

Nicotinic Acetylcholine Receptors

The nAChR is probably the neurotransmitter receptor best characterized at present. Studies on nAChRs have been favoured by the existence of a very rich natural source of these receptors: the electric organ of electric fishes such as *Torpedo californica* and *T. marmorata*. This led to the purification and partial amino acid sequencing of nAChRs from those organs. Synthetic oligonucleotides based on those peptide sequences were used to clone the different subunits of the nAChRs from electric organs (for reviews see Hucho, 1986; McCarthy *et al.*, 1986; Maelicke, 1988). Similarly, nAChRs from mammalian muscle have been purified and several subunits have been cloned from different species (see Maelicke, 1988), showing high similarity to those from electric fishes. nAChRs from electric organs and muscle are pentameric and contain four different types of subunits with the stoichiometry $\alpha_2\beta\gamma\delta$ (see Hucho, 1986; Maelicke, 1988). Neuronal nAChRs have different properties from those of muscle and electric organ. Purified nAChRs from chicken (Whiting and Lindstrom, 1986) and rat (Whiting and Lindstrom, 1987) brain were shown to contain two types of subunit, α and β, with probable stoichiometry of $\alpha_2\beta_2$ or $\alpha_3\beta_2$. These receptors do not bind α-bungarotoxin, a specific probe for muscle and electric organ nAChRs. Additionally, an α-bungarotoxin binding component has also been purified from rat brain (Whiting and Lindstrom, 1987) and has been shown to consist of four types of subunit with apparent molecular weights very similar to those of the four subunits from muscle and electric organ receptors. The physiological relevance of this α-bungarotoxin binding component is unclear.

A number of cDNA and genomic clones have been isolated which code for different α and β subunits in the CNS, thus suggesting the existence of a family of related nAChRs in mammalian brain. Four distinct neuronal α subunit genes have been isolated, which are related to the $\alpha 1$ gene encoding the α subunit found in muscle nAChRs: $\alpha 2$, isolated from rat brain (Wada *et al.*, 1988); $\alpha 3$, obtained from the PC12 cell line (Boulter *et al.*, 1986); and $\alpha 4$, isolated from cDNA libraries from rat hypothalamus and hippocampus (Goldman *et al.*, 1987). In chick brain $\alpha 2$, $\alpha 3$, $\alpha 4$ and non-alpha subunits have also been identified (Nef *et al.*, 1988). As for the β subunit, three neuronal clones related to the $\beta 1$ gene encoding the muscle nAChR β subunit have been isolated: $\beta 2$ (Deneris *et al.*, 1988), $\beta 3$ (Deneris *et al.*, 1989) and $\beta 4$ (Duvoisin *et al.*, 1989). For more information on the nomenclature of the various subunits reported see Steinbach and Ifune (1989).

Several ISHH studies have been carried out by Patrick, Heinemann and co-workers, to examine the expression of the different subunits of neural nAChRs. Among the α subunits, $\alpha 2$ shows the most restricted distribution, with the highest levels of hybridization observed in the interpeduncular nucleus (Wada *et al.*, 1988, 1989a). $\alpha 3$ and $\alpha 4$ transcripts show a much wider distribution, with high levels of signal detected in the medial habenula and several other thalamic nuclei, and in substantia nigra pars compacta (SNC) and ventral tegmental area (VTA) (Boulter *et al.*, 1986; Goldman *et al.*, 1986, 1987; Wada *et al.*, 1989a). High levels of $\alpha 3$ transcripts in the hippocampus have been reported in some studies (Boulter *et al.*, 1986; Goldman *et al.*, 1986) whereas in others (Wada *et al.*, 1988, 1989a) much lower and much more restricted hybridization signals are shown. $\alpha 4$ transcripts are also abundant in neocortex and hippocampal formation (Goldman *et al.*, 1987; Wada *et al.*, 1989a). Transcripts for the $\beta 2$ subunit present a widespread distribution, which overlaps with that of $\alpha 2$, $\alpha 3$ and $\alpha 4$ subunits, thus suggesting that $\beta 2$ subunits may contribute to the formation of most of the nAChRs in brain (Deneris *et al.*, 1988; Wada *et al.*, 1989a). In contrast, both $\beta 3$ and $\beta 4$ display much more restricted distributions. $\beta 3$ mRNA is present in the medial and lateral habenula, SNC and VTA, the reticular nucleus of the thalamus and the mesencephalic nucleus of the trigeminal nerve. All these areas also contain transcripts for one or more of the $\alpha 3$, $\alpha 4$ and $\beta 2$ subunits (Deneris *et al.*, 1989). $\beta 4$ transcripts are only detected in the medial habenula (Duvoisin *et al.*, 1989). The overlapping distributions of many of the mRNAs for the different subunits raise the possibility that individual neurons express more than one subtype of α or β subunit (Wada *et al.*, 1989a). Double-labelling studies will be required in order to establish this point. In general, these ISHH studies are in good agreement with autoradiographic studies with nicotinic ligands such as [^{3}H]acetylcholine and [^{3}H]nicotine (Clarke *et al.*, 1985) and with immunological detection of nAChRs (Deutch *et al.*, 1987; Swanson *et al.*, 1987). However, some cell groups which showed hybridization signal were not detected with radioligands or antibodies. These discrepancies, as discussed by Wada *et al.* (1989a), may be due to a higher sensitivity of ISHH when compared with immunohistochemical methods, or to the fact that the complementary RNA probes used in the ISHH studies might also recognize heterogeneous nuclear RNA which is not processed to cytoplasmic mRNA.

In the case of nAChRs, hybridization studies have shown that a great diversity of receptors might be obtained in brain by combining the multiple isoforms of the different subunits. However, the limited number of available ligands, as well as the lack of information on the exact nature of their binding sites, makes it difficult to establish whether the genetic diversity observed in brain nAChRs is paralleled by a similar functional diversity. In this respect, a novel type of nAChR has recently been characterized functionally in neurons of the medial habenula (Mulle and Changeux, 1990) and further functionally distinct variants are likely to be found in the future.

GABA$_A$ Receptors

GABA$_A$ receptors mediate the action of GABA (the major inhibitory neurotransmitter in the brain) in the vast majority of neurons in the mammalian brain. Binding of GABA to this type of receptor results in the opening of an integral chloride channel. In addition to the GABA binding site, the receptor contains several other binding sites for a variety of classes of drugs, among them the benzodiazepines (see Barnard *et al.*, 1987).

The receptor was purified from bovine brain and was shown to contain two classes of subunits, α and β, with a stoichiometry of $\alpha_2\beta_2$. The β subunits contain the binding sites for GABA, whereas benzodiazepines bind to the α subunits (Mamalaki *et al.*, 1987). Oligonucleotides derived from partial amino acid sequences were used to screen cDNA libraries from bovine brain, and clones encoding the $\alpha 1$ and $\beta 1$ subunits were isolated. These subunits showed significant homology with each other and with the different subunits of the nAChR, thus suggesting the existence of the wide superfamily of ligand-gated ion channels (Schofield *et al.*, 1987). The same group later reported the isolation of two additional α subunits, $\alpha 2$ and $\alpha 3$ (Levitan *et al.*, 1988). The α1 subunit has also been cloned from rat (Khrestchatisky *et al.*, 1989; Lolait *et al.*, 1989) and human (Garrett *et al.*, 1988; Hirouchi *et al.*, 1989; Schofield *et al.*, 1989), and a further α4 subunit has been reported in rat (Khrestchatisky *et al.*, 1989). Diversity of β subunits is also evident, with β2 and β3 cloned from bovine and rat brain (Ymer *et al.*, 1989). Expression in *Xenopus* oocytes of any of the three α subunits with the β subunit resulted in functional GABA$_A$ receptors with many properties of native receptors. However, these receptors did not display the benzodiazepine potentiation observed in native receptors. This suggested the existence of further components of the receptor necessary for this potentiation (Levitan *et al.*, 1988). This theory was confirmed by the cloning of a novel type of subunit, γ2 (Pritchett *et al.*, 1989b). When this subunit is coexpressed with α1 and β1 subunits, functional receptors with the expected benzodiazepine pharmacology are obtained. The previous assignment of the benzodiazepine binding site to the α subunits may be due to the fact that α and γ subunits have similar molecular mass, which leads to comigration of both species (Pritchett *et al.*, 1989b). A fourth subunit class, δ, has been cloned from rat brain. Coexpression of δ with α1 and β1 subunits yields functional receptors lacking benzodiazepine binding sites (Shivers *et al.*, 1989).

Several reports on the localization of the transcripts for the different forms of subunits of GABA$_A$ receptors have been published. Initial ISHH studies (Séquier *et al.*, 1988; Siegel, 1988), when heterogeneity of α and β subunits was not yet identified, showed patterns of hybridization for the α and β subunits that correlated fairly well with the distribution of the benzodiazepine binding sites for [^{3}H]flumazenil and with immunohistochemical patterns obtained with a monoclonal antibody specific for the β subunit (Séquier *et al.*, 1988). However, in some regions the hybridization intensities detected for one of the subunits were not paralleled by similar intensities for the other subunit, suggesting that variants could exist. This was confirmed later, as summarized above, for both the α and β subunits. The differential patterns of hybridization observed for the different α subunits (Wisden *et al.*, 1988; Khrestchatisky *et al.*, 1989) suggest the existence in the brain of a multiplicity of GABA$_A$ receptor subtypes. The pattern of hybridization for the α1 subunit shows a significant overlap with the distribution of the pharmacologically defined GABA$_A$–benzodiazepine receptors of type I. Thus, it is suggested that this subunit could be present in that type of GABA$_A$ receptor (Wisden *et al.*, 1989). Support for this hypothesis was presented by Pritchett *et al.* (1989a). Expression in mammalian cells of GABA$_A$ receptors resulting from the combination of either α1, α2 or α3 with β1 and γ2 subunits showed that α1-containing receptors displayed binding characteristics consistent with those of type I GABA$_A$–benzodiazepine receptors, whereas the characteristics of α2- and α3-containing receptors were more consistent with type II receptors. The expression of β2 and β3 subunits has only been studied by Northern analysis (Ymer *et al.*, 1989), showing that transcripts for these two subtypes are in fact more abundant than those for the β1 subunit and providing a basis for the explanation of some of the previously reported imbalances of signal (Séquier *et al.*, 1988; Siegel, 1988). The isolation of the two novel classes of subunits, γ2 and δ, together with studies on transfected receptors containing these subunits and with their patterns of mRNA distribution, have led Shivers and co-workers (Shivers *et al.*, 1989) to propose the existence of two major classes of GABA$_A$ receptors. The γ2-subunit-containing subtype could represent the subset of GABA$_A$ receptors which are coupled to benzodiazepine receptor sites. This idea is supported by the overlapping distributions of transcripts for the γ2 subunit (Shivers *et al.*, 1989) and benzodiazepine binding sites (Young and Kuhar, 1979; Unnerstall *et al.*, 1981) and by the requirement for the presence of the γ2 subunit in transfected recombinant receptors in order to obtain a typical benzodiazepine pharmacology (Pritchett *et al.*, 1989b). This γ2-subunit-containing subtype would include the reported type I and type II GABA$_A$–benzodiazepine receptors (Shivers *et al.*, 1989). Less information is available for the δ-subunit-containing subtype, which could represent (Shivers *et al.*, 1989) the subset of GABA$_A$ receptors that lack benzodiazepine binding sites and are selectively labelled by [^{3}H]muscimol (Palacios *et al.*, 1980, 1981; Unnerstall *et al.*, 1981).

It is clear from the previous paragraphs that the GABA$_A$ receptor system is difficult to understand, owing to the multiplicity of subunits, and to the fact that several ligands exist which recognize different subpopulations of receptors (e.g. muscimol versus benzodiazepines). To illustrate this difficulty, we show in Figure 1 the distribution of hybridization signal obtained with probes derived from the sequence of the α1 chain of the bovine GABA$_A$ receptor (Schofield *et al.*, 1987), and in Figure 2 the distribution of binding sites for various GABA$_A$ receptor ligands at some of the anatomical levels shown in Figure 1. These results clearly show that there is no perfect overlapping between any of the binding sites and that of the cells expressing the α1 chain

---

Figures 1 and **2** Comparison of the distribution of the mRNA coding for the α1 subunit of the GABA$_A$ receptor and that of several ligand binding sites of the GABA$_A$ receptor in the rat brain. Figure 1A–D shows the distribution of mRNA for the α1 subunit of the GABA$_A$ receptor. The oligonucleotide probe used was derived from the bovine α1 subunit sequence. White regions represent areas rich in hybridization signal. This photograph was kindly provided by Dr M. R. Brann, from the Laboratory of Molecular Biology, National Institute of Neurological Disorders and Stroke, National Institutes of Health, Bethesda, USA. Figure 2 shows the distribution of binding sites for different GABA$_A$ receptor radioligands. A, B: Distribution of high-affinity GABA$_A$ binding sites labelled by [^{3}H]muscimol. C, D: Benzodiazepine binding sites labelled by [^{3}H]flunitrazepam. E, F: Convulsant sites labelled by the channel blocker [^{35}S]*t*-butyl bicyclophosphorothionate (TBPS). These pictures illustrate the lack of a complete correspondence between the different distributions. Thus, the thalamus (Th) contains high densities of [^{3}H]muscimol binding sites (Figure 2B), but shows low levels of [^{3}H]flunitrazepam binding (Figure 2D). In contrast, the globus pallidus (GP) shows high densities of binding sites for both [^{3}H]flunitrazepam (Figure 2D) and [^{3}H]TBPS (Figure 2F) but is practically devoid of [^{3}H]muscimol binding (Figure 2B). Interestingly, mRNA for the α1 subunit is highly abundant in both structures (Figure 1C,D). See text for further details. Bars = 3 mm

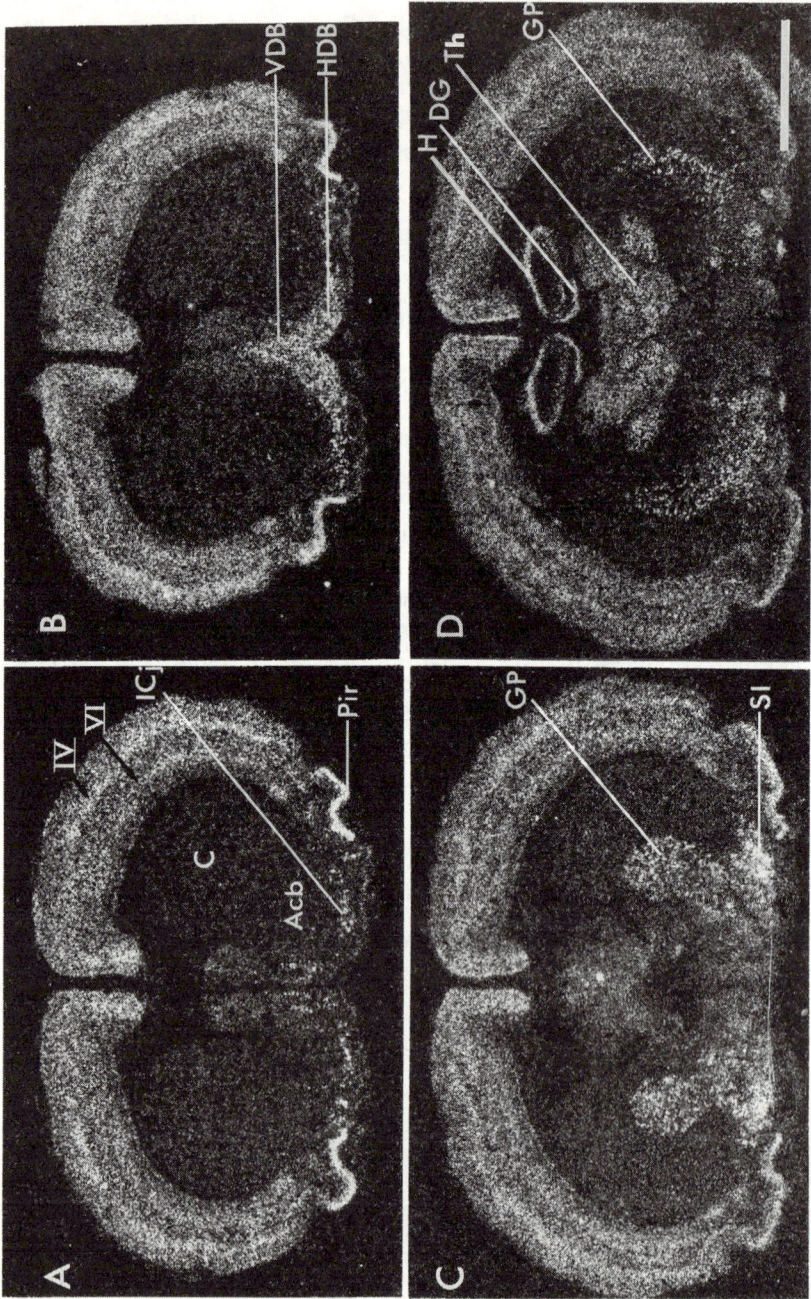

Figure 1   See main caption on p. 13

of the receptor. Thus, while high levels of mRNA for this chain are expressed by cells in the globus pallidus (Figure 1C, D), high densities of benzodiaze-pine binding sites (Figure 2D) and convulsant sites (Figure 2F) but not of muscimol binding sites (Figure 2B) are seen in this region. In contrast, the opposite situation can be seen in several thalamic nuclei that contain high densities of muscimol binding sites (Figure 2B) but not benzodiazepine sites (Figure 2D), although they do express high levels of the alpha chain (Figure 1D) (see also Olsen *et al.* (1990)). This could be interpreted as an indication that this particular α chain is a part of both the receptor type binding benzodiazepines and the type binding muscimol, but is probably different from the subunit actually binding muscimol. Interestingly, the distribution of the δ chain mRNA (see above, Shivers *et al.*, 1989) shows an excellent correlation with that of muscimol binding sites. This example illustrates how, with the available information, it is still very difficult to establish clearly the

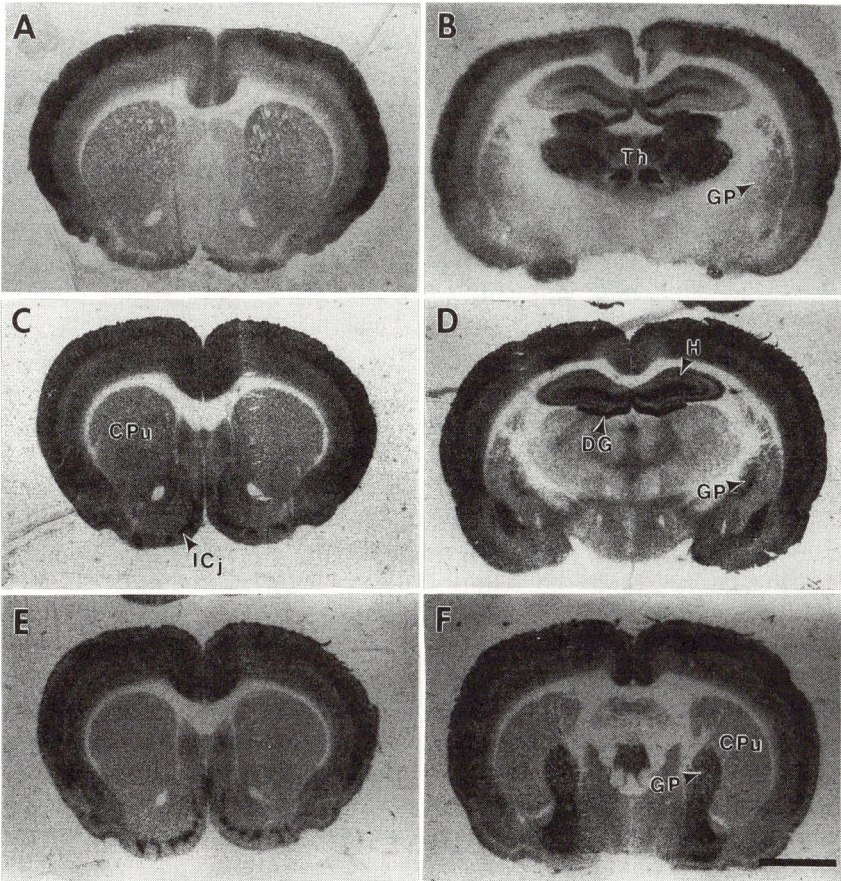

16   *M. T. Vilaró, M. I. Martinez-Mir, M. Sarasa,* et al.

possible subunit isoform combination and stoichiometry of the different
GABA$_A$ receptors.

Glycine Receptor

Glycine is, together with GABA, a major inhibitory amino acid in the central
nervous system, predominantly in spinal cord and brainstem. The glycine
receptor, a ligand-gated chloride channel, has been purified from spinal cord
by chromatography through analogues of its potent natural antagonist, the
convulsant strychnine. Purified receptors contain three different
polypeptides, of 48, 58 and 93 kD. Strychnine binding occurs to the 48 kD
subunit (for a review see Betz, 1987). Partial amino acid sequence of the
purified 48 kD subunit was determined and oligonucleotides based on this
sequence were used to isolate a cDNA clone for this subunit (Grenningloh *et
al.*, 1987). The deduced protein is similar, both in sequence and in putative
transmembrane organization, to the various nAChR and GABA$_A$ receptor
subunits (Stevens, 1987).

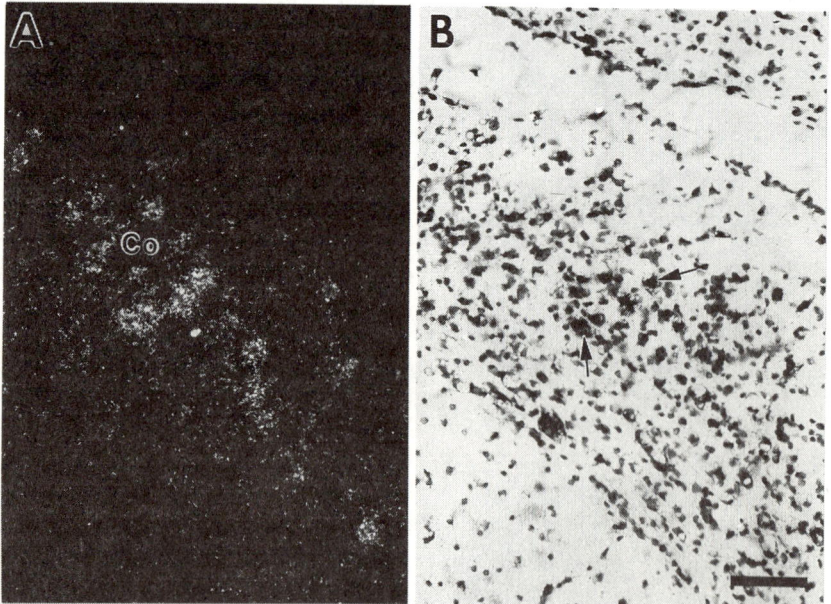

Figure 3 Cellular localization of the mRNA coding for the strychnine binding subunit
of the glycine receptor in the cochlear nucleus of the rat brain. A is a dark field image
of a tissue section hybridized with the glycine receptor probe and dipped in nuclear
track emulsion. Autoradiographic grains are seen as bright points. B corresponds to
the same section counterstained with Giemsa. Arrows in B point to some of the cells
which show an enrichment of grains in A. Bar = 0.1 mm

We have studied the distribution in the rat brain of the cells containing mRNA coding for the strychnine binding subunit of the glycine receptor. The hybridization signal clearly shows a rostro-caudal increasing gradient, with the highest levels in spinal cord and several nuclei of the pons and medulla, namely hypoglossus and facial nuclei; the dorsal column nuclei; the trigeminal, vestibular and cochlear nuclei; the nucleus olivaris; and nuclei of the reticular formation. Significant levels of signal are also observed in the red nucleus of the midbrain, the parafascicular nucleus of the thalamus, the zona incerta and the hypothalamus. Figure 3 illustrates the high degree of cellular resolution that can be attained with ISHH. A tissue section at the level of the cochlear nucleus hybridized with the glycine receptor oligonucleotide probe was dipped in nuclear track emulsion. Figure 3(A) shows the enrichment of silver grains over the cell bodies which express that particular mRNA.

In contrast to the results for the nAChR and GABA$_A$ receptors, we have observed an extensive overlap of the distribution of the transcripts for this subunit and that of the [^{3}H]strychnine binding sites (Figure 4). Most of the work carried out so far with autoradiography and antibodies raised against this protein have resulted in distributions that, excluding possible problems of interpretation of the nuclei labelled, are generally in very good agreement. It could be proposed that, in contrast to the GABA$_A$ receptors mentioned above, the degree of diversity of the glycine receptor is much lower. However, there are indications of diversity in the forms of the strychnine-sensitive glycine receptor, but these appear to be developmentally regulated and absent from the adult rat brain (Akagi and Miledi, 1988; Hoch *et al.*, 1989).

Much work is still necessary for a full understanding of the relationship between binding sites and subunit composition of the receptors of class I. The development of subunit-specific antibodies as well as of new ligands appears to be particularly important.

5. *Class II Neurotransmitter Receptors:* In situ *Hybridization Histochemistry Studies*

While nearly two dozen of class II receptors have been cloned to date (see Table 1), detailed studies of the distribution of their mRNAs have been carried out, to our knowledge, only for the five MChRs, dopamine D2 and the three cloned 5-HT receptors.

Muscarinic Cholinergic Receptors

While pharmacological data generated using different selective antagonist molecules, particularly pirenzepine (Hammer *et al.*, 1980) and the compound AF-DX 116 (Hammer *et al.*, 1986), provided evidence for the existence of

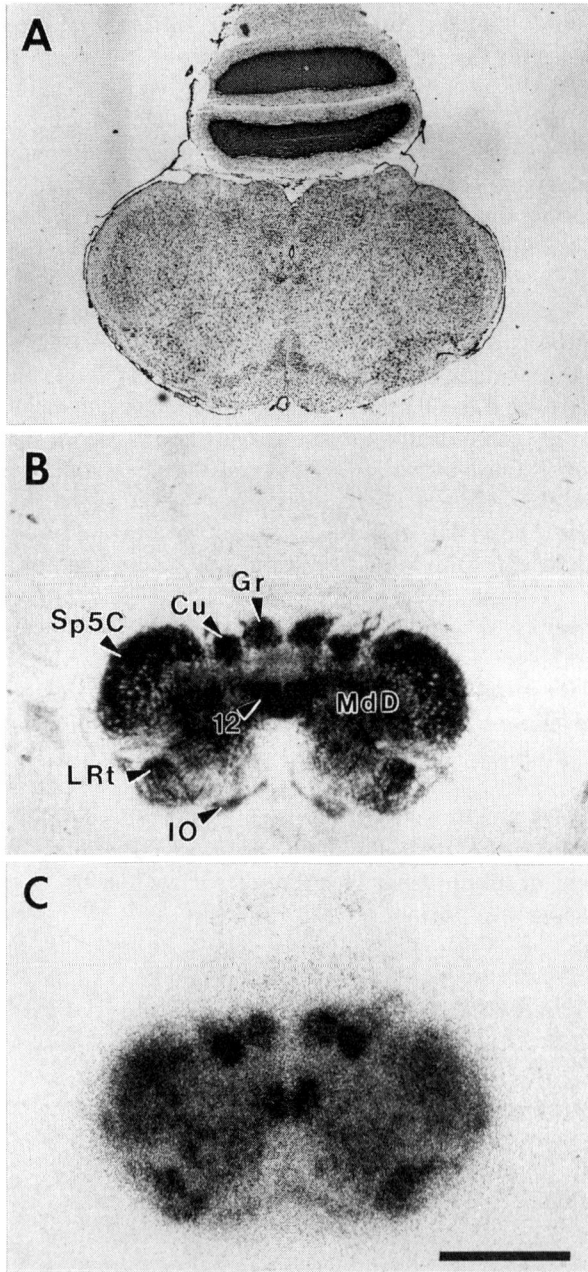

Figure 4 Distribution in the rat brainstem of mRNA coding for the strychnine binding subunit of the glycine receptor (C) and of binding sites for [³H]strychnine (B). A corresponds to the same section as in B stained with cresyl violet. Note the very good overlapping of the binding (B) and hybridization (C) patterns of signal. In this and subsequent figures, dark areas correspond to regions rich in hybridization signal.
Bar = 2 mm

three (de Jonge *et al.*, 1986) and perhaps four (Michel *et al.*, 1989b) different MChR subtypes, molecular cloning has clearly established the existence of five different subtypes of this receptor (Bonner, 1989). The first MChR to be cloned was the receptor from porcine brain. After purification and partial amino acid sequencing, oligonucleotide probes were synthesized and used to screen a cDNA library from porcine cerebrum. The cDNA clone obtained (Kubo *et al.*, 1986a) was shown to encode the *m1* MChR subtype. Using similar strategies, two groups independently cloned the porcine cardiac MChR (Kubo *et al.*, 1986b; Peralta *et al.*, 1987b). The cloned cDNA was assigned to the *m2* subtype. Bonner and co-workers used probes derived from a highly conserved region of the porcine brain MChR to screen a rat cerebral cortex cDNA library. Three different clones were isolated, one of them being the rat homologue of the porcine cerebral *m1*. The other two clones were related to, but distinct from, the brain and cardiac MChRs. Thus, they were called *m3* and *m4* receptors (Bonner *et al.*, 1987). The rat *m2* subtype was also cloned from a cardiac cDNA library (Gocayne *et al.*, 1987). A human genomic library was screened with porcine probes, and the *m2* and *m4* genes were isolated (Bonner *et al.*, 1987). Simultaneously, cloning of four human MChR genes was reported by another group (Peralta *et al.*, 1987a), again using probes derived from the porcine receptors. Finally, the human and rat genes for a fifth MChR have been cloned (Bonner *et al.*, 1988).

We and others (Buckley *et al.*, 1988; Vilaró *et al.*, 1989; Palacios *et al.*, 1990) have examined the regional distribution of the mRNAs coding for these receptors in the rat brain, using ISHH. Our results show that the five MChR mRNAs present a differential regional and cellular distribution in the rat brain. Figure 5 shows that all five subtypes are expressed in the hippocampal formation. Both the distribution and cellular localization of these receptors appear to differ in this brain region. Thus, while *m1* mRNA is abundant in the pyramidal cell layer of Ammon's horn and the granule cell layer of the dentate gyrus (Figure 5B), the other four receptor subtype mRNAs are much less abundant or absent in the latter region but present at different levels in the pyramidal cell layer of Ammon's horn (Figure 5 C–F). Differences inside this layer were also observed. For example, the *m5* receptor mRNA was more abundant in the caudal–ventral aspects of the posterior hippocampus than in the anterior parts of this structure. Differences in the distribution of the mRNAs for the MChRs were also seen in the basal ganglia and associated structures. In the striatum *m4* and, of lower abundance, *m1* messages predominated. In contrast, in the pars compacta of the substantia nigra, the site of origin of the nigrostriatal dopaminergic projection, an enrichment in *m5* mRNA was observed, whereas no transcripts for the other four subtypes were detected (Vilaró *et al.*, 1990a). An interesting observation was obtained with probes for the *m2* receptor mRNA. Figure 6 illustrates the localization of *m2* mRNA in some areas where cholinergic cell bodies of neurons projecting to the hippocampus, such as the septal neurons, or cholinergic motoneurons of some cranial nerves are located. Transcripts for *m2* MChR were also

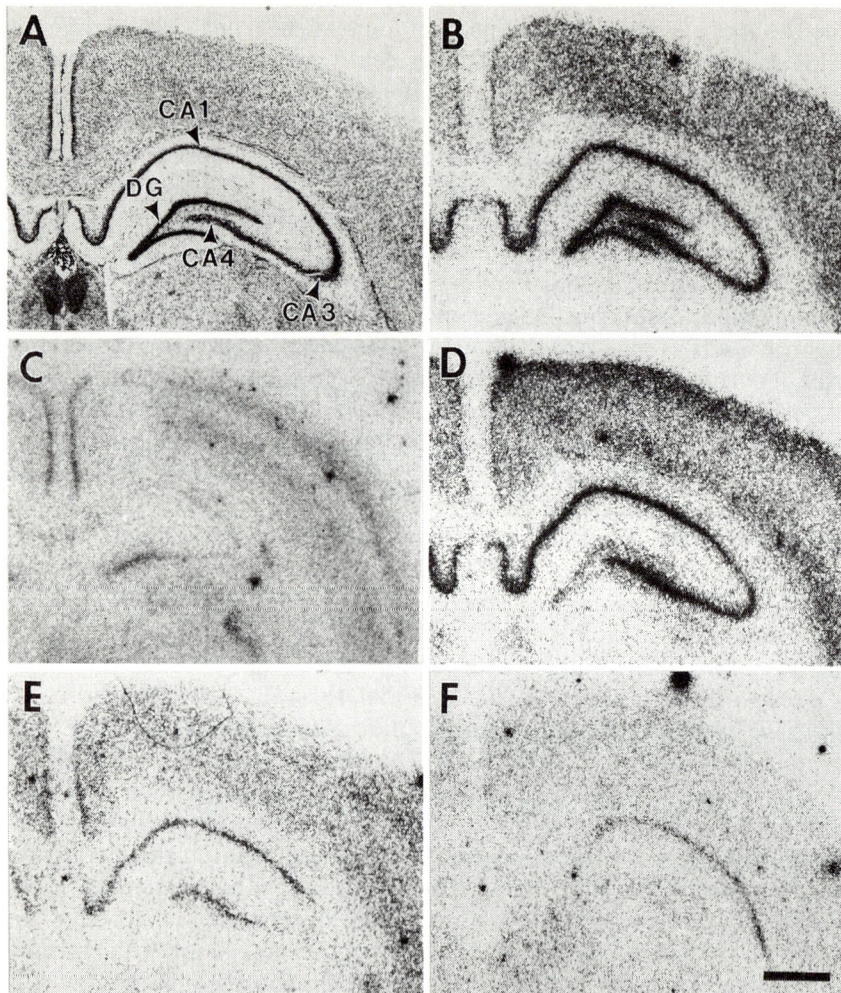

Figure 5 Distribution of transcripts for the five subtypes of MChRs in the rat hippocampal formation. A is a cresyl violet staining of a tissue section close to that seen in B. B, C, D, E and F illustrate the distribution of mRNAs for *m1*, *m2*, *m3*, *m4* and *m5* MChRs. Section in C is more anterior than in A, whereas section in F is more caudal than in A. Note high levels of *m1* MChR mRNA in the pyramidal cell layer of the cornu ammonis (CA) and in the granule cells of the dentate gyrus (DG). In contrast, in the latter cell population, transcripts for the other four subtypes are much less abundant or indetectable. *m2* transcripts are enriched in the CA4 subfield of the anterior hippocampus, whereas *m5* transcripts are detected in the CA1 subfield and more abundant in the caudal aspects of this structure. Bar = 1 mm

detected in the olfactory bulb, cortex, various thalamic nuclei and pontine nuclei. Thus, the distribution of *m2* transcripts is more extensive than that previously reported (Buckley *et al.*, 1988). Interestingly, we observed the expression of *m2* message not only in the cholinergic cell bodies projecting to

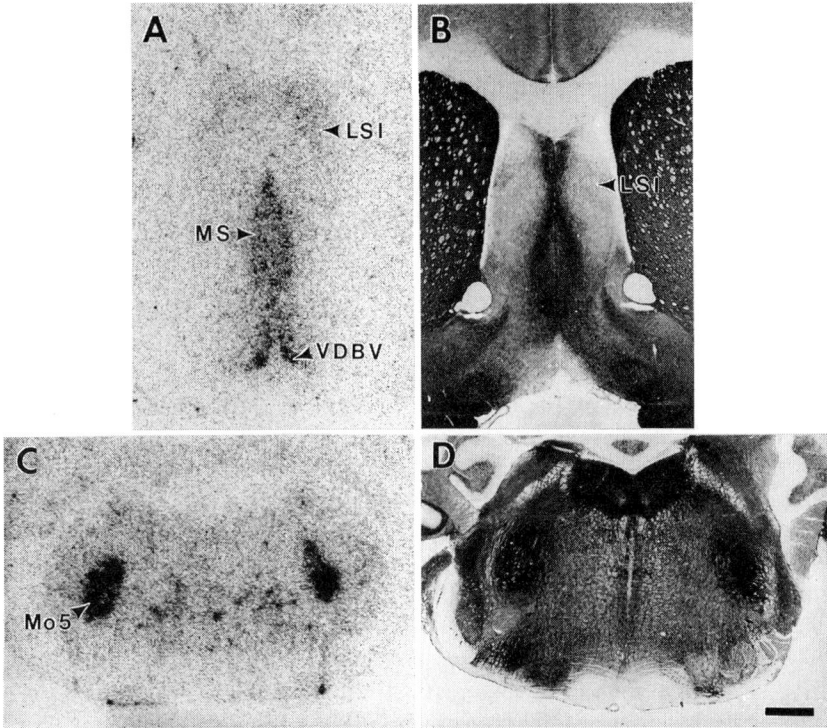

Figure 6 A, C: Distribution of mRNA coding for the *m2* MChR subtype at two levels of the rat brain where cholinergic neurons are localized. B, D: Acetylcholinesterase activity in sections close to those seen in A and C. The presence of *m2* transcripts in those cholinergic cell populations indicates that this particular subtype represents a MChR presynaptically located. Bar = 1 mm

the hippocampus (Figure 6A), but also in the hippocampus itself (Figure 5C). These results suggest that M2 receptors can be localized not only presynaptically on cholinergic terminals, a notion generally accepted and supported by pharmacological evidence, but also postsynaptically in the hippocampal target cells.

In order to examine the correlation between the distribution of mRNAs for the different MChR subtypes and that of the corresponding binding sites, we used receptor autoradiographical techniques. Liganus such as [³H]N-methylscopolamine ([³H]NMS), which do not differentiate between the various subtypes, were used to obtain a general picture of the distribution of MChRs. Unlabelled ligands which are reported to differentiate between the MChR subtypes were used in a concentration-dependent manner to separate these subtypes. In this way, we constructed concentration-dependent inhibition curves, and, using computer-assisted quantitative image analysis, we examined the pharmacological characteristics of the MChRs in different brain areas.

In general, a good agreement was found between the regional pharmacological analysis and the distribution of the mRNAs for the different subtypes.
Thus, for example [³H]NMS binding was readily displaced by the M2 selective
antagonist AF-DX 116 in regions such as the pontine nuclei and the
superficial layer of the superior colliculus. Accordingly, these regions are
enriched in transcripts for the *m2* subtype. Similarly, the pharmacological
profile obtained with several antagonists in the caudate putamen and olfactory tubercle (Vilaró *et al.*, 1990b) is not consistent with any of the
well-defined pharmacological subtypes M1, M2 or M3, but is similar to the
profile shown by the atypical MChR present in the PC12 and NG108-15 cell
lines (Michel *et al.*, 1989a,b). Consistently, *m4* mRNA predominates in these
two regions, and has also been detected in the NG108-15 cells (Peralta *et al.*,
1987a). However, the agreement is not complete throughout the rat brain.
Thus, whereas the pyramidal cells of the hippocampus express mRNAs for
the *m1*, *m3*, *m4* and, at lower abundance, *m2* and *m5* subtypes, the properties
of the sites labelled by [³H]NMS are consistent with a nearly homogeneous
population of M1 sites. This example illustrates the necessity for the
development of more selective ligands and of specific antibodies against the
different subtypes in order to establish clearly the nature of the MChRs in
some areas of the brain.

Several autoradiographic studies have been reported with radiolabelled
subtype-selective muscarinic agonists or antagonists. The distribution of
binding sites labelled by [³H]pirenzepine ([³H]PZ), an M1-selective antagonist (Cortés and Palacios, 1986; Spencer *et al.*, 1986) agrees well with the
hybridization pattern observed for the *m1* subtype (Buckley *et al.*, 1988;
Vilaró *et al.*, 1989). It should be noted that high densities of [³H]PZ binding
sites were observed in the caudate putamen and olfactory tubercle, regions
where *m4* transcripts predominate. Given the fact that cloned *m4* receptors,
when expressed in mammalian cells, show an affinity for PZ only fivefold
lower than that shown by cloned *m1* receptors (Buckley *et al.*, 1989), it could
be that, under certain conditions, binding of [³H]PZ to these two brain
regions in fact reflects binding to both M1 and M4 receptors. The autoradiographic distribution of sites labelled by [³H]AF-DX 116 (Regenold *et al.*,
1989), an M2-selective antagonist, correlates very well with the distribution of
m2 mRNA, with the highest densities of both binding sites and hybridization
signal in pontine nuclei, motor nuclei of the brainstem and some thalamic
nuclei. The distribution of transcripts for the *m2* subtype is also paralleled by
the distribution of binding sites for two putative M2-selective agonists:
[³H]acetylcholine (Quirion *et al.*, 1989) and [³H]oxotremorine-M (Spencer *et
al.*, 1986). However, there are some brain areas, such as the cortex and the
caudate putamen, where rather high densities of binding sites for both
radioligands are observed, although few or no transcripts are detected for the
m2 receptor. In contrast, *m4* transcripts are relatively or highly abundant in
these two regions. Again these discrepancies can be explained by the fact that
these two agonists display very similar efficacies for cloned *m2* and *m4*

receptors transfected in mammalian cells (Novotny and Brann, 1989; M. R. Brann, personal communication).

In the case of MChRs, ISHH studies have provided a detailed image of the distribution of transcripts for the five different subtypes. However, the picture will not be complete until subtype-specific antibodies and more subtype-selective ligands are available, which will allow the localization of the different receptor proteins.

Dopamine D2 Receptors

Two types of dopamine receptor mediate the effects of this neurotransmitter in the central nervous system and in the periphery, the so-called D1 and D2 receptor subtypes (Kebabian and Calne, 1979). A cDNA coding for the rat dopamine D2 receptor has been cloned (Bunzow *et al.*, 1988), by cross-hybridization with a probe derived from the hamster β_2-adrenergic receptor gene. On the basis of this sequence, we and others (Meador-Woodruff *et al.*, 1989; Mengod *et al.*, 1989; Najlerahim *et al.*, 1989; Weiner and Brann, 1989; Le Moine *et al.*, 1990) have examined the regional distribution of the cells containing mRNA coding for the dopamine D2 receptor in the rat brain and pituitary gland. We have compared this distribution with that of the dopamine D2 receptor sites as visualized by autoradiography with the selective dopamine D2 agonist [^{3}H]SDZ 205-502 (Mengod *et al.*, 1989). In the majority of the brain areas examined (Figure 7) and in the pituitary gland there was a qualitatively good anatomical correlation between the distribution of dopamine D2 receptor mRNA and the binding of [^{3}H]SDZ 205-502. Regions of good agreement between the distribution of the hybridization signal and receptor binding include the nuclei caudate putamen and accumbens and the dopaminergic cell bodies of the SNC and VTA. These results indicate that, in the striatum, dopamine, D2 receptors are expressed by cells intrinsic to this nucleus and also localized to presynaptic dopaminergic terminals arising in mesencephalic regions, thus providing direct anatomical evidence to support previous functional studies.

However, dopamine D2 receptor binding is also found in other brain areas where no hybridization signal was detected with our probes. These areas could be grouped in several anatomically different systems: the olfactory bulb (Figure 7A,B); the visual system, including the superficial grey layer of the superior colliculus (Figure 7I,J) and olivary pretectal nucleus (Figure 7G,H); a third group of brain areas comprising the lateral septum (Figure 7E,F), the hippocampus (Figure 7G,H), the entorhinal cortex and other cortical areas; and, finally, the molecular layer of lobules 9 and 10 of the cerebellum (Figure 7K,L). Several explanations could be advanced to account for these discrepancies. It could be that our hybridization probes are not sensitive enough to detect the very low levels of expression in those areas where receptor binding is low, such as the neocortex. However, other areas including the olfactory bulb, the hippocampus, components of the visual pathways and the cerebellum, contain levels of receptor binding which are as high as those seen in areas where good correlation between binding and hybridization signal was observed. Alternatively, it could be postulated that the turnover rate is different and, consequently, mRNA transcripts will be below our detection level. However, for some areas, a simpler explanation could be that these receptors visualized by binding autoradiography are synthesized in cell bodies located outside the areas examined in this study. Receptors in the olfactory and visual systems are probably synthesized by cells in, for example, the nasal epithelium and retina, respectively, and transported to the brain, where they

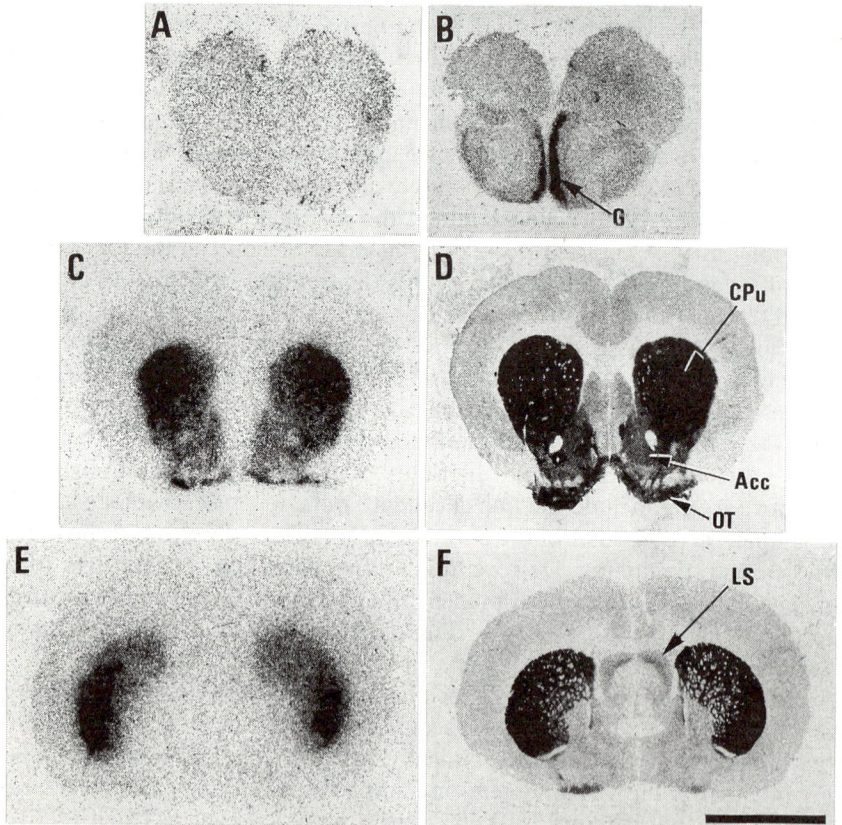

Figure 7 Distribution of the dopamine D2 receptor mRNA in the rat brain (left column). Comparison with the distribution of dopamine D2 receptor binding visualized with [³H]SDZ 205-502 (right column). Note the overlapping distributions of both patterns of signal in structures such as the caudate putamen (CPu), substantia nigra compacta (SNC) and ventral tegmental area (VTA), contrasting with the lack of correspondence in other structures—e.g. olfactory bulb (A,B), superior colliculus (I,J) and cerebellum (K,L). See text for details. Bars = 5 mm. From Mengod *et al.*, 1989, with permission

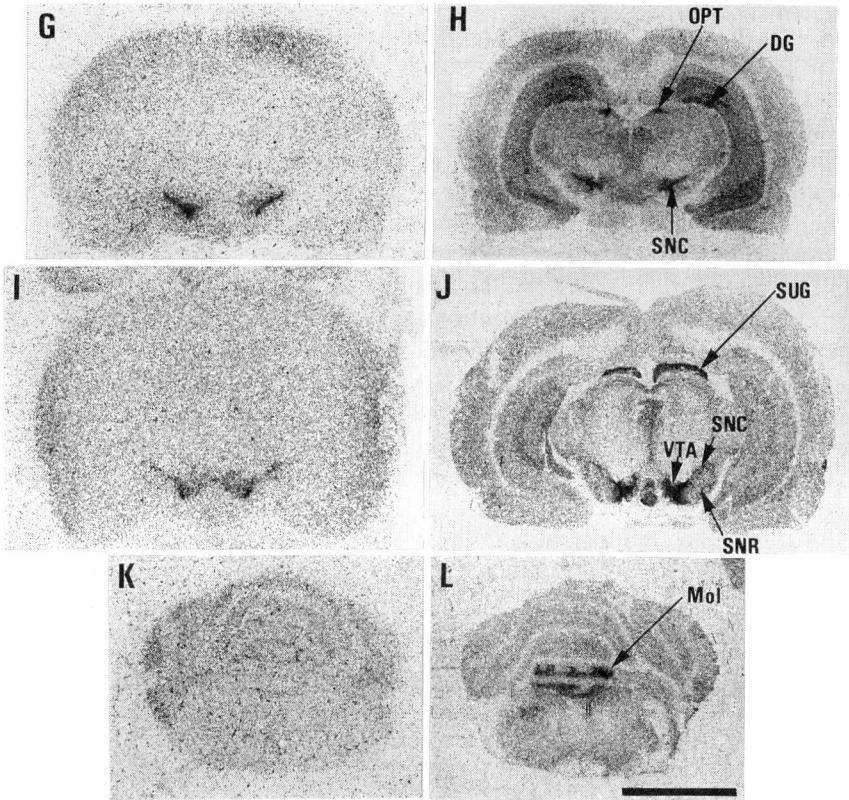

Figure 7 (*continued*)

may be presynaptically located. However, this hypothesis does not account for the lack of correlation between hybridization and binding in neocortex, hippocampal formation and cerebellum, where the intrinsic and extrinsic sources of innervation were examined. No hybridization could be observed in any cell population in cortex, septum, thalamus, hypothalamus, cerebellar cortex or inferior olive, to mention some of the possible sources. The only remaining alternative, excluding the lack of sensitivity, is that these receptors are encoded by mRNAs which are not recognized by our probes, thus suggesting the possible existence of multiple subtypes of dopamine D2 receptors.

Such diversity has, indeed, been recently reported, but, as it will become clear below, it cannot account for the lack of correlation mentioned above. Six different groups (Dal Toso *et al.*, 1989; Giros *et al.*, 1989; Grandy *et al.*, 1989; Monsma *et al.*, 1989; Selbie *et al.*, 1989; Chio *et al.*, 1990) have reported almost simultaneously the cloning of a second form of dopamine D2 receptor cDNA. When compared with the form previously isolated (Bunzow *et al.*, 1988), this novel form contains an insert sequence encoding an additional fragment of 29 amino acids in the putative third cytoplasmic loop. When the corresponding genomic clones were isolated (Dal Toso *et al.*, 1989; Giros *et al.*, 1989; Grandy *et al.*, 1989), they were shown to contain several exons within the coding region, one of them encoding the 29 amino acids which differentiate both receptor isoforms. Therefore, isoforms of the dopamine D2 receptor are generated by alternative splicing of exons contained in the same gene. This is a novel mechanism of generation of diversity for the neurotransmitter receptors of class II, most of which lack introns in their coding regions (O'Dowd *et al.*, 1989). In our ISHH studies discussed above (Mengod *et al.*, 1989) we used oligonucleotide probes corresponding either to the amino or to the carboxy terminal regions of the receptor. Therefore, these probes do in fact recognize both variants of mRNA. In order to study whether the two isoforms of dopamine D2 receptor are differentially expressed in brain, we have synthesized oligonucleotides which recognize exclusively one or other of the forms. Preliminary results indicate that both forms display overlapping patterns of distribution, in both brain and pituitary gland, although the longer form seems to be more abundant, in agreement with other reports (Dal Toso *et al.*, 1989; Giros *et al.*, 1989; Monsma *et al.*, 1989; Selbie *et al.*, 1989; Chio *et al.*, 1990). A more detailed study is currently in progress.

Serotonin Receptors

The cDNAs coding for the rat 5-HT$_{1A}$ (Albert *et al.*, 1990), 5-HT$_{1C}$ (Julius *et al.*, 1988) and 5-HT$_2$ (Pritchett *et al.*, 1988) receptors as well as the gene for the human 5-HT$_{1A}$ (Kobilka *et al.*, 1987; Fargin *et al.*, 1988) have been cloned and sequenced. While the 5-HT$_{1A}$ receptor is encoded by an intronless gene in both man (Kobilka *et al.*, 1987) and rat (Albert *et al.*, 1989), the genes coding for mouse 5-HT$_{1C}$ and rat 5-HT$_2$ receptors contain several introns in their coding regions (Lübbert *et al.*, 1990). On the basis of these sequences, we have visualized by ISHH the regional and cellular distribution of the mRNAs for these receptors. Preliminary results in our laboratory have demonstrated the presence of high levels of 5-HT$_{1A}$ mRNA in the rat hippocampal formation (Figure 8A), particularly in the granule cells of the dentate gyrus and the pyramidal cells of Ammon's horn, and in the dorsal raphe nucleus (Pompeiano, Palacios and Mengod, in preparation). These results are in good agreement with lesion studies which suggested that the great majority of hippocampal 5-HT$_{1A}$ receptors were expressed by cells intrinsic to this brain region which degenerated after local kainic acid or colchicine injections (Palacios and Dietl, 1988). Moreover, they strongly suggest that postsynaptic 5-HT$_{1A}$ receptors in the hippocampus and presynaptic 5-HT$_{1A}$ receptors in the serotoninergic cell bodies of the dorsal raphe nucleus could be encoded by the same gene (Pompeiano, Palacios and Mengod, in preparation). The distribution of 5-HT$_{1A}$ mRNA correlates well

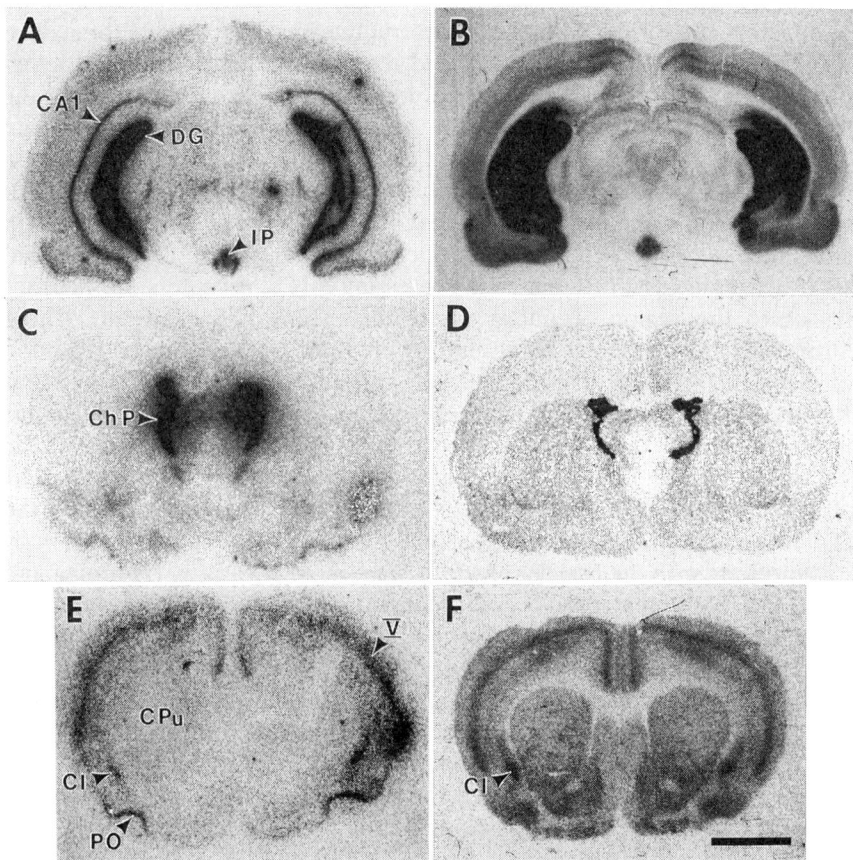

Figure 8 Distribution of transcripts and binding sites for different 5-HT receptor subtypes at some levels of the rat brain. A, B: Distribution of 5-HT$_{1A}$ mRNA and of 5-HT$_{1A}$ binding sites visualized with [^{3}H]8OH-DPAT. 5-HT$_{1C}$ mRNA (C) and 5-HT$_{1C}$ binding sites (D) labelled by [^{3}H]mesulergine in the presence of spiperone are both highly abundant in the choroid plexus (ChP). Distribution of 5-HT$_2$ mRNA (E) and of 5-HT$_2$ binding sites (F) visualized by [^{3}H]mesulergine. Bar = 3 mm

with that of 5-HT$_{1A}$ receptor binding sites, as visualized with [^{3}H]8OH-DPAT (Figure 8A,B).

More detailed studies have been carried out on the 5-HT$_{1C}$ (Hoffman and Mezey, 1989; Molineaux *et al.*, 1989; Mengod *et al.*, 1990a) and 5-HT$_2$ (Mengod *et al.*, 1990b) receptor mRNAs. Using oligonucleotide probes complementary to the 5-HT$_2$ receptor mRNA, the highest levels of hybridization were observed in the frontal cortex (Figure 8E). The rest of the neocortex, the piriform cortex and the entorhinal cortex, were also rich in 5-HT$_2$ receptor transcripts, as well as some subcortical areas, such as the claustrum and the endopiriform nucleus. Positive signals were also present in the olfactory bulb, the anterior olfactory nucleus and several brainstem nuclei, including the pontine nuclei and motor trigeminal, facial and hypoglossal nuclei. Intermediate densities of hybridization signal were seen in the lateral and dorsal part of the caudate nucleus, in the nucleus accumbens and in the olfactory tubercle. In contrast, the cerebellum and several brainstem and thalamic areas did not show any specific signal (Mengod *et al.*, 1990b). This distribution compares well with that of 5-HT$_2$ binding sites labelled with ligands such as $(\pm)[^{125}I]DOI$, [^{3}H]mesulergine (Figure 8F) or [^{3}H]ketanserin. This overlap suggests that the cells expressing 5-HT$_2$ receptors are neurons intrinsic to the region or nuclei where the receptors are present. These neurons are most probably interneurons involved in local circuits (Sheldon and Aghajanian, 1990). This applies to 5-HT$_2$ receptors in the forebrain but not in the cranial nerve nuclei, where 5-HT$_2$ receptors are expressed by motor neurons, although there is no information on the presence of presynaptic receptors in the terminals of the hypoglossal or facial nerves. Thus, the results of ISHH for the 5-HT$_2$ receptor mRNA have provided new insight into the cellular localization of these receptors.

The results with the 5-HT$_{1C}$ receptor were more surprising (Hoffman and Mezey, 1989; Molincaux *et al.*, 1989; Mengod *et al.*, 1990a). As expected, the highest densities of hybridization signal were found in the choroid plexus (Figure 8C). However, and rather unexpectedly, because of the low density of receptors, high levels of hybridization were also seen in many areas of the brain. These include the anterior olfactory nucleus; the piriform cortex; the amygdala; some thalamic nuclei, especially the lateral habenula; the CA3 area of the hippocampal formation; the cingulate cortex and some components of the basal ganglia and associated areas, particularly the subthalamic nucleus, and the substantia nigra. The midbrain and the brainstem showed moderate levels of hybridization, although some nuclei such as the locus coeruleus were found to contain 5-HT$_{1C}$ receptor mRNA. Because of the widespread distribution of its mRNA, we re-examined the presence of 5-HT$_{1C}$ binding sites in the mouse and rat brain. In general, the distribution of 5-HT$_{1C}$ mRNA corresponded well with that of the 5-HT$_{1C}$ receptors visualized with [^{3}H]mesulergine (Figure 8D). Nevertheless, exceptions were seen, particularly in the lateral habenula and in the subthalamic nucleus. In these two brain nuclei the density of 5-HT$_{1C}$ binding sites was much lower than that expected from the high levels of mRNA. An explanation for these discrepancies is not available at the present time. These results suggest the existence of different receptor turnover rates in different cell populations and/or pathways.

6.   Conclusions

As is often the case with a new technique, the application of ISHH to the study of the regional and cellular localization of the mRNAs for neurotransmitter receptors, although still in its infancy, has already generated interesting information and new data, and has raised a number of new questions. For several receptors, such as glycine, dopamine D2, 5-HT$_2$ and 5-HT$_{1A}$, the results obtained using this technique clearly point to the neuronal cell populations expressing these receptors or the particular subunit being studied. These results confirm previous deductions from lesion studies. Furthermore in at least two instances—i.e. dopamine D2 and 5-HT$_{1A}$ receptors—these studies suggest that both pre- and postsynaptic receptors could be encoded by the same gene. Preliminary studies in our laboratory also indicate that this type of approach can be used to study the regulation of receptor expression in response to lesions, drug treatment or other physiological and pharmacological manipulations.

Among the problems raised by these ISHH studies, three deserve mention.

The first is the demonstration of a diversity of receptors much larger than suspected. This concept has already been formulated by those directly involved in the cloning of the various receptors, but it is confirmed and extended by ISHH results. The example we have provided is that of dopamine D2 receptors, where the receptors cloned to date do not, in our opinion, account for all the recognized D2 sites visualized using different ligands.

A second aspect of this problem is the clear inadequacy of the tools, ligands and antibodies at present available to account for the different possible receptors deduced from cloning studies. Paramount examples are those of the nAChRs and GABA$_A$ receptors.

Finally, the correlation between mRNA abundance and densities of binding sites appears to be a complex one. We have mentioned the cases of the MChRs and that of the 5-HT$_{1C}$ receptor as examples where the establishment of such a correlation is difficult from the comparison of the available binding and hybridization data.

In spite of all these problems, it is evident (and we hope this chapter demonstrates this) that the use of ISHH techniques has quickly become an essential tool in the study of neurotransmitter receptors. Future technical improvements will allow better anatomical resolution, an improvement in quantitative aspects and its application to the study of pathologies of receptors in diseases of the human brain.

Acknowledgements

The photos in Figure 2 are taken from unpublished work by M. Sanchez and J. M. Palacios. The authors wish to thank W. S. Young III and J. G. Richards for a critical reading of the manuscript and K. H. Wiederhold for his expert help with photography.

Note added in proof: A human D1 dopamine receptor gene has recently been cloned by Suhanara *et al.* (1990).

Supported by fellowships from: (M.I.M.-M.) Conselleria de Cultura, Educació i Ciència de la Generalitat Valenciana, Spain; (M.S.) Fundación Juan March, Spain; (M.P.) C.N.R. Rome, Italy. M.I.M.-M.'s permanent address is Department Farmacologia i Farmacotècnia, Universitat de València, Spain.

Abbreviations Used in Illustrations

12	hypoglossal nucleus
Acb	accumbens nucleus
CA1	field CA1 of Ammon's horn
CA3	field CA3 of Ammon's horn
CA4	field CA4 of Ammon's horn
ChP	choroid plexus
Cl	claustrum
Co	cochlear nucleus
CPu	caudate putamen
Cu	cuneate nucleus
DG	dentate gyrus
G	glomerular layer of the olfactory bulb
GP	globus pallidus
Gr	gracile nucleus
H	hippocampus
HDB	horizontal limb of the diagonal band
ICj	islands of Calleja
IO	inferior olive
IP	interpeduncular nucleus
LRt	lateral reticular nucleus
LS	lateral septum nucleus
LSI	lateral septum nucleus, intermediate
MdD	reticular nucleus of the medulla, dorsal
Mo5	motor trigeminal nucleus
Mol	molecular layer of the cerebellar lobules 9 and 10
MS	medial septum nucleus
OPT	olivary pretectal nucleus
OT	olfactory tubercle
Pir	piriform cortex
PO	primary olfactory cortex
SI	substantia innominata
SNC	substantia nigra compacta
SNR	substantia nigra reticulata
Sp5C	nucleus of spinal tract of trigeminal nerve, caudal
SUG	superficial grey layer of the superior colliculus
Th	thalamus
VDB	vertical limb of the diagonal band
VDBV	vertical limb of the diagonal band, ventral
VTA	ventral tegmental area

References

Akagi, H. and Miledi, R. (1988). Heterogeneity of glycine receptors and their messenger RNAs in rat brain and spinal cord. *Science, N.Y.*, **242**, 270–273

Albert, P., Zhou, Q. Y., Van Tol, H. H. M., Bunzow, J. R. and Civelli, O. (1990). Cloning, functional expression and mRNA tissue distribution of the rat 5-hydroxytryptamine$_{1A}$ receptor gene. *J. Biol. Chem.*, **265**, 5825–5832

Angerer, L. M., Stoler, M. H. and Angerer, R. C. (1987). In situ hybridization with RNA probes: an annotated recipe. In *In situ Hybridization. Applications to Neurobiology* (ed. K. L. Valentino, J. H. Eberwine and J. D. Barchas). Oxford University Press, Oxford

Ariëns, E. J. (1979). Receptors: from fiction to fact. *Trends Pharmacol. Sci.*, **1**, 11–15

Barnard, E. A., Darlison, M. G. and Seeburg, P. (1987). Molecular biology of the GABA_A receptor: the receptor/channel superfamily. *Trends Neurosci.*, **10**, 502–509

Betz, H. (1987). Biology and structure of the mammalian glycine receptor. *Trends Neurosci.*, **10**, 113–117

Bonner, T. I. (1989). The molecular basis of muscarinic receptor diversity. *Trends Neurosci.*, **12**, 148–151

Bonner, T. I., Buckley, N. J., Young, A. C. and Brann, M. R. (1987). Identification of a family of muscarinic acetylcholine receptor genes. *Science, N.Y.*, **237**, 527–532

Bonner, T. I., Young, A. C., Brann, M. R. and Buckley, N. J. (1988). Cloning and expression of the human and rat m5 muscarinic acetylcholine receptor genes. *Neuron*, **1**, 403–410

Boulter, J., Evans, K., Goldman, D., Martin, G., Treco, D., Heinemann, S. and Patrick, J. (1986). Isolation of a cDNA clone coding for a possible neural nicotinic acetylcholine receptor α-subunit. *Nature*, **319**, 368–374

Brimblecombe, R. W. (1974). Historical introduction. In *Drug Actions on Cholinergic Systems* (Pharmacological Monographs) (ed. P. B. Bradley). Macmillan Press, London, pp. 1–18

Buckley, N. J., Bonner, T. I. and Brann, M. R. (1988). Localization of a family of muscarinic receptor mRNAs in rat brain. *J. Neurosci.*, **8**, 4646–4652

Buckley, N. J., Bonner, T. I., Buckley, C. M. and Brann, M. R. (1989). Antagonist binding properties of five cloned muscarinic receptors expressed in CHO-K1 cells. *Molec. Pharmacol.*, **35**, 469–476

Bunzow, J. R., Van Tol, H. H. M., Grandy, D. K., Albert, P., Salon, J., Christie, M., Machida, C. A., Neve, K. A. and Civelli, O. (1988). Cloning and expression of a rat D_2 dopamine receptor cDNA. *Nature*, **336**, 783–787

Chio, C. L., Hess, G. F., Graham, R. S. and Huff, R. M. (1990). A second molecular form of D_2 dopamine receptor in rat and bovine caudate nucleus. *Nature*, **343**, 266–269

Clarke, P. B. S., Schwartz, R. D., Paul, S. M., Pert, C. B. and Pert, A. (1985). Nicotinic binding in rat brain: autoradiographic comparison of [^{3}H]acetylcholine, [^{3}H]nicotine, and [^{125}I]-α-bungarotoxin. *J. Neurosci.*, **5**, 1307–1315

Coghlan, J. P., Aldred, P., Haralambidis, J., Niall, H. D., Penschow, J. D. and Tregear, G. W. (1985). Hybridization histochemistry. *Anal. Biochem.*, **149**, 1–28

Cortés, R. and Palacios, J. M. (1986). Muscarinic cholinergic receptor subtypes in the rat brain. I. Quantitative autoradiographic studies. *Brain Res.*, **362**, 227–238

Dal Toso, R., Sommer, B., Ewert, M., Herb, A., Pritchett, D. B., Bach, A., Shivers, B. D. and Seeburg, P. H. (1989). The dopamine D_2 receptor: two molecular forms generated by alternative splicing. *EMBO Jl*, **8**, 4025–4034

de Jonge, A., Doods, H. N., Riesbos, J. and van Zwieten, P. A. (1986). Heterogeneity of muscarinic binding sites in rat brain, submandibular gland and atrium. *Br. J. Pharmacol.*, **89**, Suppl., 551P

Deneris, E. S., Boulter, J., Swanson, L. W., Patrick, J. and Heinemann, S. (1989). β3: a new member of nicotinic acetylcholine receptor gene family is expressed in brain. *J. Biol. Chem.*, **264**, 6268–6272

Deneris, E. S., Connolly, J., Boulter, J., Wada, E., Wada, K., Swanson, L. W., Patrick, J. and Heinemann, S. (1988). Primary structure and expression of β2: a novel subunit of neuronal nicotinic acetylcholine receptors. *Neuron*, **1**, 45–54

Deutch, A. Y., Holliday, J., Roth, R. H., Chun, L. L. Y. and Hawrot, E. (1987). Immunohistochemical localization of a neuronal nicotinic acetylcholine receptor in mammalian brain. *Proc. Natl Acad. Sci. USA*, **84**, 8697–8701

Dohlman, H. G., Caron, M. G. and Lefkowitz, R. J. (1987). A family of receptors coupled to guanine nucleotide regulatory proteins. *Biochemistry*, **26**, 2657–2664

Duvoisin, R. M., Deneris, E. S., Patrick, J. and Heinemann, S. (1989). The functional diversity of the neuronal nicotinic acetylcholine receptors is increased by a novel subunit: β4. *Neuron*, **3**, 487–496

Fargin, A., Raymond, J. R., Lohse, M. J., Kobilka, B. K., Caron, M. G. and Lefkowitz, R. J. (1988). The genomic clone G-21 which resembles a β-adrenergic receptor sequence encodes the 5-HT_{1A} receptor. *Nature*, **335**, 358–360

Garrett, K. M., Duman, R. S., Saito, N., Blume, A. J., Vitek, M. P. and Tallman, J. F. (1988).

Isolation of a cDNA clone for the alpha subunit of the human GABA-A receptor. *Biochem. Biophys. Res. Commun.*, **156**, 1039–1045

Giros, B., Sokoloff, P., Martres, M.-P., Riou, J.-F., Emorine, L. J. and Schwartz, J. C. (1989). Alternative splicing directs the expression of two D_2 dopamine receptor isoforms. *Nature*, **342**, 923–926

Gocayne, J., Robinson, D. A., Fitzgerald, M. G., Ghung, F.-Z., Kerlavage, A. R., Lentes, K.-U., Lai, J., Wang, Ch.-D., Fraser, C. M. and Venter, J. C. (1987). Primary structure of rat cardiac β-adrenergic and muscarinic cholinergic receptors obtained by automated DNA sequence analysis: Further evidence for a multigene family. *Proc. Natl Acad. Sci. USA*, **84**, 8296–8300

Goldman, D., Deneris, E., Luyten, W., Kochhar, A., Patrick, J. and Heinemann, S. (1987). Members of a nicotinic acetylcholine receptor gene family are expressed in different regions of the mammalian central nervous system. *Cell*, **48**, 965–973

Goldman, D., Simmons, D., Swanson, L. W., Patrick, J. and Heinemann, S. (1986). Mapping of brain areas expressing RNA homologous to two different acetylcholine receptor α-subunit cDNAs. *Proc. Natl Acad. Sci. USA*, **83**, 4076–4080

Grandy, D. K., Marchionni, M. A., Makam, H., Stofko, R. E., Alfano, M., Frothingham, L., Fischer, J. B., Burke-Howie, K. J., Bunzow, J. R., Server, A. C. and Civelli, O. (1989). Cloning of the cDNA and gene for a human D_2 dopamine receptor. *Proc. Natl Acaꓹ. Sci. USA*, **86**, 9762–9766

Gregor, P., Mano, I., Maoz, I., McKeown, M. and Teichberg, V. I. (1989). Molecular structure of the chick kainate-binding subunit of a putative glutamate receptor. *Nature*, **342**, 689–692

Grenningloh, G., Rienitz, A., Schmitt, B., Methfessel, C., Zensen, M., Beyreuther, K., Gundelfinger, E. D. and Betz, H. (1987). The strychnine-binding subunit of the glycine receptor shows homology with nicotinic acetylcholine receptors. *Nature*, **328**, 215–220

Hall, Z. W. (1987). Three of a kind: The β-adrenergic receptor, the muscarinic acetylcholine receptor, and rhodopsin. *Trends Neurosci.*, **10**, 99–101

Hamel, E. and Beaudet, A. (1984). Electron microscopic autoradiographic localization of opioid receptors in rat neostriatum. *Nature*, **312**, 155–157

Hammer, R., Berrie, C. P., Birdsall, N. J. M., Burgen, A. S. V. and Hulme, E. C. (1980). Pirenzepine distinguishes between different subclasses of muscarinic receptors. *Nature*, **283**, 90–92

Hammer, R., Giraldo, E., Schiavi, G. B., Monferini, E. and Ladinsky, H. (1986). Binding profile of a novel cardioselective muscarine receptor antagonist, AF-DX 116, to membranes of peripheral tissues and brain in the rat. *Life Sci.*, **38**, 1653–1662

Henderson, R. and Unwin, P. N. T. (1975). Three-dimensional model of purple membrane obtained by electron microscopy. *Nature*, **257**, 28–32

Hirouchi, M., Kuwano, R., Katagiri, T., Takahashi, Y. and Kuriyama, K. (1989). Nucleotide and deduced amino acid sequences of the $GABA_A$ receptor α-subunit from human brain. *Neurochem. Int.*, **15**, 33–38

Hoch, W., Betz, H. and Becker, C.-M. (1989). Primary cultures of mouse spinal cord express the neonatal isoform of the inhibitory glycine receptor. *Neuron*, **3**, 339–348

Hoffman, B. J. and Mezey, E. (1989). Distribution of serotonin 5-HT_{1C} receptor mRNA in adult rat brain. *FEBS Lett.*, **247**, 453–462

Hollmann, M., O'Shea-Greenfield, A., Rogers, S. W. and Heinemann, S. (1989). Cloning by functional expression of a member of the glutamate receptor family. *Nature*, **342**, 643–648

Hucho, F. (1986). The nicotinic acetylcholine receptor and its ion channel. *Eur. J. Biochem.*, **158**, 211–226

Julius, D., MacDermott, A. B., Axel, R. and Jessel, T. (1988). Molecular characterization of a functional cDNA encoding the serotonin 1c receptor. *Science, N.Y.*, **241**, 558–564

Kebabian, J. W. and Calne, D. B. (1979). Multiple receptors for dopamine. *Nature*, **277**, 93–96

Khrestchatisky, M., MacLennan, A. J., Chiang, M.-Y., Xu, W., Jackson, M. B., Brecha, N., Sternini, C., Olsen, R. W. and Tobin, A. J. (1989). A novel α subunit in rat brain $GABA_A$ receptors. *Neuron*, **3**, 745–753

Kobilka, B. K., Frielle, T., Collins, S., Yang-Feng, T., Kobilka, T. S., Francke, U., Lefkowitz, R. J. and Caron, M. G. (1987). An intronless gene encoding a potential member of the family of receptors coupled to guanine nucleotide regulatory proteins, *Nature*, **329**, 75–79

Kubo, T., Fukuda, K., Mikami, A., Maeda, A., Takahashi, H., Mishina, M., Haga, T., Haga, K., Ichiyama, A., Kangawa, K., Kojima, M., Matsuo, H., Hirose, T. and Numa, S. (1986a). Cloning, sequencing and expression of complementary DNA encoding the muscarinic acetylcholine receptor. *Nature*, **323**, 411–416

Kubo, T., Maeda, A., Sugimoto, K., Akiba, I., Mikami, A., Takahashi, H., Haga, T., Haga, K., Ichiyama, A., Kangawa, K., Matsuo, H., Hirose, T. and Numa, S. (1986b). Primary structure of porcine cardiac muscarinic acetylcholine receptor deduced from the cDNA sequence. *FEBS Lett.*, **209**, 367–372

Kuhar, M. J., De Souza, E. B. and Unnerstall, J. R. (1986). Neurotransmitter receptor mapping by autoradiography and other methods. *Ann. Rev. Neurosci.*, **9**, 27–59

Le Moine, C., Normand, E., Guitteny, A. F., Fouque, B., Teoule, R. and Bloch, B. (1990). Dopamine receptor gene expression by enkephalin neurons in rat forebrain. *Proc. Natl Acad. Sci. USA*, **87**, 230–234

Levitan, E. S., Schofield, P. R., Burt, D. R., Rhee, L. M., Wisden, W., Köhler, M., Fujita, N., Rodriguez, H. F., Stephenson, A., Darlison, M. G., Barnard, E. A. and Seeburg, P. H. (1988). Structural and functional basis for GABA$_A$ receptor heterogeneity. *Nature*, **335**, 76–79

Lewis, M. E., Krause II, R. G. and Roberts-Lewis, J. M. (1988). Recent developments in the use of synthetic oligonucleotides for *in situ* hybridization histochemistry. *Synapse*, **2**, 308–316

Lolait, S. J., O'Carroll, A.-M., Kusano, K., Muller, J.-M., Brownstein, M. J. and Mahan, L. C. (1989). Cloning and expression of a novel rat GABA$_A$ receptor. *FEBS Lett.*, **246**, 145–148

Lübbert, H., Foguet, M., Hartikka, J., Merguin, L. and Staufenbiel, M. (1990). Molecular biology of the serotoninergic system in the rodent brain. *J. Cell. Biochem.*, Suppl., **14F**, CP 205

McCarthy, M. P., Earnest, J. P., Young, E. F., Choe, S. and Stroud, R. M. (1986). The molecular neurobiology of the acetylcholine receptor. *Ann. Rev. Neurosci.*, **9**, 383–413

Maelicke, A. (1988). Structure and function of the nicotinic acetylcholine receptor. In *Handbook of Experimental Pharmacology*, Vol. 86, *The Cholinergic Synapse* (ed. V. P. Whittaker). Springer-Verlag, Berlin, Heidelberg

Mamalaki, C., Stephenson, F. A. and Barnard, E. A. (1987). The GABA$_A$/benzodiazepine receptor is a heterotetramer of homologous α and β subunits. *EMBO Jl.*, **6**, 561–565

Meador-Woodruff, J. H., Mansour, A., Bunzow, J. R., Van Tol, H. H. M., Watson, S. J. Jr. and Civelli, O. (1989). Distribution of D$_2$ dopamine receptor mRNA in rat brain. *Proc. Natl Acad. Sci. USA*, **86**, 7625–7628

Mengod, G., Martinez-Mir, M. I., Vilaró, M. T. and Palacios, J. M. (1989). Localization of the mRNA for the dopamine D$_2$ receptor in the rat brain by *in situ* hybridization histochemistry. *Proc. Natl Acad. Sci. USA*, **86**, 8560–8564

Mengod, G., Nguyen, H., Le, H., Waeber, C., Lübbert, H. and Palacios, J. M. (1990a). The distribution and cellular localization of 5-HT$_{1C}$ receptor mRNA in the rodent brain examined by *in situ* hybridization histochemistry. Comparison with receptor binding distribution. *Neuroscience*, **35**, 577–591

Mengod, G., Pompeiano, M., Martinez-Mir, M. I. and Palacios, J. M. (1990b). Localization of the mRNA for the 5-HT$_2$ receptor by *in situ* hybridization histochemistry. Correlation with the distribution of receptor sites. *Brain Res.* (in press)

Michel, A. D., Delmendo, R., Stefanich, E. and Whiting, R. L. (1989a). Binding characteristics of the muscarinic receptor subtype of the NG108-15 cell line. *Arch. Pharmacol.*, **340**, 62–67

Michel, A. D., Stefanich, E. and Whiting, R. L. (1989b). PC12 phaeochromocytoma cells contain an atypical muscarinic receptor binding site. *Br. J. Pharmacol.*, **97**, 914–920

Mishina, M., Takai, T., Imoto, K., Noda, M., Takahashi, T., Numa, S., Methfessel, C. and Sakmann, B. (1986). Molecular distinction between fetal and adult forms of muscle acetylcholine receptor. *Nature*, **321**, 406–411

Molineaux, S. M., Jessell, T. M., Axel, R. and Julius, D. (1989). 5-HT1C receptor is a prominent serotonin receptor subtype in the central nervous system. *Proc. Natl Acad. Sci. USA*, **86**, 6793–6797

Monsma, F. J. Jr, McVittie, L. D., Gerfen, C. R., Mahan, L. C. and Sibley, D. R. (1989). Multiple D$_2$ dopamine receptors produced by alternative splicing. *Nature*, **342**, 926–929

Mulle, C. and Changeux, J.-P. (1990). A novel type of nicotinic receptor in the rat central nervous system characterized by patch-clamp techniques. *J. Neurosci.*, **10**, 169–175

Najlerahim, A., Barton, A. J. L., Harrison, P. J., Heffernan, J. and Pearson, R. C. A. (1989). Messenger RNA encoding the D$_2$ dopamine receptor detected by *in situ* hybridization histochemistry in rat brain. *FEBS Lett.*, **255**, 335–339

Nef, P., Oneyser, C., Alliod, C., Couturier, S. and Ballivet, M. (1988). Genes expressed in the brain define three distinct neuronal nicotinic acetylcholine receptors. *EMBO Jl*, **7**, 595–601

Novotny, E. A. and Brann, M. R. (1989). Agonist pharmacology of cloned muscarinic receptors. Abstracts from the *Fourth International Symposium on Subtypes of Muscarinic Receptors*, Wiesbaden, No. 69, *Trends Pharmacol. Sci.* supplement

O'Dowd, B. F., Lefkowitz, R. J. and Caron, M. G. (1989). Structure of the adrenergic and related receptors. *Ann. Rev. Neurosci.*, **12**, 67–83

Olsen, R. W. (1990). Molecular biology of GABA$_A$ receptors. *FASEB J.*, **4**, 1469–1480

Olsen, R. W., McCabe, R. T. and Wamsley, J. K. (1990). GABA$_A$ receptor subtypes: autoradiographic comparison of GABA, benzodiazepine, and convulsant binding sites in rat central nervous system. *J. Chem. Neuroanat.*, **3**, 59–76

Ovchinnikov, Y. A. (1982). Rhodopsin and bacteriorhodopsin: structure–function relationships. *FEBS Lett.*, **148**, 179–189

Palacios, J. M. and Dietl, M. M. (1988). Autoradiographic studies of serotonin receptors. In *The Serotonin Receptors* (ed. E. Sanders-Bush). Humana Press, Clifton, New Jersey, pp. 89–138

Palacios, J. M., Mengod, G., Vilaró, M. T., Wiederhold, K. H., Boddeke, H. W. G. M., Alvarez, F. J., Chinaglia, G. and Probst, A. (1990). Cholinergic receptors in the rat and human brain. Microscopic visualization. *Progr. Brain. Res.*, **84**, 343–353

Palacios, J. M., Probst, A. and Cortés, R. (1986). Mapping receptors in the human brain. *Trends Neurosci.*, **9**, 284–289

Palacios, J. M., Wamsley, J. K. and Kuhar, M. J. (1981). High affinity GABA receptors— autoradiographic localization. *Brain Res.*, **222**, 285–307

Palacios, J. M., Young, W. S. III and Kuhar, M. J. (1980). Autoradiographic localization of γ-aminobutyric acid (GABA) receptors in the rat cerebellum. *Proc. Natl Acad. Sci. USA*, **77**, 670–674

Parascandola, J. (1980). Origins of the receptor theory. *Trends Pharmacol. Sci.*, **1**, 189–192

Peralta, E. G., Ashkenazi, A., Winslow, J. W., Smith, D. H., Ramachandran, J. and Capon, D. J. (1987a). Distinct primary structures, ligand-binding properties and tissue-specific expression of four human muscarinic acetylcholine receptors. *EMBO Jl*, **6**, 3923–3929

Peralta, E. G., Winslow, J. W., Peterson, G. L., Smith, D. H., Ashkenazi, A., Ramachandran, J., Schimerlik, M. I. and Capon, D. J. (1987b). Primary structure and biochemical properties of an M$_2$ muscarinic receptor. *Science, N.Y.*, **236**, 600–605

Persohn, E., Malherbe, P., Pritchett, D. B., Bach, A. W. J., Wozny, M., Taleb, O., Dal Toso, R., Shih, J. C. and Seeburg, P. H. (1988). Structure and functional expression of cloned rat serotonin 5-HT-2 receptor. *EMBO Jl*, **7**, 4135–4140

Pritchett, D. B., Lüddens, H. and Seeburg, P. H. (1989a). Type I and Type II GABA$_A$-benzodiazepine receptors produced in transfected cells. *Science, N.Y.*, **245**, 1389–1392

Pritchett, D. B., Sontheimer, H., Shivers, B. D., Ymer, S., Kettenmann, H., Schofield, P. R. and Seeburg, P. H. (1989b). Importance of a novel GABA$_A$ receptor subunit for benzodiazepine pharmacology. *Nature*, **338**, 582–585

Quirion, R., Araujo, D., Regenold, W. and Boksa, P. (1989). Characterization and quantitative autoradiographic distribution of [^{3}H]acetylcholine muscarinic receptors in mammalian brain. Apparent labelling of an M$_2$-like receptor subtype. *Neuroscience*, **29**, 271–289

Regenold, W., Araujo, D. M. and Quirion, R. (1989). Quantitative autoradiographic distribution of [^{3}H]AF-DX 116 muscarinic-M$_2$ receptor binding sites in rat brain. *Synapse*, **4**, 115–125

Richards, J. G. (1990). *In situ* hybridization histochemistry reveals a diversity of GABA$_A$ receptor subunit mRNAs in neurons of the rat spinal cord and dorsal root ganglia. *J. Neurosci.* (in press)

Richards, J. G., Schoch, P., Häring, P., Takacs, B. and Möhler, H. (1987). Resolving GABA$_A$/benzodiazepine receptors: Cellular and subcellular localization in the CNS with monoclonal antibodies *J. Neurosci.*, **7**, 1866–1886

Schofield, P. R., Darlison, M. G., Fujita, N., Burt, D. R., Stephenson, F. A., Rodriguez, H., Rhee, L. M., Ramachandran, J., Reale, V., Glencorse, T. A., Seeburg, P. H. and Barnard, E. A., (1987). Sequence and functional expression of the GABA$_A$ receptor shows a ligand-gated receptor super-family. *Nature*, **328**, 221–227

Schofield, P. R., Pritchett, D. B., Sontheimer, H., Kettenmann, H. and Seeburg, P. H. (1989). Sequence and expression of human GABA$_A$ receptor α1 and β1 subunits. *FEBS Lett.*, **244**, 361–364

Schofield, P. R., Shivers, B. D. and Seeburg, P. H. (1990). The role of receptor diversity in the CNS. *Trends Neurosci.*, **13**, 8–11

Selbie, L. A., Hayes, G. and Shine, J. (1989). The major dopamine D2 receptor: molecular analysis of the human D2$_A$ subtype. *DNA*, **8**, 683–689

Séquier, J. M., Richards, J. G., Malherbe, P., Price, G. W., Mathews, S. and Möhler, H. (1988). Mapping of brain areas containing RNA homologous to cDNAs encoding the α and β subunits of the rat GABA$_A$ γ-aminobutyrate receptor. *Proc. Natl Acad. Sci. USA*, **85**, 7815–7819

Sheldon, P. W. and Aghajanian, G. K. (1990). Serotonin (5-HT) induces IPSPs in pyramidal layer cells of rat piriform cortex: evidence for the involvement of a 5-HT$_2$-activated interneuron. *Brain Res.*, **506**, 62–69

Shivers, B. D., Killisch, I., Sprengel, R., Sontheimer, H., Köhler, M., Schofield, P. R. and Seeburg, P. H. (1989). Two novel GABA$_A$ receptor subunits exist in distinct neuronal subpopulations. *Neuron*, 3, 327–337

Siegel, R. E. (1988). The mRNAs encoding GABA$_A$/benzodiazepine receptor subunits are localized in different cell populations of the bovine cerebellum. *Neuron*, 1, 579–584

Singer, R. H., Bentley Lawrence, J. and Rashtchian, R. N. (1987). Toward a rapid and sensitive in situ hybridization methodology using isotopic and nonisotopic probes. In *In situ Hybridization. Applications to Neurobiology.* (ed. K. L. Valentino, J. H. Eberwine and J. D. Barchas). Oxford University Press, Oxford

Spencer, D. G. Jr., Horváth, E. and Traber, J. (1986). Direct autoradiographic determination of M1 and M2 muscarinic acetylcholine receptor distribution in the rat brain: relation to cholinergic nuclei and projections. *Brain Res.*, **380**, 59–68

Steinbach, J. H. and Ifune, C. (1989). How many kinds of nicotinic acetylcholine receptor are there? *Trends Neurosci.*, 12, 3–6

Stevens, C. F. (1987). Channel families in the brain. *Nature*, **328**, 198–199

Suhanara, R. K., Niznik, H. B., Weiner., D. M., Storman, T. M., Brann, M. R., Kennedy, J. L., Gelernter, J. E., Rozmahell, R., Yang, Y., Israel, Y., Seeman, P. and O'Dowd, B. F. (1990). The human dopamine D1 receptor locus to an intronless gene on chromosome 5. *Nature*, in press

Swanson, L. W., Simmons, D. M., Whiting, P. J. and Lindstrom, J. (1987). Immunohistochemical localization of neuronal nicotinic receptors in the rodent central nervous system. *J. Neurosci.*, 7, 3334–3342

Tecott, L. H., Eberwine, J. H., Barchas, J. D. and Valentino, K. L. (1987). Methodological considerations in the utilization of in situ hybridization. In *In situ Hybridization. Applications to Neurobiology* (ed. K. L. Valentino, J. H. Eberwine and J. D. Barchas). Oxford University Press, Oxford

Unnerstall, J. R., Kuhar, M. J., Niehoff, D. L. and Palacios, J. M. (1981). Benzodiazepine receptors are coupled to a subpopulation of γ-aminobutyric acid (GABA) receptors: evidence from a quantitative autoradiographic study. *J. Pharmacol. Exp. Ther.*, **218**, 797–804

Vilaró, M. T., Boddeke, H. W. G. M., Wiederhold, K.-H., Kischka, U., Mengod, G. and Palacios, J. M. (1989). Regional expression of muscarinic receptor (MChR) subtypes in rat brain: an *in situ* hybridization/receptor autoradiography study. Abstracts from the *Fourth International Symposium on Subtypes of Muscarinic Receptors*, Wiesbaden, No. 68, *Trends Pharmacol. Sci.* supplement

Vilaró, M. T., Palacios, J. M. and Mengod, G. (1990a). Localization of m5 muscarinic receptor mRNA in rat brain examined by *in situ* hybridization histochemistry. *Neurosci. Lett.*, **114**, 154–159

Vilaró, M. T., Wiederhold, K.-H., Palacios, J. M. and Mengod, G. (1990b). Muscarinic cholinergic receptors in the rat caudate putamen and olfactory tubercle belong predominantly to the *m4* class: *In situ* hybridization and receptor autoradiography evidence. *Neuroscience*, in press

Wada, K., Ballivet, M., Boulter, J., Connolly, J., Wada, E., Deneris, E. S., Swanson, L. W., Heinemann, S. and Patrick, J. (1988). Functional expression of a new pharmacological subtype of brain nicotinic acetylcholine receptor. *Science, N.Y.*, **240**, 330–334

Wada, K., Dechesne, C. J., Shimasaki, S., King, R. G., Kusano, K., Buonanno, A., Hampson, D. R., Banner, C., Wenthold, R. J. and Nakatani, Y. (1989). Sequence and expression of a frog brain complementary DNA encoding a kainate-binding protein. *Nature*, **342**, 684–689

Wada, E., Wada, K., Boulter, J., Deneris, E., Heinemann, S., Patrick, J. and Swanson, L. W. (1989). Distribution of alpha2, alpha3, alpha4, and beta2 neuronal nicotinic receptor subunits mRNAs in the central nervous system: a hybridization histochemical study in the rat. *J. Comp. Neurol.*, **284**, 314–335

Watson, S. J., Sherman, T. G., Kelsey, J. E. Burke, S. and Akil, H. (1987). Anatomical localization of mRNA: in situ hybridization of neuropeptide systems. In *In situ Hybridization. Applications to Neurobiology* (ed. K. L. Valentino, J. H. Eberwine and J. D. Barchas), Oxford University Press, Oxford

Weiner, D. M. and Brann, M. R. (1989). The distribution of a dopamine D2 receptor mRNA in rat brain. *FEBS Lett.*, **253**, 207–213

Whiting, P. J. and Lindstrom, J. M. (1986). Purification and characterization of a nicotinic acetylcholine receptor from chick brain. *Biochemistry*, **25**, 2082–2093

Whiting, P. and Lindstrom, J. (1987). Purification and characterization of a nicotinic acetylcholine receptor from rat brain. *Proc. Natl Acad. Sci. USA*, **84**, 595–599

Wisden, W., Morris, B. J., Darlison, M. G., Hunt, S. P. and Barnard, E. A. (1988). Distinct $GABA_A$ receptor α subunit mRNAs show differential patterns of expression in bovine brain. *Neuron*, **1**, 937–947

Wisden, W., Morris, B. J., Darlison, M. G., Hunt, S. P. and Barnard, E. A. (1989). Localization of $GABA_A$ receptor α-subunit mRNAs in relation to receptor subtypes. *Molec. Brain Res.*, **5**, 305–310

Ymer, S., Schofield, P. R., Draguhn, A., Werner, P., Köhler, M. and Seeburg, P. H. (1989). $GABA_A$ receptor β subunit heterogeneity: functional expression of cloned cDNAs. *EMBO Jl*, **8**, 1665–1670

Young, W. S. III and Kuhar, M. J. (1979). Autoradiographic localisation of benzodiazepine receptors in the brains of humans and animals. *Nature*, **280**, 393–395

2

In Vivo Methods for the Rate of Serotonin Synthesis and Axonal Transport Measurements in the Brain

MIRKO DIKSIC

Montreal Neurological Institute and Hospital, and Department of Neurology and Neurosurgery, McGill University, 3801 University St, Montreal, Quebec, H3A 2B4

Contents

Current Aspects of the Neurosciences, Vol. 3. Edited by N. N. Osborne. © The Macmillan Press Ltd 1991

1. Introduction

For more than twenty years researchers have been searching for a method of measuring the rate of brain serotonin synthesis which is both convenient and anatomically precise. Serotonin (5-hydroxytryptamine; 5-HT) is a neurotransmitter widely distributed in the brain. It has been implicated in many brain functions (e.g. sleep cycle: Jouvet, 1967; food intake: Blundell and Hill, 1987) and in disorders ranging from migraine (e.g. Andersen and Dafny, 1983) to schizophrenia (e.g. Sedvall, 1981) and depression (e.g. Young et al., 1981). To date it has been impossible to measure serotonin synthesis rate in living human brain, although it has often been determined in laboratory animals in a 'normal' state and under the influence of various drugs. All procedures developed to date are fatal and therefore obviously not useful in humans. Attempts have been made to measure the neurotransmitter concentration in post-mortem human brain (e.g. Dodd et al., 1988). However, although these measurements might provide information on the steady state concentration of 5-HT, they cannot give any information about the 5-HT synthesis rate. And, of course, there is always the possibility of post-mortem changes.

The development of an antibody specific for 5-HT (Steinbush et al., 1978) and tryptophan hydroxylase (Weissman et al., 1987) has made it possible to obtain information on the neurotransmitter and/or enzyme distribution, but, again, use of this antibody does not give any direct information on the 5-HT serotonin synthesis rate. In addition, since immunochemical methods cannot be quantitative, it is impossible to make quantitative comparisons of distributions obtained with these two antibodies. A recently developed push–pull perfusion method used in conjunction with high-performance liquid chromatography (HPLC) separation permits determination of the 'locally' released neurotransmitter (e.g. 5-HT) and its metabolite (e.g. 5-HIAA) (Petersen et al., 1989; Sharp et al., 1989). If certain conditions are fulfilled (that is, if the presence of a cannula causes no artefacts and the released 5-HT is directly proportional to the synthesis rate), these methods can yield information on the average synthesis rate. It takes about 20 min to collect a sample containing enough material for analysis. Unfortunately, there are no good animal models for many diseases in which the 5-HT system is involved (e.g. depression, migraine), requiring that the rate of serotonin synthesis be determined in the neurotransmitter's natural setting. If we are to study these diseases in their natural settings, a method applicable to humans must be developed.

As is the case with all research and eventually diagnostic methods that are used in humans (e.g. Yamamoto et al., 1977; Phelps et al., 1979), the methods and underlying biological model must first be evaluated and confirmed in animals (Sokoloff et al., 1977), where we are able to make direct measurements at different stages and at different times of metabolic conversion of the tracer into a final metabolite. Measurement in animals allows us to investigate and quantify the relationship between tracer and tracee. The work in animals permits detailed evaluation and confirmation of a hypothesis made in the development of an *in vivo* autoradiographic method. All biological models, regardless of how elaborate they might be, rest on several underlying assumptions and approximations that must be confirmed, as much as possible, before the model can be used in an *in vivo* autoradiographic method. *In vivo* autoradiographic methods—including positron emission tomography (PET)—measure only total tissue radioactivity (precursor plus metabolite(s)). A biological model must be used to separate the amount of tracer present in the precursor pool from that present in the metabolic pool, because only the amount found in the metabolic pool can be related to the synthesis rate. Positron emission tomography, which can be termed an *in vivo* 'autoradiographic' method used in humans, has an additional advantage over the *in vivo* autoradiographic method in laboratory animals: it allows us to observe the entire tissue time–radioactivity curve (using external radioactivity measurements) in the same subject. PET with an ^{11}C-labelled radiopharmaceutical also permits repeated measurements in the same subject approximately 1.5 h apart (this time is a function of the radionuclide's physical half-life), which is very important in tests evaluating the influence of a drug on the biological system. The use of the tryptophan analogue described here as a tracer for determining the serotonin synthesis rate is also advantageous, because it will permit determination of the synthesis rate in human brain before and during therapy.

Essential nutrients (e.g. oxygen and glucose in totality, amino acids in large part) are delivered to the brain via the circulation. By means of the blood–brain barrier (BBB), the cerebral vasculature can selectively exclude, retard or facilitate the influx of a substrate from the blood into the brain. Several of the facilitated transport systems have been identified for the essential amino acids (Oldendorf and Szabo, 1976; Christensen and Handlogten, 1979). The same transport system makes the influx of one amino acid dependent on the plasma concentration of others (e.g. L-tryptophan shares the same transporter with L-Val, L-Leu, L-Ilu, L-Phe and L-Met). It must be emphasized that a very complex relationship exists between the brain's different nutritional requirements and the supply of substrates. This relationship is the result of a variety of controls and regulations, and each of these can be affected differently by a pathological or pharmacological treatment. The best assessment of these interrelationships is obtained by studying cerebral metabolism *in vivo*, because *in vitro* studies bypass the influence of the BBB and the cerebral circulation in a particular process under study.

The object of this review is not to criticize the methods used in the determination of the brain serotonin synthesis rates (see reviews, Neckers, 1982; Korf, 1985). Rather, we outline briefly the deficiencies in the methods at present in use and describe, with the user in mind, the *in vivo* autoradiographic method we developed. We describe two different uses of the tracer (labelled α-MTrp). We discuss experimental data on the basis of which the methods are developed and outline a derivation of the equations used in the calculation of the serotonin synthesis rates. Since two types of serotonin synthesis rate measurements are described, 'X-ray' autoradiographic and PET (which could be considered *in vivo* autoradiography), the two methods of calculation are also presented. We discuss the two different uses of labelled α-MTrp, namely to determine the rate of anterograde axonal transport of newly synthesized neurotransmitter and to determine the steady state rate of serotonin synthesis. These methods should give us, for the first time, direct information on the influence, if any, of drugs used to date in the determination of the serotonin synthesis rates (Neckers, 1982; Korf, 1985). Extending the method to measurement in humans will certainly allow us to obtain direct measurements of the serotonin synthesis rate in the human brain, information which to date was acquired only by indirect measurements of tryptophan and its metabolites in the CSF obtained by lumbar puncture (e.g. Young *et al.*, 1981).

Methods used to determine the brain serotonin synthesis rate can be divided into steady state methods (the steady state of tryptophan metabolism is not altered) and non-steady-state methods (concentration of some of the tryptophan metabolites is deliberately altered) using drugs to interrupt the tryptophan metabolic pathway at a certain stage, or to block removal of 5-HIAA, the end metabolite of tryptophan, through the serotonin pathway (see reviews, Neckers, 1982; Korf, 1985). The steady state methods used to date employ radioactively labelled tryptophan and HPLC separation in conjunction with radioactivity measurements to determine the specific activity of metabolites at different times after injection of the tracer. The change in the specific activity with time is used in the estimation of the rate of serotonin synthesis (Neckers, 1982; Korf, 1985).

Non-steady-state methods use drugs (e.g. pargyline, aromatic amino acid decarboxylase inhibitor) to inhibit an enzymatic step or probenecid to inhibit an acid carrier mechanism (Neckers, 1982; Korf, 1985). These methods are open to criticism because the measurements are done in animals with constantly changing conditions. In addition, other neurotransmitter systems that might influence the serotoninergic synthesis (e.g. the dopaminergic system) are also disturbed with this treatment. However, these measurements do provide some very important information on the serotoninergic system. They have basic problems in that they are both labour-intensive and the non-steady state requires the use of drugs that inhibit some of the enzymes used in the conversion of tryptophan into serotonin or serotonin metabolite. Since all these methods are based on tissue sampling, the resolution and structure heterogeneity are limited by the method of dissection. A micro-puncture of certain brain structures could be used to increase anatomical resolution, but samples from different animals must then be pooled together to obtain samples large enough for HPLC analysis. The microdissection methods (Palkovits *et al.*, 1976) can yield information on relatively small structures, but the tissue heterogeneity might have an even more serious influence on some small structures (e.g. raphe mediamus).

Definitions

A few definitions may prove helpful.

The endogenous compound undergoing biochemical transformation is called the tracee and the radioactive compound introduced into the system is referred to as a tracer (the tracer can be of the same chemical form as the tracee but this is not necessarily so). In this presentation labelled α-methyl-L-tryptophan (α-MTrp), an analogue of the essential amino acid L-Trp, is used as the tracer. This tracer is converted in brain (Missala and Sourkes, 1988; Diksic *et al.*, 1990b) into α-methylserotonin (α-M-5-HT). α-M-5-HT stays in the brain for a long time (Diksic *et al.*, 1990b; Nagahiro *et al.*, 1990a) because it is not a substrate of the monoamine oxidase (MAO), unlike the equivalent metabolite of tryptophan (serotonin). Since α-M-5-HT (the end metabolite of the tracer being discussed) does not diffuse in any substantial amount through the membrane (at least during the experimental time used in our studies), we shall consider the movement of labelled α-MTrp in the brain as being within a three-compartment model without any loss from the third (metabolic) compartment.

A compartment is defined as the volume or the region of space in which a substrate and tracer distribute, and within which a specific activity is uniform. The tracer and tracee move between compartments with distinguishable kinetics. The concept of a chain chemical reaction, which could be envisioned as a sequence of compartments, was first introduced to biology by Burton (1936). A compartmentation of the biological system was introduced by Teorell (1937) for the *in vivo* transport of drugs. Historically, the multicompartmental theory using radioactive tracers was first described by Sheppard (1948). The boundary of a compartment may correspond to anatomical structures, or, more precisely, to part of a structure (e.g. extracellular space), but this is not essential. Compartments should preferably have clearly identifiable biological counterparts, but this also is not essential (e.g. the compartments might be simply identified by their kinetic characteristics without real biological counterpart). Movement of the tracer between compartments is described by the first-order differential equations with constant coefficients. All rate constants for the tracer are first-order rate constants. It must be clearly understood that any compartment in this respect is more a mathematical creation than a biological/biochemical reality, and as long as it is treated as such, it can be implemented in data analysis.

2.   In Vivo *Serotonin Synthesis Rate*

Background

Serotonin used in the brain for neurotransmission is synthesized in that organ
from an essential amino acid, L-Trp (e.g. Tozer *et al.*, 1966). (Serotonin does
not cross the blood–brain barrier and therefore cannot be delivered to the
brain via the circulation.) Tryptophan enters the brain by a branched-chain
amino acid transport system, indicating that the brain tissue concentration of
this amino acid is influenced by the plasma concentration of other amino acids
sharing the same carrier system (Oldendorf, 1971; Yudilevich *et al.*, 1972;
Pardridge, 1977). In addition, L-Trp is the only amino acid that is partially
bound to the plasma proteins and, as such, not all plasma L-Trp is available
for transport to the brain (Curzon *et al.*, 1973; Etienne *et al.*, 1976).
   In the first step, the conversion of L-Trp is catalysed by tryptophan-5-
monoxygenase (E.C. 1.14.16.4), also known as tryptophan-5-hydroxylase,
into 5-hydroxy-L-tryptophan (e.g. Osborne, 1982). The *in vivo* activity of this
enzyme is believed to be the rate-limiting step in the 5-HT synthesis. In
addition, the enzyme is present only in the serotoninergic neurons (Kuhar *et
al.*, 1972). L-Trp, used as a precursor for this reaction, must enter serotoninergic neurons from the extracellular space and/or glial cells. We must
remember that L-Trp is also used for the brain protein synthesis (Barondes,
1974). Assuming that at a steady state L-Trp is supplied from the brain L-Trp
compartment and that all of it is 'available' for the hydroxylation, the
concentration (10–30 μM: Young and Sourkes, 1977) is still below that of
tryptophan hydroxylase (K_m between 50 μM and 120 μM: Friedman *et al.*,
1972; Green, 1989). Probably not all of this L-Trp is available for the
hydroxylation with the tryptophan hydroxylase, because it is also used in the
protein synthesis in the areas where this enzyme is not present. This suggests
that the enzyme is not saturated with this substrate and that an increase in the
brain L-Trp concentration should increase the rate of 5-HT synthesis (e.g.
Fernstrom, 1983). The latter has been confirmed experimentally in laboratory
animals (Green *et al.*, 1962; Curzon and Marsden, 1975; Sarna *et al.*, 1985)
and humans (Kopin, 1959; Coppen *et al.*, 1963; Young and Teff, 1989), and it
is the basis for using L-Trp as a drug. The enzyme also requires molecular
oxygen and a cofactor, L-erythro-tetrahydrobiopterin (Friedman *et al.*, 1972).
The K_m of tryptophan hydroxylase for tetrahydrobiopterin is about 31 μM,
substantially higher than its estimated concentration of 1 μM in the brain
(Friedman *et al.*, 1972). There is a similar situation with the K_m for oxygen
The K_m is about 2.5%, which is again lower than the brain tissue concentration of oxygen under normal conditions (Katz, 1980). These data suggest that
tryptophan hydroxylase is not saturated with any substrate or cofactor.
   Conversion of 5-hydroxy-L-tryptophan (5-H-Trp) into 5-HT is accomplished by action of the aromatic amino acid decarboxylase (AAAD; E.C.

4.1.1.28), the enzyme present in serotoninergic, dopaminergic, noradrenergic and adrenergic neurons (Bowsher and Henry, 1986), and requires pyridoxal-5′-phosphate. Since tryptophan hydroxylase is present only in the serotoninergic neurons (Kuhar *et al.*, 1972), and the brain concentration of 5-H-Trp is low (Tappaz and Pujol, 1980), its conversion into 5-HT probably occurs only in 5-HT neurons. The 5-HT formed is immediately stored into synaptosomes, and in part is bound to a specific serotonin-binding protein (Tamir *et al.*, 1976; Kirchgessner *et al.*, 1988). Both of these processes protect 5-HT from degradation by monoamine oxidase (E.C. 1.4.3.4). A steady-state concentration of 5-H-Trp in brain is very low (Tappaz and Pujol, 1980; Duda and Moore, 1985), permitting us, at least in the first approximation, to accept hydroxylase as a truly rate-limiting enzyme in the 5-HT synthesis. (By analogy with the chain radioactive decay, one can see that, even if the rate of decarboxylation is substantially higher, some 5-H-Trp can be found if the reactions are abruptly stopped. Similarly, short-lived radionuclides (daughter) are found in uranium (parent), which has a very long half-life (Friedlander *et al.*, 1955).) This fact is also important in the development of our model, because it permits the assumption that there is no loss of 5-H-Trp from the compartment (neurons) where it is synthesized. Note that 5-H-Trp does cross the BBB, and if there were any substantial amounts present, the modelling would become more complicated, because its loss into blood and/or the influx from blood would need to be accounted for.

The steady state concentration of 5-HT in different brain structures is, under normal conditions, kept at a closely controlled level. It has been proposed that the brain 5-HT is stored in two different neuronal pools, one mostly used in 5-HT transmission (Kleven *et al.*, 1983). The concentration of 5-HT is kept at a constant level by controlling the rate of synthesis and oxidation of part of the once-released 5-HT. The oxidation of 5-HT can occur within the neurons and without (Kelder *et al.*, 1989). Oxidation of 5-HT into 5-HIAA is a two-step process. The first step is catalysed by monoamine oxidase (primary MAO-A; however, 5-HT has some affinity towards MAO-B: Johnston, 1968; Fowler and Tipton, 1982). The second step (oxidation of aldehyde) is catalysed by aldehyde dehydrogenase (ALDH; E.C.1.2.1.3). Some 5-HIAA is also reduced by aldehyde reductase (E.C.1.1.1.2) to the 5-hydroxytryptophol (Davis *et al.*, 1966; Bulat *et al.*, 1970). However, it has been accepted that the first step (an MAO-catalysed reaction) is the rate-limiting step in the oxidation of 5-HT. The final metabolite, 5-HIAA, is removed from the brain into the CSF and the half-life of this removal process was estimated to be about 45 min in rat (Neff and Tozer, 1968) and about 130 min in mouse (our analysis of kinetic data of Tracqui *et al.*, 1983a). As a result of this, the steady state regional distribution of 5-HIAA in the brain resembles the distribution of 5-HT. Other pathways of the serotonin metabolism have been suggested (Gal and Sherman, 1978; Susilo *et al.*, 1989), but it seems that none of these have substantial importance in the brain metabolism of 5-HT in relation to the matters discussed in this review. Minor metabolism of tryptophan and 5-HT in the brain results in the formation of tryptamine (Philips *et al.*, 1974) and 5-methoxytryptamine (Green *et al.*, 1973), respectively.

In the pineal gland, which is outside the blood–brain barrier, 5-HT is converted into melatonin (5-methoxy-N^{α}-acetylserotonin), the first step being catalysed by serotonin-*N*-acetyltransferase and the second (*O*-methylation) by hydroxyindole-*O*-methyltransferase.

Non-steady-state Methods

The methods generally used in the estimation of the 5-HT synthesis rate target one of the enzymes catalysing metabolism of L-Trp or the acid carrier system which removes 5-HIAA from the brain into the CSF. In the non-steady-state methods, one of the enzymes or the 5-HIAA carrier system is inhibited with a drug and the rate of accumulation and/or disappearance is converted into the 5-HT synthesis rate, assuming, perhaps incorrectly, that there is no alteration of the synthesis rate by the drug(s) used (e.g. Korf, 1985). The non-steady-state methods can also be divided further into isotopic (which use radioactive L-tryptophan) and non-isotopic (which do not). Non-isotopic methods estimate the rate of 5-HT synthesis from the accumulation rate of 5-H-Trp (Carlsson *et al.*, 1976) after inhibition of the central AAAD (e.g. changes in the concentration of dopamine also occur when AAAD inhibitors are used), or from the rate of accumulation of 5-HT after MAO inhibition (Neff and Tozer, 1968). It is also possible to estimate the rate of 5-HT synthesis from the rate of 5-HIAA disappearance after pretreatment with MAO inhibitors (Tozer *et al.*, 1966) or from the rate of accumulation of 5-HIAA after probenecid pretreatment (Neff *et al.*, 1967). The use of *p*-chlorophenylalanine (PCPA) (Koe and Weissmann, 1966) or 6-fluorotryptophan, a tryptophan hydroxylase inhibitor (Miwa *et al.*, 1987), also permits estimation of the 5-HT synthesis rate from measurements of the disappearance rate of 5-HT after pretreatment with PCPA or 6-fluorotryptophan. Of course, if there is any control (through feedback mechanisms) of the 5-HT synthesis rate by any of the L-Trp metabolites (Hamon *et al.*, 1973, 1979; van Wijk *et al.*, 1979), the rate estimated by these methods will not yield correct results. The influence of L-Trp metabolites on the serotonin synthesis rate has been suggested by several investigators (Macon *et al.*, 1971; Hamon *et al.*, 1973; Curzon and Marsden, 1975; Carlsson *et al.*, 1976; Hamon *et al.*, 1979). The use of probenecid as the drug which inhibits 5-HIAA efflux from the brain might be complicated by the observation that it also enhances 5-HT synthesis (Schubert, 1974). The possibility of post-mortem changes in the brain metabolite concentration (van Wijk and Korf, 1981) could influence the final estimate of the synthesis rate. However, the rates obtained by different non-steady-state methods are similar (Korf, 1985), suggesting that there might not be a serious problem with these methods or that the different pharmacological manipulations used in measurements produce similar artefacts. At this time there are no conclusive answers to these questions, but the method we have developed might eventually supply a few.

Steady State Methods

The serotonin synthesis rate can also be estimated by measuring the change in the specific activity of different L-Trp metabolites after introducing a pulse of radioactively labelled L-Trp into the circulation (Curzon and Green, 1969; Neff *et al.*, 1971; Curzon *et al.*, 1972; Lane and Aprison, 1978), or injecting labelled 5-H-Trp (Baumann, 1975) intravenously or intracisternally. The use of labelled 5-H-Trp can be criticized on the grounds that there has been no identification of a specific uptake system on the serotoninergic neurons for 5-H-Trp, meaning that the conversion into 5-HT would not be done exclusively in the 5-HT neurons (Ng *et al.*, 1972; Awazi and Guldberg, 1978). As mentioned earlier, since the activity of hydroxylase is considered to be a rate-limiting step in the 5-HT synthesis, labelled 5-H-Trp cannot be good for the estimation of the 5-HT synthesis rate: it bypasses the rate-limiting step.

The use of labelled L-Trp for serotonin synthesis rate measurements was based on measurement of the specific activity of tryptophan and different metabolites in the brain tissue. These methods are usually simple but are very labour-intensive (as are non-steady-state methods) and have, like the steady state methods, a very limited anatomical resolution. Since L-Trp is also incorporated into proteins, one cannot use autoradiography, because, in general, after about 30 min only half the total brain radioactivity remains in the protein pool. Isotopic methods use the plasma or the brain specific radioactivity as an indication of the precursor pool specific activity (Neff *et al.*, 1971). This can be justified on the grounds that there is fast equilibrium between plasma and brain free-tryptophan pools. Of course, the immediate precursor for the neurotransmitter synthesis is the neuronal tryptophan pool. Measurement of the specific radioactivity of the intraneuronal pool is difficult, and in the first approximation the assumption that the specific radioactivity of that pool is closely related to the specific radioactivity of the brain free-tryptophan is probably satisfactory. Direct comparison of the specific radioactivity of these two pools (brain free-tryptophan and neuro-transmitter pools) also disregards the fact that there is a lag time (e.g. Neff *et al.*, 1971) between this equilibration, as well as the fact that only comparisons between integrated specific radioactivities are correct (Sokoloff *et al.*, 1977).

The time course of the specific activities of L-Trp and 5-HT measured after i.v. injection revealed that the changes of their specific radioactivities were very similar, suggesting to the authors that cerebral 5-HT is in the one compartment (Schute, 1976; Lane and Aprison, 1978). In addition to these data, there is pharmacological evidence that brain 5-HT exists in multiple functional pools (Kleven *et al.*, 1983). However, the time course of the specific radioactivity of 5-HIAA has been found to be different (Schubert, 1974; Tracqui *et al.*, 1983b). The model proposed by Tracqui *et al.* (1983a,b) is quite complex and indicates that there are three Trp compartments (plasma, brain free-tryptophan and tryptophan incorporated into proteins) and two 5-HT compartments. Of the three Trp compartments, only one serves as the precursor for the central Trp compartment which is the precursor for the 5-HT synthesis. It is probably possible to simplify the model, reducing the number of compartments and the rate constants to a more workable number, and still obtain satisfactory estimates of the 5-HT synthesis rate.

3.   Metabolism of α-Methyl-L-tryptophan

The metabolism of α-methyltryptophan has been studied by Sourkes and collaborators for the past 20 years (Sourkes, 1971; Roberge *et al.*, 1972; Missala and Sourkes, 1988). α-MTrp has been shown to be a substrate for tryptophan hydroxylase (Sourkes, 1971; Gal and Christiansen, 1975), and the product of this hydroxylation, 5-hydroxy-α-methyltryptophan, is a substrate for AAAD in the brain (Sourkes, 1971). The product of these biochemical reactions is α-M-5-HT. The Michaelis–Menten kinetical constants for these enzymes have been determined with different cofactors (Gal and Christensen, 1975; Schirlin *et al.*, 1988). The enzymes have a somewhat lower affinity for a α-MTrp and α-M-5-H-Trp than for Trp and 5-H-Trp. However, *in vivo*, a reasonable amount of compound is converted into α-methylserotonin when α-MTrp at a tracer level is injected into rats (Diksic *et al.*, 1990b). We have evaluated the conversion of labelled α-MTrp into α-M-5-HT at the tracer level, using a micropuncture technique in conjunction with HPLC separation. We found that the conversion is time-dependent and that 120 min after the tracer injection 50% and 85% of total radioactivity is present in the raphe dorsalis and pineal body in the form of α-M-5-HT. We also found about 2% of total radioactivity to be present as 5-hydroxy-α-methyl-L-tryptophan (Diksic, Nagahiro and Sourkes, unpublished observation). The latter observation agrees well with other biochemical measurements and indicates that hydroxylation can be assumed as the rate-limiting step in the *in vivo* conversion. (In effect, the transport to the enzyme site from the precursor pool could also be a rate-limiting step; the final outcome is the same.) This is equivalent to the situation of tryptophan conversion into 5-HT, suggesting that labelled α-MTrp could be used as a tracer for the measurement of the brain serotonin synthesis rate. Extracerebral metabolism of α-MTrp is outside the scope of this review, because it does not have any relevance to the brain metabolism when α-MTrp is used at a tracer level. At a pharmacological dose, α-MTrp has a complex effect on the central neurotransmitter levels (Missala and Sourkes, 1988).

Labelled α-MTrp is even better than tryptophan, because its product, α-M-5-HT, is not a substrate for MAO and, as such, the label gets trapped in the brain. Madras and Sourkes (1965) reported that α-MTrp is incorporated very little into proteins in the liver. Our own evaluation of the protein incorporation in the brain showed that less than 2% of radioactivity is found in proteins (Diksic *et al.*, 1990b) when labelled α-MTrp is used as a tracer, in contrast to labelled L-Trp, where about 50% of total radioactivity in tissue is found in the protein fraction about 30–40 min after introduction of the tracer (Diksic and Nagahiro, unpublished data). All of these observations suggest that labelled α-MTrp is a very good compound for use as a tracer when studying the serotonin synthesis rate. Since this tracer is converted *in vivo* into α-M-5-HT, a compound being identified with some biological actions similar to 5-HT when used at a pharmacological dose (Missala and Sourkes, 1988; Montine and Sourkes, 1989), it is also possible to use radioactively labelled α-MTrp for measurement of the axonal transport of serotonin (Nagahiro *et al.*, 1990a).

4. *Principles of Radioisotopic Assays of Biochemical Reaction In Vivo*

The use of mathematical models is becoming increasingly important in the study of biological systems, providing additional information to many scientific areas, including medicine. These models permit a better understanding of complex biological processes.

In principle, the rate of any chemical/biochemical reaction can be estimated from measurements of the rate of the formation of the reaction product(s) or from disappearance of reactant(s). These measurements are made easier by the addition of a radioactively labelled reactant as a tracer (meaning that the amount of radioactive compound does not change the concentration of that reactant), because the measurement of radioactivity is very sensitive. Selection of a tracer to be used in a biological system is often complicated by the competing/parallel reactions carrying the label into two or more products (e.g. labelled tryptophan). This could greatly complicate *in vivo* analysis, especially when there is a very limited number of metabolic products that can be directly measured (e.g. autoradiography and emission tomography). Both of these methods can obtain information only on the total tissue concentration of the tracer (Sokoloff *et al.*, 1977; Phelps *et al.*, 1979). However, in special cases it is possible to remove the free label from slices by washing them with an appropriate solvent and obtaining tracer concentration incorporated into a product (e.g. brain proteins: Kirikae *et al.*, 1989). To avoid this complexity, it is beneficial to have a tracer that follows the biochemical process but does not enter other competing metabolic pathways to any great extent, nor does its final metabolite leave the compartment under evaluation. It is also desirable to have a tracer for which it is possible to devise experimental conditions that would, at the time of measurement, have most of the label present in the final metabolite (Sokoloff *et al.*, 1977). These conditions greatly reduce the errors introduced by approximations made and incorporated into a biological model.

In vivo study of a biological system is further complicated by the dynamic nature of the system under study, and its interconnection and interdependence with parts of the system or with other systems within the organ under evaluation or the body as a whole that affect the system under study. The latter might have special relevance when drugs are used as auxiliary tools in a study (e.g. determination of the rate of brain serotonin synthesis).

In general, a dynamic system is defined as one in which the current value of a variable of the system depends not only on the present value of the input to the system, but also on the history of the system. In other words, the system will have a lag time between input and response, because the response originates in a compartment other than the one into which the input was introduced. This concept, in conjunction with the use of a tracer, allows us to study the dynamics of a biological system and at the same time does not change the steady state of the system under consideration or the system as a whole. Most biological systems operate by a feedback mechanism which actually ensures that a biological system is in a steady state (e.g. plasma glucose levels, body temperature, neurotransmitter concentrations).

An example of these processes can be found in the use of labelled glucose and deoxyglucose as tracers for glucose utilization measurements (Sokoloff *et al.*, 1977). Deoxyglucose is greatly beneficial, because it follows the brain glucose metabolic process only to the level of 6-phosphate. (Any discussion of the influence of the brain dephosphatase in the deoxyglucose model is outside the scope of this chapter—see, e.g. Nelson *et al.*, 1987; Redies and Diksic, 1989.) Labelled α-MTrp has been successfully used for measurement of the brain serotonin synthesis rate (Diksic *et al.*, 1990b; Nagahiro *et al.*, 1990b) and as a tracer to the neuronal serotonin pool (Nagahiro *et al.*, 1990a). The latter permits us to study the rate of neuronal transport of serotonin, which has to date been possible only through exogeneously introduced serotonin (Beaudet and Descarries, 1976). Exogenous introduction of labelled 5-HT into brain structures or ventricles (Aghajamian *et al.*, 1966) has a major disadvantage, because 5-HT is taken up into other than serotoninergic neurons (e.g. Doucet *et al.*, 1988). The uptake into other neurons, even if partially blocked, complicates analysis of the data (see below).

5. *Rate of Serotonin Synthesis by α-MTrp Method*

Theory

The method for measuring the serotonin synthesis rate is based on the biological model shown schematically in Figure 1. In this context the

a-MTrp Model

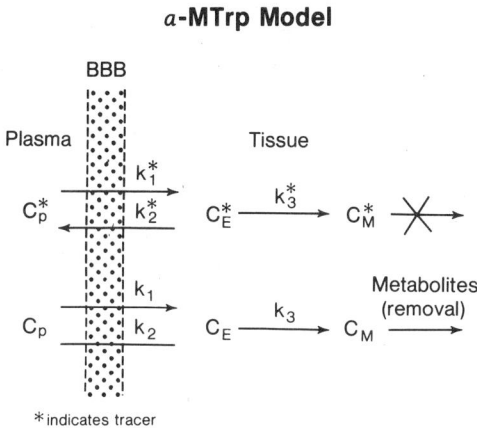

*indicates tracer

Figure 1 A schematic presentation of the α-MTrp biological model identifying the transfer coefficients for the movement of the tracer between different compartments. All coefficients are first-order rate constants. K_1^* governs transfer from plasma into brain; k_2^* governs transfer back. The coefficient for the transfer from the precursor pool into the irreversible pool is k_3^*. The coefficients with a star are those for endogenous tryptophan. Note that in the equations, K_1^* (actually the product of the plasma volume, ml, in the unit weight of brain, g, and the k_1^*) is used and represents the unidirectional clearance of the tracer from the plasma to the brain

biological model is actually a set of differential equations that describe this or any other biological system. Figure 1 is a pictorial representation of the proposed compartmental arrangement from which differential equations (see below) are derived. This biological model is based on the biochemical properties of α-MTrp and its metabolites formed in the brain (see review above) and on the applicability of tracer kinetics. After labelled α-MTrp has been introduced into the system (e.g. a 'pulse' intravenous injection), it is transported bidirectionally between the blood and brain precursor compartment by the BBB amino acid carrier (Diksic *et al.*, 1988), the same one that transports L-Trp and some other essential amino acids (Oldendorf, 1971; Yudilevich *et al.*, 1972). From the precursor compartment (probably extracellular space, glia and neurons other than serotoninergic neurons), it enters the serotoninergic neurons, probably mainly via the high-affinity uptake system (Knapp and Mandell, 1972; Mandell and Knapp, 1977). Some tryptophan possibly enters the precursor pool (compartment) from the protein degradation. However, some experimental measurements of brain specific radioactivity after i.v. injection of labelled L-Trp would suggest that the amount is small in comparison with the amounts entering from plasma (Neff *et al.*, 1971; Tracqui *et al.*, 1983a,b).

As mentioned earlier, the conversion of L-Trp into 5-H-Trp and 5-HT occurs exclusively in the serotoninergic neurons. As far as this model is concerned, the rate constant k_3^* (Figure 1) could be associated with the high-affinity neuronal transport of L-Trp, with *in vivo* activity of tryptophan hydroxylase or, as a matter of fact, with any other process that might, in actuality, control the access of L-Trp from the precursor pool to the enzyme site. Since there are no data on the free-tryptophan concentration at the enzyme site, we shall assume that in this model k_3^* represents the rate-limiting step in the 5-HT synthesis. As described earlier, the conversion of labelled α-MTrp into α-M-5-HT has been established in the brain structure known to be rich in serotoninergic cell bodies (raphe nucleus) and the pineal body (Nagahiro *et al.*, 1990b). Our data also suggest that α-MTrp and L-Trp share the same carrier at the BBB level (Diksic *et al.*, 1988, 1990a). Therefore,

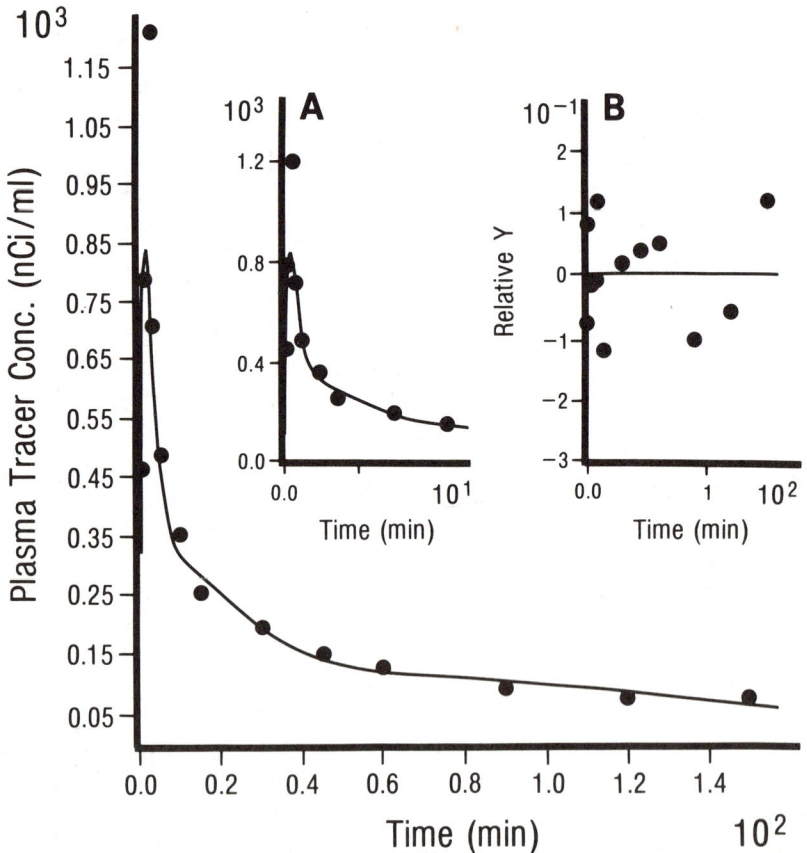

Figure 2   A representative plasma time–radioactivity curve (input function) obtained in a 150 min experiment (Li-treated rat). This curve was fitted to a function of form $Y(t) = \sum_{i=1}^{3} A_i \cdot t \cdot e^{-\lambda_i t}$, where $Y(t)$ represents the value of function at time t (plasma radioactivity), and A_i and λ_i are constants. Insert A presents the peak of the input function; dots are experimental points and the solid line is the fitted curve. In insert B, relative errors of the fit are presented as a function of time

α-MTrp and L-Trp are competitive substrates for the BBB transport and the rate-limiting process mentioned above. Unlike the neurotransmitter serotonin, α-M-5-HT gets trapped in the brain tissue (Nagahiro *et al.*, 1990a,b), permitting use of the three-compartmental model in which the end metabolic product accumulates with time (example of a distribution after 24 h is shown in Figure 2).

In devising a biological model that can represent brain serotonin synthesis, we must make certain assumptions and accept a degree of approximation, since the actual forces governing the transfer of metabolites from one compartment to another are disregarded. It is assumed that: (1) tracer kinetics are applicable; (2) all transfer coefficients are of the first order; (3) the transfer coefficients permit us to describe the process with a set of ordinary differential equations with constant coefficients; (4) tryptophan metabolism is in a steady state and remains in a steady state during the experiment, unchanged by the tracer injection; (5) mixing of the tracer and the tracee is 'instantaneous' in all compartments; (6) only the rate-limiting steps are considered; (7) the plasma is the only source of tryptophan for the neurotransmitter synthesis (i.e. an appreciable amount is not coming from protein degradation); (8) incorporation of the tracer into brain proteins or alternative metabolic pathways in brain is negligible; and (9) the loss of α-methylserotonin, the end metabolite of the tracer or α-M-5-H-Trp, from the metabolic pool is also negligible during the experiment. Assumptions (8) and (9) have been confirmed, at least in part, by data presented in Diksic *et al.* (1990b) and Nagahiro *et al.* (1990b).

Let us imagine that a unit impulse was introduced (e.g. a bolus intravenous injection) at time $t = 0$ to the whole biological 'system' (body). The unit impulse of a radioactively labelled tracer into a dynamic system will produce a characteristic arterial plasma time–radioactivity curve. This arterial plasma time–radioactivity curve is an input function into other parts of the body (e.g. brain). In dynamic biological systems this input function has a characteristic shape, and, when 'accurate' estimates of kinetic constants of a biological model are contemplated, this function must be well known (e.g. Kato *et al.*, 1984b; Evans *et al.*, 1986). Since the introduction of a bolus into a biological system is not a pure δ function, the input function (arterial plasma time–radioactivity curve) has a value of zero for $t = 0$ and the maximum at some time greater than $t = 0$ (Finkelstein and Carson, 1985). This clearly implies that accurate estimates of the kinetic parameters cannot be made when the plasma curve is approximated by the sum of exponentials (the value is not zero at time zero).

Considering the schematics in Figure 1, this biological model can be represented by a set of differential equations with constant coefficients (Sokoloff *et al.*, 1977; Kato *et al.*, 1984b). This set of differential equations can be solved by several methods (Ritger and Rose, 1968). The solution of this system by the Laplace transformation method gives the total radioactivity in respective compartments at time T as

$$C_E^*(T) = f_F^* K_1^* \int_0^T e^{-(k_2^*+k_3^*)(T-t)} \cdot C_p^*(t) \cdot dt \qquad (1)$$

$$C_M^*(T) = \frac{f_F^* \cdot K_1^* \cdot k_3^*}{k_2^* + k_3^*} \int_0^T [1 - e^{(k_2^*+k_3^*)(T-t)}] \cdot C_p^*(t) \cdot dt \qquad (2)$$

$$C_i^*(T) = \left[K^* + K^* \cdot \frac{k_2^*}{k_3} e^{-(k_2^*+k_3^*)t} \right] \otimes C_p^*(t) + V_c \cdot C_p^*(T) \qquad (3)$$

where $C_p^*(t)$ is the plasma tracer concentration (input function) as a function of time (nCi/ml), and $C_E^*(t)$ and $C_M^*(t)$ are time-dependent tracer amounts in the precursor and metabolic compartments (nCi/g), respectively.

Taking into account that the total tissue radioactivity ($C_i^*(T)$) is the sum of the radioactivity present in precursor and metabolic pools and the radioactivity found in the vascular compartment, the total tissue radioactivity measured at time T is described by Equation 3. The vascular compartment fraction is identified by V_c. The symbol $\otimes$ identifies the operation for convolution. The kinetic constant K_1^* is actually the first-order rate constant k_1^* (min^{-1}; Figure 1) multiplied by the plasma volume in the unit weight of the brain (ml/g). K_1^* could be thought of as the rate of unidirectional transfer of tracer from plasma to brain. k_2^* and k_3^* are the first-order rate constants for the transfer of tracer from the precursor compartment back to the plasma and into the metabolic (irreversible) compartment, respectively. The tracer-free fraction (not protein-bound) in the plasma is identified by f_F^*. (Note that there is no need to know this fraction (Diksic *et al.*, 1990b).) It is assumed that, once the tracer is in the metabolic compartment, there is no loss during the experimental period, the kill time in the experiments involving laboratory animals or up to the end of a PET scanning sequence (T).

Here K^* (ml g^{-1} min^{-1}) is equal to $(K_1^* \cdot k_3^* \cdot f_F^*)/(k_2^*+k_3^*)$ and represents the rate of the net unidirectional transfer of the tracer into the irreversible (metabolic) compartment. Using one of the optimization techniques allows us to estimate variables in Equation 3. It is also possible to have a vascular compartment as a variable if the first few minutes of the tissue uptake curve and the plasma input function are well defined. As discussed elsewhere (Diksic *et al.*, 1990b; Nagahiro *et al.*, 1990b), knowing the constant K^*, the lumped constant (LC) and the plasma free-tryptophan concentration (C_p; nmol g^{-1}) is all that is required to estimate the rate of serotonin synthesis (R; nmol g^{-1} min^{-1}):

$$R = K^* \cdot \frac{C_p}{LC} \qquad (4)$$

Estimation of K^* using Equation 3 is possible if there is a good sampling (number of different animals) for times T up to about 150 min after the tracer injection when experiments are done in rats (the curve is composed of a large number of distinct points representing different animals). The reason for this is a slight but real animal-to-animal difference, which introduces additional noise into the data. However, for PET measurements it is possible to use this equation, because the entire time tissue–radioactivity curve is obtained in the same animal (or human) and from the same tracer injection (Phelps *et al.*, 1979; Evans *et al.*, 1986; Diksic *et al.*, 1990a). In PET measurements it is sufficient to sample the tissue time–radioactivity curve up to about 70–80 min after the tracer injection.

To overcome the need to cover the large time period in the autoradiographic measurement, we have devised an alternative and more practical experimental protocol (Nagahiro *et al.*, 1990b). It is based on the biochemical characteristics of α-MTrp, the amount of its conversion into α-M-5-HT and some kinetic considerations. It has been shown (Patlak *et al.*, 1983; Kato *et al.*, 1984a) that the tissue distribution volume ($DV(T)$) is a linear function of the exposure time $\Theta(T) = [\int_0^T C_p^*(t) \cdot dt]/C_p^*(T)$ after an apparent (or actual) steady state has been reached. (A steady state characteristic requires that the change in the precursor compartment be zero: $dC_E^*(t)/dt = 0$.) The slope of this linear relation is equal to K^* (the rate of the undirectional net trapping), and the intercept is the apparent volume of the tracer distribution (V_{app}):

$$DV(T) = \frac{C_i^*(T)}{C_p^*(T)} = K^* \cdot \Theta(T) + V_{app} \qquad (5)$$

We have shown (Diksic *et al.*, 1990b) that 1 h after an i.v. injection of ^{14}C-labelled α-MTrp into rats, it was reasonable to assume that an apparent steady state is reached. The protocol that uses this relation (Equation 5) in the estimation of the serotonin synthesis rate requires that the rats be killed at two different times after injection of the tracer—e.g. 60 min and 150 min. (An example of tracer distribution in the brain of Li-treated rats killed at these two time intervals is shown in Figure 3.) It should be noted that, even though the rats are killed at the same time after injection of the tracer, different exposure times ($\Theta(T)$) are usually obtained. This fact indicates that previous measurements where rats were simply killed at a certain time after injection and the kill time was used in the serotonin synthesis rate estimation might be erroneous (e.g. Neff *et al.*, 1971). This, in practice, makes better sampling of the straight line (Equation 5), because a set of different $\Theta(T)$s are obtained (Nagahiro *et al.*, 1990b; Diksic and Sourkes, 1990). In general, when experiments are done in rats that are on the same diet and receive equivalent treatment before and during the experiment, the plasma free-tryptophan concentration does not differ greatly between animals. The ratio between plasma free-tryptophan and the sum of all amino acids sharing the same carrier is also constant (Diksic and Takada, to be published). However, if there is any indication that the plasma free-tryptophan concentration varies substantially between animals, Equation 5 could be multiplied by C_p and then the slope of the line calculated (Equation 3 in Nagahiro *et al.*, 1990b). The latter requires an assumption that the brain tryptophan concentration in the

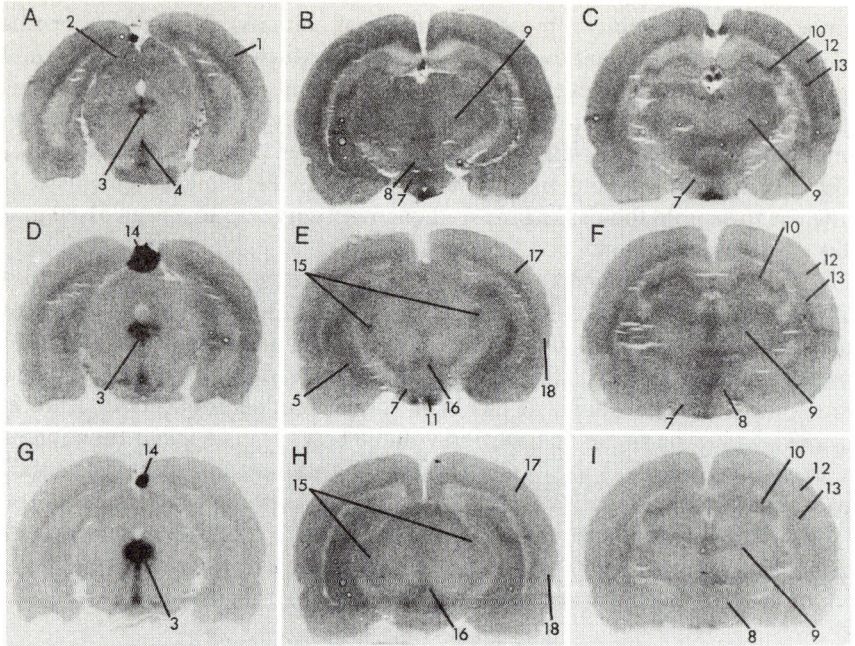

Figure 3 A representative set of autoradiograms obtained in brains of rats injected with 50 μCi and killed at 1 h (A–C), 2.5 h (D,E) and 6 h (G–I). Several structures are identified by numbers: (1) occipital cortex; (2) superior colliculus; (3) raphe dorsalis; (4) raphe mediamus; (5) hippocampus (neutral); (6) medial forebrain bundle; (7) hypothalamus; (8) medial forebrain bundle; (9) thalamus; (10) hippocampus (dorsal); (11) mamillary body; (12) parietal cortex; (13) parietal cortex (layer VI); (14) pineal body; (15) medial geniculate nucleus; (16) ventral tegmental area; (17) temporal cortex; and (18) perirhinal area

precursor pool be the same in different animals. Since the underlying hypothesis of the experiments in animals is that all animals have the same rate of serotonin synthesis and, as discussed above, since the rate is related to the concentration of tryptophan in the precursor pool, this assumption is probably reasonable because it is based on the use of different animals for measurements.

The LC is actually the ratio between the ratios of several other constants, namely the Michaelis–Menten constants for tracer (K_m^* and V_{max}^*) and tracee (K_m and V_{max}) and the volumes of distribution of tracer (V_D^*) and tracee (V_D),

$$LC = \frac{V_D^*}{V_D} \cdot (K_m/V_{max})/(K_m^*/V_{max}^*)$$

LC was calculated from the measurement of the distribution volumes in rat brain (Missala and Sourkes, 1988) and *in vitro* measurements of the Michaelis–Menten constants (details are given in Diksic *et al.*, 1990b). The lumped constant was estimated to be 0.46 (Diksic *et al.*, 1990b) and is assumed to be uniform throughout the brain. Certainly the Michaelis–Menten constants vary from region to region, but probably the ratio between those for tracer and tracee would not change; in other words, if the ratio for tracer increases by a factor, the ratio for tracee will increase by the same factor. A similar reasoning probably holds true for the volume of distribution. This assumption is at present under active investigation in the α-MTrp model. However, this assumption is true in another brain system: glucose–deoxyglucose (Kuwabara *et al.*, 1990).

Experimental Procedures

Autoradiographic Measurement of the Synthesis Rate

The animals are housed in the animal quarters at 22 °C for at least 3 days before being used in experiments. To avoid any influence of circadian rhythm, known to affect brain serotonin synthesis and the plasma tryptophan concentration, the animals are kept on a regular day–night cycle (7 a.m. to 7 p.m., light) for at least 3 days, and killed between 1300 h and 1400 h. Since food intake affects the plasma concentration of amino acids, and could thereby affect the brain serotonin synthesis, the animals were deprived of food the night before being used in experiments but given water *ad libitum*. This procedure produces animals that have a very closely reproducible ratio between plasma-free tryptophan and the sum of other amino acids using the same uptake system (Takada and Diksic, unpublished observation). Under light halothane anaesthesia (1–1.5%), the femoral artery and vein are catheterized with a PE-50 polyethylene catheter. The animals are placed in loose-fitting plaster casts (Sokoloff *et al.*, 1977; Sako *et al.*, 1984) and allowed to wake up. The tracer is injected at least 2 h after the animals waken. To avoid serious disturbance of the steady state, 30 µCi of the tracer (specific radioactivity ≈50 mCi/mmol) is injected over 2 min. Most of our experiments have been done with 50 µCi. In autoradiographic measurements the animals are killed at 60 min and 150 min after tracer injection. Usually there are six rats per time point. During the experimental period, about twelve 20 µl plasma samples are taken at increasing time intervals for the input function determination (radioactivity measurement: Nagahiro *et al.*, 1990b). In addition to these samples, two plasma samples (20 µl each) are taken for determination of plasma total and free-tryptophan concentration. Determination of the plasma free-tryptophan fraction is done in the plasma filtered through an Ultrafree-MC filter (Catalogue No. UF3LGCOO, Millipore Canada) with a 10 000 MW cutoff point. After the animals have been decapitated, the brain is removed, frozen, and cut into 30 µm sections for exposure to X-ray film (SB-5; Eastmont Kodak Co., Rochester, N.Y.) along standards calibrated to the tissue equivalent. Four to five weeks of exposure will produce autoradiograms of very good quality. The autoradiograms are quantified by using the functional relation between optical density and radioactivity (in standards calibrated as 30 μm tissue equivalent), and the tissue radioactivity (nCi/g) is converted into tissue distribution volume (Equation 5; Nagahiro *et al.*, 1990b). The last plasma sample is taken immediately before the animal is killed. To reduce a small but occasional real scatter in the plasma radioactivity curve, this curve is fitted to a function given in the caption of Figure 2. In general, the total plasma integrals calculated by integration of the fitted function (Figure 2) or by interpolation between actual data points are very similar. The plasma tracer concentration, $C_p^*(T)$, used in Equation 5, is calculated from the fitted function (an example given in Figure 4). The slope of this relation (Equation 5) is then estimated by the least-squares method and the serotonin synthesis rate is calculated according to Equation 4.

Plasma gases and haematocrit levels should be assessed periodically, and if they are substantially outside the physiological range, the animals should be excluded from the group. Body temperature should also be kept within the physiological range. In rat experiments this is usually accomplished by using a regular light bulb (e.g. Sako *et al.*, 1984). Care must be taken to ensure that the animals are not exposed to any differential stress, because this will make interpretation of the data more difficult.

PET Measurement with ^{11}C-labelled α-MTrp

Animals for PET studies are handled in a manner similar to that described above for rats. The major difference is that they are imaged under anaesthesia (e.g. Redies *et al.*, 1989). However, humans are awake during the scanning procedure. In both humans and animals used for PET scanning, the food intake is controlled as mentioned above for rats. PET imaging has an advantage over the experiments in rats (discussed above) because the entire tissue time–radioactivity curve is obtained after a single injection of the tracer and it permits repeated measurements in the same subject (Diksic *et al.*, 1987, 1988). Unfortunately, ^{11}C-labelled α-MTrp must be synthesized in close proximity to the PET scanner, because the half-life of ^{11}C is only 20 min. This tracer can be synthesized by a method we described earlier (Chaly and Diksic, 1988), using ^{11}C-labelled methyl iodide as the reagent to introduce the label into the final molecule. To determine K^* (Equation 3), the serotonin synthesis rate is best estimated by fitting Equation 3 to the experimental tissue time–radioactivity curve (possibly on a regional basis if the region is large enough to give reasonable statistics) and then using Equation 4 for calculation of the synthesis rate. During scanning, plasma samples are taken at progressively increasing time intervals to obtain the plasma input function. Two to three plasma samples should also be taken for measurement of the plasma total tryptophan concentration and the free-tryptophan fraction in the plasma. Special care should be taken to keep plasma physiological parameters within the physiological range; otherwise the plasma free-tryptophan fraction and the brain serotonin synthesis rate could be influenced.

Rate of 5-HT Axonal Transport
The rate of axonal transport is determined in laboratory animals, using
radioactively labelled α-MTrp (^{14}C or ^{3}H), which is *in situ* transformed into
α-M-5-HT, a serotonin analogue (structural and functional: see, e.g., Missala
and Sourkes, 1988). As discussed above, α-M-5-HT is probably stored in the
brain in the same place that endogenous 5-HT is stored. (This storage space
may be the vesicles. We are currently carrying out experiments with Dr A.
Beaudet to determine whether there is co-storage in vesicles.) An advantage
of this method to determine the rate of axonal transport is that the tracer is
synthesized *in situ* and does not require any other pharmacological treatment
or invasive introduction of tracer into the brain (e.g. intracerebral or
intraventricular injection). Animals are injected intravenously with 50 μCi of
^{14}C-labelled α-MTrp in these experiments over 2–5 min. ^{3}H-labelled compound can also be used, in which case the amount should be 1–1.5 mCi. An
intraperitoneal injection could also be used, but this will spread the input
function to the brain considerably. Rats are killed about 6–8 h after tracer
injection and 30–50-μm-thick slices obtained as above. It is good practice to
get an accurate count of the slices taken for use in the estimation of the
distance to which the tracer has travelled (Nagahiro *et al.*, 1990a), but the
distance can also be estimated on the basis of stereotaxic coordinates.
The distance to which the radioactivity has travelled from the raphe dorsalis
along the medial forebrain bundle (MFB) is determined by measuring the
ratio of the radioactivity in the MFB and hypothalamus, the terminal field of
these projections (Takagi *et al.*, 1980). By plotting this ratio as a function of
the distance, the length of travel is determined. The ratio between these two
structures found in rats killed 60 min after tracer injection is taken as being
the measurement of the background radioactivity. It is assumed that, once
this ratio is observed, there is no tracer contribution from the anterograde
transport (Nagahiro *et al.*, 1990a).

6. *Autoradiographic Measurements of the Regional Synthesis Rate*

Normal Rats

A set of autoradiograms presented in Figure 3 shows brain tracer distribution
at 60 min (A–C), 150 min (D–F) and 6 h (G–I) after injection. The
distribution observed 24 h after injection is presented in Figure 4.
Regional rates of cerebral serotonin synthesis determined by the α-MTrp
method in normal conscious adult female Wistar rats are presented in Table
1. Data show that the rate of serotonin synthesis varies greatly between
different brain structures. Unfortunately, there are no other measurements of
the synthesis rate that can be, without reservation, directly compared with

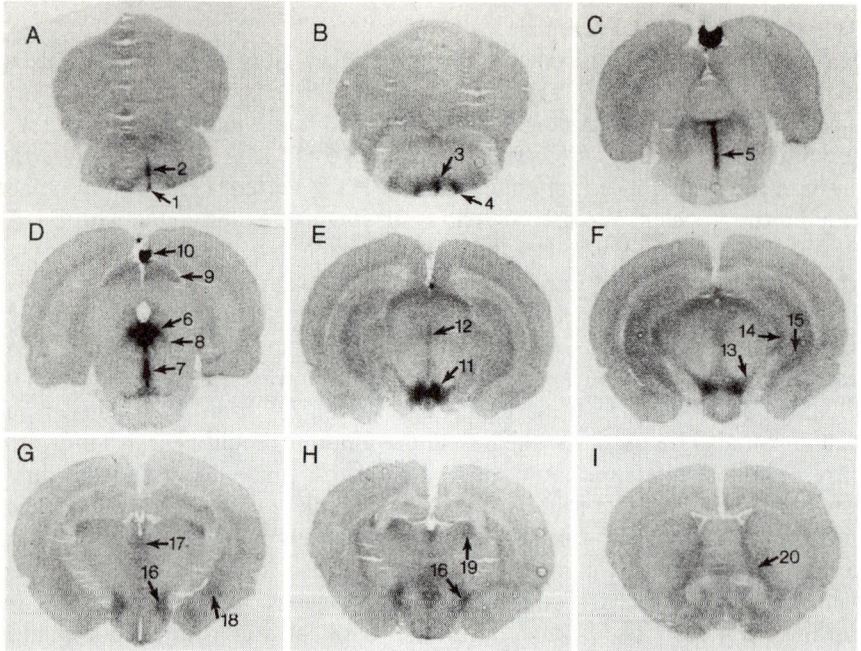

Figure 4 A set of representative autoradiograms displaying rat brain distribution of radioactivity 24 h after injection of 50 μCi of ^{14}C-labelled α-MTrp. The structures especially identified are: (1) raphe pallidus; (2) raphe obscurus; (3) raphe magnus; (4) group of cells ventral to n. facialis; (6) raphe pontis; (5) raphe dorsalis; (7) raphe mediamus; (8) decussation of superior cerebellar peduncles; (9) superior colliculus; (10) pineal body; (11) ventral tegmental area; (12) periaqueductal grey matter; (13) substantia nigra; (14) lateral geniculate body; (15) hippocampus; (16) medial forebrain bundle; (17) periventricular thalamic nuclei; (18) amygdala; (19) lateral thalamic nuclei; (20) caudate putamen

these measurements. The synthesis rates obtained by this autoradiographic method are calculated from the radioactivity measured in a 30-μm-thick section of a particular structure. To estimate the rate of synthesis in the whole rat brain, the rates in all brain structures should be added and the appropriate weights used for each structure. Since this is not really practical, the measurements obtained by other biochemical methods (using tissue sampling) should not be directly compared with data obtained by this method; only a rough comparison can be made. Another problem of comparing data obtained by the biochemical method is the use of drugs as an integral part of these methods (see above). To get an idea of what kind of synthesis rate was obtained by biochemical methods, synthesis rates between 16.7 pmol g^{-1} min^{-1} and 41.7 pmol g^{-1} min^{-1} were reported for the whole rat brain (Korf, 1985).

From the data presented in Table 1, it is obvious that the rate of serotonin synthesis is about 5–6 times greater in the brain area rich in serotoninergic cell

Table 1   Rate of serotonin synthesis in representative discrete structures of normal (untreated) rat brain and in pineal body: evaluation of the two-time-point method

Structure	R (pmol g^{-1} min^{-1})[a]
Parietal cortex; layer VI	37 ± 13
Thalamus	33 ± 13
Caudate (medial part)	58 ± 14
Accumbens nucleus	67 ± 19
Hypothalamus	26 ± 10
Hippocampus	47 ± 13
Raphe dorsalis	166 ± 37
Medial raphe nucleus	95 ± 20
Pineal body	251 ± 31

[a] Rates are given as an estimate $\pm$ s.d. (Uncertainty was calculated from the standard deviation of the slope ($K^{C_p} = K^* \cdot C_p$) in Equation 5, estimated from the least-squares fit: Bevington, 1969.)

bodies (e.g. raphe dorsalis) compared with those measured in the terminal areas (e.g. hypothalamus, cortex). It must be emphasized that these measurements represented the rates of serotonin synthesis in awake rats, but the rates might be influenced by the fact that the lower part of the rats' bodies were restrained (a form of stress) for at least 3 h before they were killed. Acute and chronic stress (Curzon *et al.*, 1972; Čulman *et al.*, 1984; Adell *et al.*, 1988) have different effects on the rate of serotonin synthesis. The fact that rats have to be partially restrained, at least for 3 h, must be considered when an experimental protocol is developed. If the experimental protocol is properly developed, it should not influence comparison of the synthesis rates obtained in a treated group of rats with those of a control group (an example is given later). However, the control group will most likely be exposed to a different stress compared with rats used here as normal animals (Table 1). An idea of this effect can probably be obtained by comparing rates in normal rats (Table 1) with those in controls for the Li-treatment protocol (Table 2).

An interesting relative comparison might be made between the synthesis rates (Table 1) and measurements of the tryptophan hydroxylase activity (Ehret *et al.*, 1987). The ratios between the rates in several structures are quite close to the ratios between enzyme activities (e.g. pineal/raphe dorsalis; pineal/raphe medianus; raphe dorsalis/hippocampus). However, comparison of absolute values (enzyme activity–rate of serotonin synthesis) suggests that the rates presented here (Table 1) are appreciably lower than those expected from the non-activated enzyme activity measurements (e.g. Ehret *et al.*, 1987). This suggests that the activity of tryptophan hydroxylase is not fully expressed *in vivo* and that it possesses a substantial reserve which probably can be called upon in certain situations when there is a high demand for the synthesis of the neurotransmitter. For example, reserpine treatment has been shown to increase the activity of tryptophan hydroxylase (Sze, 1981).

Serotonin Synthesis Rates in Lithium-treated Rats

Data in the literature indicate that the lithium ion increases the brain serotonin synthesis rate (Perez-Cruet *et al.*, 1971; Stewart *et al.*, 1988). Since serotonin levels are low in depressed patients, lithium was introduced for the treatment of depression (e.g. Goodnick and Gershon, 1985; Ghadirian *et al.*, 1989). The data we present here clearly support the role of lithium in the increase of brain serotonin synthesis and show that the increase in the rate is differential.

In this experimental protocol, rats were divided into two groups. One group of rats received an injection of LiCl solution (85 mg/kg and a constant volume 5 ml/kg: Perez-Cruet *et al.*, 1971), and a second (control) group, normal saline (5 ml/kg: Perez-Cruet *et al.*, 1971). Injections were done twice a day for 5 days. All other preparation and handling was done as described above. The plasma lithium concentration was determined in the plasma the day following the last injection. All animals had Li concentrations well above 0.7 μmol/ml (Nagahiro *et al.*, 1990a), the level accepted as the minimum for a therapeutic effect (Stewart *et al.*, 1988). A set of autoradiograms obtained in Li-treated rats is presented in Figure 5. The rates of serotonin synthesis obtained for the control and Li-treated animals are presented in Table 2. An example of the plasma input function and the function fit to the experimental data is presented in Figure 2. All physiological parameters were within normal range and there was no difference in those parameters between the two groups of animals (Nagahiro *et al.*, 1990b). As seen from the data

Table 2 Rate of serotonin synthesis in representative discrete structures of the rat brain and in the pineal body. Results for untreated control (NaCl-treated) and LiCl-treated animals are given

| | R (pmol g^{-1} min^{-1})[a] | | |
Structure	Controls[b]	Li-treated[c]	% Differences
Parietal cortex	23 ± 7[d]	35 ± 11[d]	52
Thalamus	31 ± 13	32 ± 13	0
Caudate (medial)	37 ± 9[d]	54 ± 14[d]	46
Accumbens nucleus	53 ± 15	65 ± 16	23
Hippocampus	38 ± 10[d]	51 ± 12[d]	34
Hypothalamus	40 ± 10	43 ± 11	10
Dorsal raphe nucleus	202 ± 41[d]	258 ± 29[d]	28
Medial raphe nucleus	141 ± 55	170 ± 28	21
Pineal body	257 ± 44	273 ± 44	6

[a] Rates are given as an estimate ± s.d. (Uncertainty was calculated from the standard deviation of the slope ($K^{C_p} = K^* \cdot C_p$) in Equation 5, estimated from the least-squares fit: Bevington, 1969.)
[b] $N = 10$; NaCl-treated rats.
[c] $N = 18$.
[d] Significant effect of lithium ($p < 0.05$) by the two-tailed t-test for comparing Li-treated rats with controls.

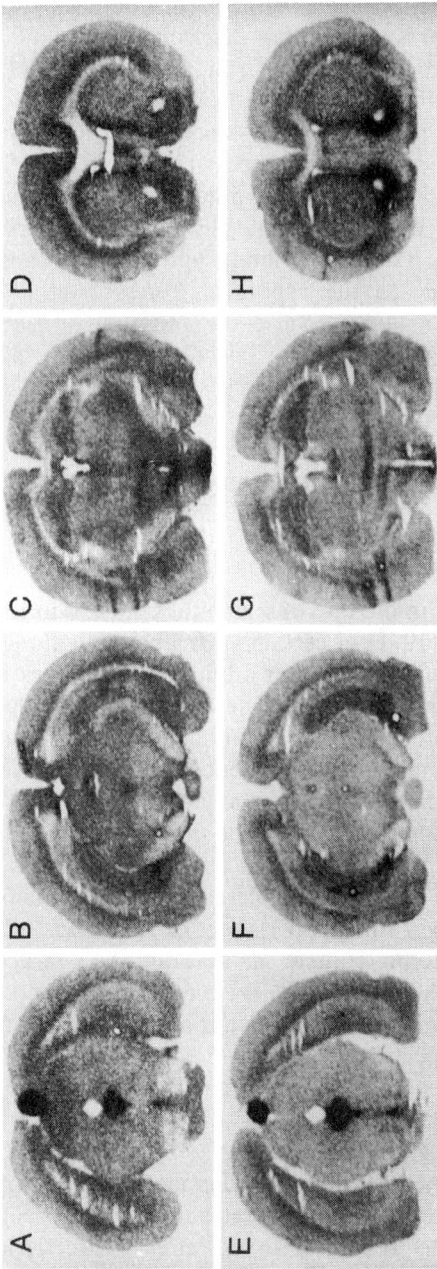

Figure 5 A set of representative autoradiograms showing the tracer distribution at 60 min (A–D) and 150 min (E–H) in Li-treated rats (the treatment protocol is described under the experimental procedure)

presented in Table 2, Li treatment as used in this protocol produces a differential change in the serotonin synthesis rate in different brain structures. However, the plasma Li concentration in the animals used in our study (Nagahiro *et al.*, 1990b) is higher than that generally found in patients of Li therapy (Goodnick and Gershon, 1985; Stewart *et al.*, 1988). For example, there was no change in the serotonin synthesis rate in the thalamus, only a 6% increase in the pineal body, but a 50% increase in the parietal cortex and caudate nucleus. For the first time it is possible to assess the effect of lithium treatment on the brain serotonin synthesis rate with good anatomical resolution (≈ 0.1 mm). In our experiments we did not observe any change in the plasma concentration of free or total tryptophan (Takada and Diksic, to be published), contrary to the report of Perez-Cruet *et al.* (1971) and Goodnick and Gershon (1985). Since the rats used in our protocol were handled for 5 days as well as before injection, one must also consider the possible influence of chronic and mild stress on these measurements. Gessa and Tagliamonte (1974) have reported an increase of 71% in the plasma free-tryptophan concentration in rats subjected to mild stress. However, our animals (even those rats used for the experiments in Table 1) have a different stress profile from that of the rats Gessa and Tagliamonte used, which might be one of the reasons that we did not observe a change in free or total plasma tryptophan concentration.

An increase of 82% in the rate of serotonin synthesis in rat brain reported by Perez-Cruet *et al.* (1971) is certainly far above anything that would be expected from our results, even after addition of the rates for the all-brain structures with appropriate weights. One explanation for this large increase observed by Perez-Cruet *et al.* (1971) could be found in their observation that the plasma free and total tryptophan concentration increased in Li-treated animals. Discounting the possibility of any other artefact in their measurements, their rats must somehow have been more stressed, and the increase in serotonin synthesis is probably more a result of the stress than of the Li treatment and could be related to the increase of the plasma free-tryptophan. An asymmetric (left/right difference) effect of LiCl and NaCl treatment on the steady state serotonin content in several brain structures has been reported (Mandell and Knapp, 1979). We have not observed any asymmetric influence on the serotonin synthesis rate nor any left to right difference in the images. (A visual inspection of Figure 5 also illustrates this.) However, although the images do not directly represent the rate of synthesis, they could give a rough indication of the content of α-MTrp and α-M-5-HT in the structures evaluated (e.g. raphe dorsalis).

Drug-effect experiments and use of this method could offer us valuable information on the serotonin synthesis rates in different brain structures. We might then be able to relate observed effects directly to a particular treatment. The method can clearly settle some of the controversy related to the possible influence of certain drugs on the measured serotonin synthesis rates used as treatment in previous methods (e.g. probenecid, AAAD inhibitors).

7. PET Measurements in Dog Brain

Positron emission tomography has the unique advantage of allowing repeated testing in the same animal. PET displays the radioactivity distribution in a volume of tissue and, after reconstruction and appropriate corrections, provides quantitative tomographic images of tissue radioactivity distribution. The mechanics of the PET scanner and image reconstruction are outside the scope of this chapter and interested readers are referred to the literature (e.g. Hoffman and Phelps, 1986). Here we describe only scanning procedures related to these particular measurements.

Since hydroxylase (a rate-limiting enzyme) is not saturated with any of the substrates (tryptophan or oxygen; see discussion above) or cofactor, the rate of serotonin synthesis can be influenced by changing the concentration of a substrate. With PET we can assess the rate of synthesis under different conditions in the same animal (e.g. change in the plasma tryptophan concentration and arterial oxygen tension), and the entire tissue time–radioactivity curve (uptake curve) is obtained from the same injection of ^{11}C-labelled tracer. Here two examples are presented to serve a double purpose—to show the use of the method and to confirm the theory mentioned above (lack of the enzyme saturation with substrates). PET results on the serotonin synthesis rates also confirm previous reports in rats of repeated measurements in the same brain under different steady-state conditions. This feature makes the method accessible to measurements in living human brain.

Table 3 The brain serotonin synthesis rates estimated under different experimental conditions[a]

Experiment (number)	Influx (nmol g^{-1} min^{-1})	Plasma tryptophan[b] (nmol/ml)	Arterial PaO$_2$ (mmHg)	R (pmol g^{-1} min^{-1})
1	3.27	16.6 (13–17.4)	90 ± 2	18.5 ± 4.5
2	19.15	191.5 (168–218)	90 ± 2	320 ± 95
3	39.7	381 (374–387)	91 ± 2	620 ± 112
4	—	75 (72–78)	76 ± 2	39 ± 8
5	—	74.6 (72–77)	106 ± 1	54 ± 10

[a]Data are presented as an average ± s.d. The uncertainty in the synthesis rate was estimated from the variance–covariance matrix of the tissue curve time–radioactivity fit to the model equation or from the error obtained from the fit to the straight line of the linear portion in the volume of distribution graph.
[b]The range of the plasma tryptophan concentration between about 30 min before tracer injection and the end of the study is given in parentheses.

Of course, PET measurements in animals can be carried out only under general anaesthesia.

In the first set of experiments, the plasma tryptophan concentration in a dog was elevated to two levels substantially above the baseline (Table 3). In the second set of experiments the plasma oxygen tensions were changed (Diksic *et al.*, 1987, 1988, 1990a). A set of PET images obtained in the dog study are presented in Plate 1(A), with enlargements of images at 30 min and 50 min after tracer injection shown in Plate 1(B) and Plate 1(C), respectively. The plasma tryptophan concentration was elevated by giving a one-time (over 5 min) i.v. injection of 200 mg of L-Trp (9.78 mg/ml) and having the dog on a continuous drip (≈ 1 ml/min) with a solution of L-Trp of the same concentration for about 1.5 h before the tracer injection. This procedure produced a plasma tryptophan concentration of a reasonably 'constant' value. (Table 3 shows that the average was within about 20% in the second study and within 5% in the third.)

The plasma oxygen tensions were altered by manipulating the stroke volume and the rate of breathing. (The dog was on a respirator under general anaesthesia.) Measurements were done at two different PaO_2 levels (Table 3). Tissue time–radioactivity curves were analysed, as discussed in the theory, and from the fit to Equation 3 the K^* was obtained and used according to Equation 4 to estimate the synthesis rate in that cross-section. (The rates in all three brain cross-sections were added together.) No attempt was made to obtain tissue time–radioactivity curves in a smaller volume of tissue. As seen from Plate 1, the limited resolution of the PET scanner probably allows us to get only whole brain tissue time–radioactivity with good statistics. It might be possible to obtain a curve for only grey matter, but for our purposes this is unnecessary, because there is no synthesis of serotonin in the glia. The inclusion of white matter probably lowers our count rate per gram but does not change the shape of the curve, and does not change the value of K^*.

The rates of serotonin synthesis estimated in dog brain with PET under different conditions (plasma Trp and oxygen changes) are given in Table 3. Data show that the plasma tryptophan increase indeed resulted in an increase of the serotonin synthesis rate. The rate of synthesis increased more than the average tryptophan plasma concentration when the plasma tryptophan increased from 16.6 nmol/ml to 191.5 nmol/ml. However, there was an equivalent increase in the synthesis rate when the plasma was increased from 191.5 nmol/ml to 381 nmol/ml. This certainly points to the fact that the synthesis rate-limiting step is almost linearly related to the increase in the plasma tryptophan concentration. In experiment No. 2 (Table 3), the plasma tryptophan was more variable and increased towards the end of the experiment. This plasma increase is probably responsible, at least in part, for the larger increase in the brain serotonin synthesis rate observed between experiments Nos 1 and 2. However, it should be pointed out that comparison of experiments Nos 1 and 3 revealed an increase in the serotonin synthesis rate by a factor of about 33.5, whereas the plasma tryptophan was increased

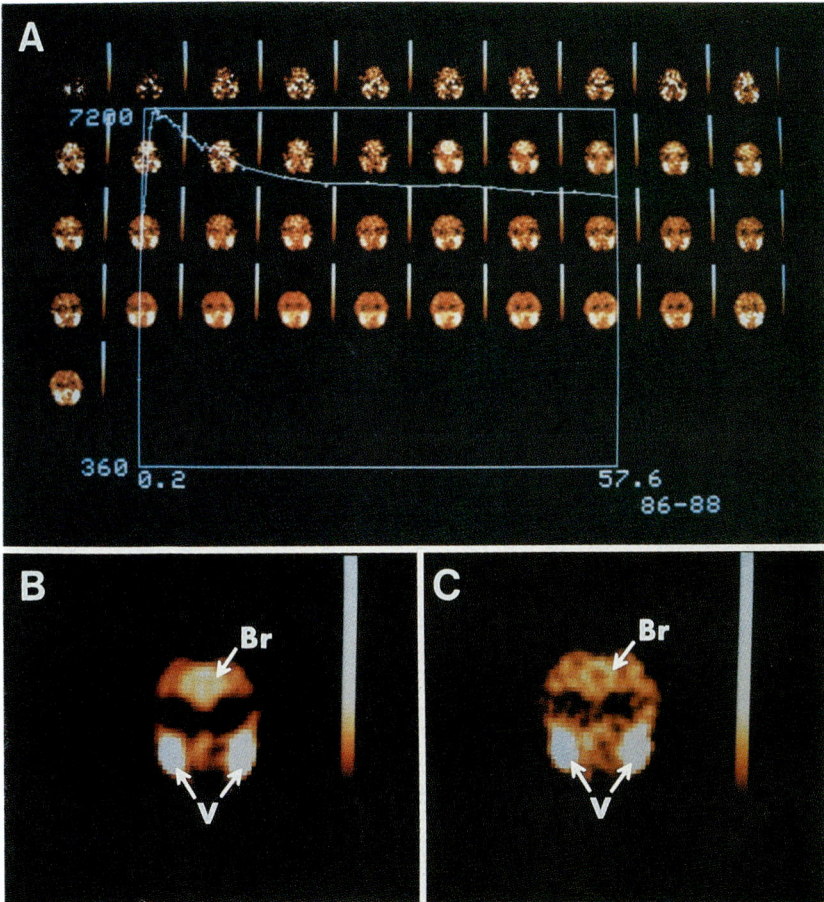

Plate 1 Images obtained in dog brain after injection of 5 mCi of α-[^{11}C]methyl-L-tryptophan with the tissue time–radioactivity curve superimposed on them (A). Two enlarged images obtained at about 30 min (B) and 50 min (C) are also shown. The brain is identified by Br and the neck vessels are marked V

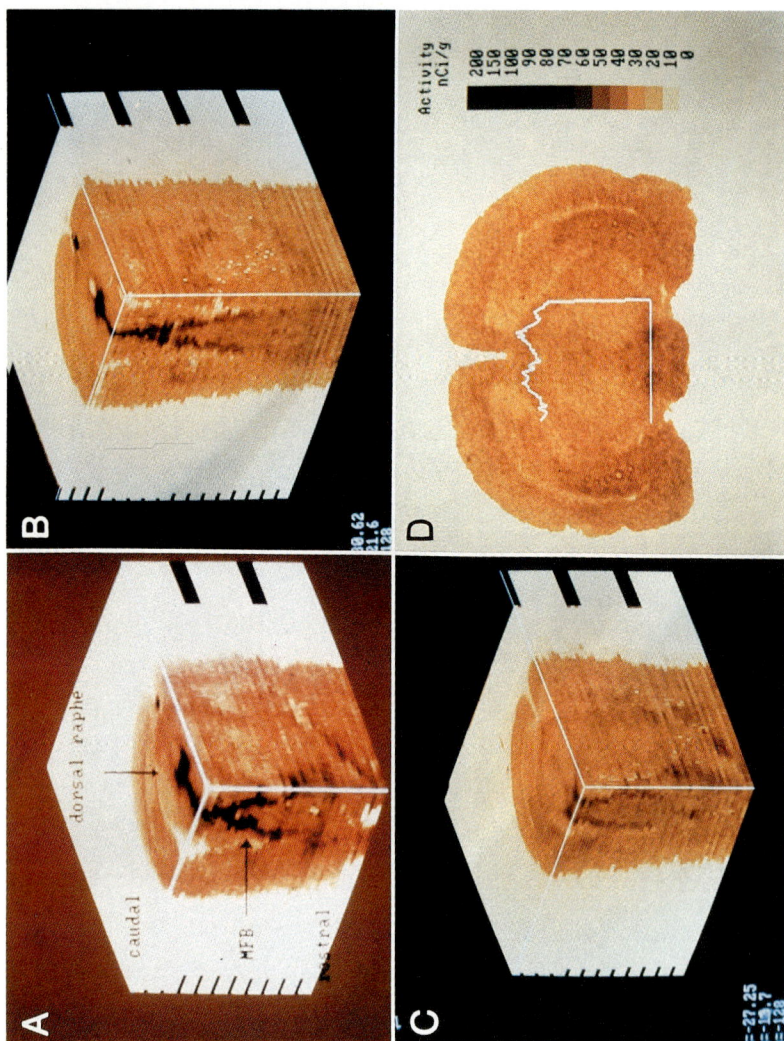

Plate 2   Three-dimensional images showing tracer distribution in the rat brain 6 h (A) and 24 h (B) after injection. Comparison of the intensity of the label in the MFB at 6 h and 24 h reveals that the tracer did not reach the terminal fields in the hypothalamus at 6 h after injection (A). In the three-dimensional image shown in C, obtained by removing a set of cross-sections from the image shown in B, one can easily see MFB. One of those cross-sections is presented in D with the profile used in the estimation of the MFB–hypothalamus ratios

by a factor of about 23. This observation would suggest that the rate-limiting step in the serotonin synthesis was 'activated', but it should be noted that this comparison is done only with a point. In our analysis we have assumed that all the tracer and tryptophan in the tissue is available for the rate-limiting step. These results were obtained by assuming that there was no difference in the plasma free-tryptophan fraction. However, the plasma free-tryptophan fraction is probably less important than the tissue free-tryptophan fraction. Experiments other than ours also assume that there is no tissue protein binding (not to be confused with protein incorporation) of tryptophan. Unfortunately, very little work has been done on this. One report indicates that the free tryptophan in the tissue precursor pool (tissue ultrafiltrate) is 7.7% of the total, less than that in plasma, where it is 11.9% (Moir, 1974). However, it should be noted that Moir's plasma free fraction is a little low, with quite a large scatter in the total plasma concentration.

There are no other measurements of the brain serotonin synthesis rate in dog brain. However, if the rates obtained by PET in dogs with plasma tryptophan and oxygen tension close to normal (experiments Nos 1 and 4, Table 3) are compared with measurements in the brain of other species, a reasonable agreement is seen. The average value for the rate in rat and mouse brain obtained from data in Korf (1985) is 31 ± 14 (range 7.7–67; $N = 14$) pmol g^{-1} min^{-1} and 73 ± 45 (range 20–133; $N = 7$) pmol g^{-1} min^{-1}, respectively. (It is more appropriate to compare PET results with the biochemical tissue sampling methods than with the autoradiographic method described above.) Taking into account the different species, the different methodologies and the divergence of data in the literature, the agreement is acceptable. The difference in the rates obtained in experiments Nos 1 and 4 results mainly from the plasma tryptophan concentration. Dogs used in our experiments were fasted overnight, but no attempt was made to keep them on a controlled diet for a long period of time in an attempt to obtain a similar plasma total tryptophan concentration. Comparison of PET data with other biochemical methods is probably easier, because from PET measurements it is not difficult to obtain the total brain synthesis rate. As discussed above, since biochemical methods use drugs as aids in experimental protocols and/or measure only the difference in the specific activities of precursor and metabolite (e.g. Neff *et al.*, 1971) in determining the serotonin synthesis rate, they should be compared with our method with caution.

From experiments Nos 1–3 one can also estimate the Michaelis–Menten constants for the BBB transport of tryptophan, assuming that α-MTrp shares the same carrier. The Michaelis–Menten (1913) equation can be transformed into the form:

$$\frac{[S]}{V} = \frac{1}{V_{max}} \cdot [S] + \frac{K_m^{app}}{V_{max}} \tag{6}$$

Here V is the influx (Table 3) calculated by multiplying the K_i^* obtained from the fit to Equation 3 and the plasma tryptophan concentration (S). (We use the variable K^* in its expanded form; note that the free fraction is included in K_1^* obtained from the fit.) Data presented in Table 3 (experiments Nos 1–3), when analysed this way, gave a K_m^{app} of 303 ± 54 μM and $V_{max} = 63 \pm 10$ nmol g^{-1} min^{-1}. The value for the K_m^{app} is in reasonable agreement with measurements in the newborn rabbit (1.6 mM: Pardridge and Mietus, 1982) and adult rat (330 μM: Smith *et al.*, 1987; 356 μM: Miller *et al.*, 1985). Since several amino acids share the same carrier, it is better to compare apparent K_m (K_m^{app}), because that is the one with which a carrier operates in a particular animal. However, real K_m can be estimated from the K_m^{app} and the concentration and the K_ms of the AA sharing the same carrier (Pardridge, 1977). A V_{max} of 63 ± 10 nmol g^{-1} min^{-1} agrees well with measurements in newborn rabbit (55 ± 10 nmol g^{-1} min^{-1}) and rat (23 ± 5 nmol g^{-1} min^{-1}).

Our measurements were done under halothane anaesthesia. It was reported that anaesthesia (pentobarbital) has an influence on the K_m (Miller *et al.*, 1985). The K_m was increased by a factor of 2.6 in pentobarbital-anaesthetized rats (Miller *et al.*, 1985) and it is possible that halothane anaesthesia used in our experiments has a similar effect.

In our analysis we have disregarded the diffusion component, which has been shown to contribute between 12% (Etienne *et al.*, 1976) and 20% (Miller *et al.*, 1985; Smith *et al.*, 1987) to the Trp influx. By disregarding this component, it is assumed that the relative amount of the diffusion component does not differ greatly at different plasma L-Trp concentrations. This notion is supported by data of Etienne *et al.* (1976), where an increase in diffusion from 12% to 17% was observed when the plasma Trp was increased from 25 μM to 100 μM. The fit with a correlation coefficient of 0.998, through three points only, can also be taken as an indication that the diffusion contribution to the tissue uptake of the tracer does not differ greatly at different plasma Trp concentrations.

8.   5-HT Axonal Transport

Since 5-HT neurons possess a system of high affinity uptake for 5-HT (Knapp and Mandell, 1972), it is possible to label the 5-HT neurons by exogeneous serotonin injected intrasticially or intraventricularly (e.g. Beaudet and Descarries, 1979). Serotoninergic neurons can also be visualized by immunocytochemistry (Steinbush *et al.*, 1978; Frankfurt and Azmitia, 1984; Weissman *et al.*, 1987). However, none of these methods can be used without concern for estimates of the 5-HT rate of transport along neurons. In experiments where labelled 5-HT is injected into a local brain area, the measured transport is not necessarily that operating in an intact brain under a steady state condition, because of the difficulty in obtaining complete mixing with endogeneous 5-HT. The immunocytochemistry is able to provide us only with information on the anatomical distribution of these neurons. There are methods described for the measurement of the protein axonal transport using [^{14}C]leucine (Bobillier *et al.*, 1975, 1976), [^{3}H]proline (Azmitia and Segal, 1978; Moore *et al.*, 1987) and neurotransmitter transport using [^{3}H]norepinephrine (Jones *et al.*, 1977) and [^{3}H]dopamine (Fibiger *et al.*, 1973). Since all these methods have a tracer that is stereotaxically injected into the brain, as mentioned above, the tracer transport is not necessarily representative of a steady state transport. The main reason for this is that the tracer does not enter the endogenous pool in a physiological manner (e.g. injection of [^{3}H]dopamine into the substantia nigra did not result in an instant equilibration of the tracer with dopamine present in the neurons and extra- and intraneuronal space).

It has been shown (Araneda *et al.*, 1980) that 5-HT is transported retrogradely from the olfactory bulb to the midbrain raphe at the rate of 0.67 mm/h and 2 mm/h. The transport rate of 5-HT in the spinal cord of 0.4–0.5 mm/h was reported (Dählström and Häggendal, 1973). In these experiments [^{3}H]5-HT was injected into the olfactory bulb, the terminal field or the spinal cord. As mentioned above, there is no proof that exogenous [^{3}H]5-HT was indeed uniformly mixed with endogenous serotonin. If the transport of [^{3}H]5-HT started before proper mixing was obtained or the transport of label occurred in a different form, the data are probably not reliable. On the basis of the biochemical data (Diksic *et al.*, 1990b) obtained after injection of this tracer, we can say that much, if not all of the radioactivity travelling from the dorsal raphe along the MFB (Nagahiro *et al.*, 1990a) is in the form of labelled α-M-5-HT, produced *in situ*. An example of the MFB labelled with this tracer at 6 h and 24 h is presented in Plate 2(A) and Plate 2(B), respectively. Visual inspection of these three-dimensional images confirms that the net transport occurs from the cell body area (dorsal and medial raphe nuclei) towards the terminal fields. An illustration in Plate 2(C) shows a cross-section where the MFB is clearly shown. A profile like the one shown in Plate 2(D) was used in the estimation of the MFB/hypothalamus ratios at different distances from the raphe. Our data clearly show that the net axonal transport of a newly synthesized neurotransmitter is from the cell bodies towards the terminals. One reason for this might be the fact that the rate of serotonin synthesis is about 6.4 times higher in the dorsal raphe than in the terminal areas (e.g. hypothalamus: Nagahiro *et al.*, 1990a). The labelling of endogenous 5-HT with *in situ* synthesized α-M-5-HT as a tracer showed an anterograde axonal transport of 0.63 mm/h (Nagahiro *et al.*, 1990a). This transport rate agrees reasonably well with the above-mentioned retrograde rates for 5-HT. Rates for the neuronal transport of other neurotransmitters are also in good agreement: dopamine in the nigrostriatal bundle, 0.8 mm/h (Fibiger *et al.*, 1973) and norepinephrine in the spinal cord, 0.7 mm/h (Häggendal and Dählström, 1969). At this time we do not know the real significance of the anterograde neurotransmitter transport.

It is generally believed that neurotransmitters such as dopamine, nore-pinephrine and 5-HT are stored in at least two different pools (Shields and

Eccleston, 1972; McMillen *et al.*, 1980; Kleven *et al.*, 1983), one containing newly synthesized and the other not so recently synthesized neurotransmitters. It has been hypothesized that newly synthesized neurotransmitters are normally used for release by neurons in normal situations. If the neurons keep the other pool of neurotransmitters, it must have some function, at least in certain situations. This 'reserve' pool could be the pool of 5-HT which is moving along the axons in both directions (retrograde and anterograde). The movement of neurotransmitters in both directions is probably a reality, because our experiments clearly show that the net transport is from the cell bodies towards the terminals and the experiments of others indicate retrograde transport as well. It is possible that the reserve pool is that for which 5-HT has been formed in the cell bodies, then transported towards terminals where it can be used as a 'reserve' pool. The neurotransmitter from the 'reserve' pool can probably be released if and when there is a large demand for the release of 5-HT. This hypothesis does not contradict the previous results, which showed retrograde transport. Certainly, in these retrograde experiments labelled 5-HT introduced at the site of the terminals did not label any one pool exclusively. Our data also suggest that there are large absolute amounts of 5-HT transported anterogradely rather than retrogradely (see visualization of the MFB at 6 h and 24 h). If this was not the case, we would not be able to visualize the MFB with the radioactivity gradient from the raphe towards the terminal fields, because all areas of the brain have the same plasma input function.

We believe that α-M-5-HT produced (synthesized *in situ*) from the precursor α-MTrp (Trp analogue), transported along MFB, measures the rate of axonal transport of 5-HT along the MFB neurons. The assumption that this analogue is only transported in 5-HT neurons must await appropriate experimental confirmation. Experiments using *in situ* synthesized α-M-5-HT should yield information on whether or not the transport rate increases with an increased rate of 5-HT release. It should also be possible to examine whether the rate of firing at a terminal (e.g. hypothalamic stimulation) increases the rate of anterograde neurotransmitter transport along the MFB, which could yield information on the possible physiological use of 5-HT transported anterogradely.

9.   *Potential Use of the α-MTrp Method*

The α-MTrp method (both [14]C- and ^{3}H-labelled tracers can be used) permits quantitative determination of the regional rate of the serotonin synthesis. It is possible to measure the rate of synthesis in all brain structures of the central nervous system and superimpose them onto histological slices (images), if necessary, to facilitate the anatomical identification. This pictorial representation might be misleading in the sense that images indirectly representing the rate of serotonin synthesis (biological function) might be mistaken for a way to identify serotonin-containing structures. The latter is probably correct, but the most important feature of the method is that it provides the means necessary to measure the dynamic biological process and the neurotransmitter synthesis rate, and as such should be accepted as a method of measuring a physiological process. This tracer can also be used in the measurement of the rate of serotonin transport along the MFB (again a biological process), from the dorsal raphe towards the terminal fields. This is, again, the way to determine a very important physiological parameter—the rate of the antero-grade transport of the CNS neurotransmitter. The importance, if any, of this transport is not known and at this time we can only speculate on the need for it. (It is hard to believe that nature would transport neurotransmitters from the cell bodies towards terminals if this movement were not required.) These methods (the rate of synthesis and transport) now provide the necessary means to measure the rate of synthesis without any pharmacological treat-ment and determine the transport rate with a neurotransmitter analogue synthesized *in situ*. *In situ* synthesis probably ensures storage of the tracer in the same way and place as endogenous serotonin (experiments are under way to test this hypothesis).

The use of ^{11}C-labelled α-MTrp and application of the method of analysis described above now provide the means for repeated measurements of the serotonin synthesis rate in the same living brain, animal or human. Measure-ments in human brain should permit the assessment of therapies in some brain diseases as well as direct testing of several hypotheses which implicate serotonin in many illnesses of the CNS.

Acknowledgements

The work described here was in part supported by grants from the MRC of Canada (SP-5, PG-41 and MA-10232). I should like to express special thanks to Drs S. Nagahiro and A. Takada for their collaboration on the research described here. The editorial help of Dr V. Lees is greatly appreciated. I also acknowledge the help of Ms Carolyn Elliot in the preparation of this chapter.

References

Adell, A., Garcia-Marquez, C., Armario, A. and Gelpi, E. (1988). Chronic stress increases serotonin and noradrenalin in rat brain and sensitizes their responses to a further acute stress. *J. Neurochem.* **50**, 1676–1681

Aghajanian, G. K., Bloom, F. E., Lovel, R., Sheard, M. and Freedman, D. X. (1966). The uptake of 5-hydroxytryptamine-^{3}H from cerebral ventricles: autoradiographic localization. *Biochem. Pharmacol.*, **15**, 1401–1403

Andersen, E. and Dafny, N. (1983). An ascending serotonergic pain modulation pathway from the dorsal raphe nucleus to the parafascicularis nucleus of the thalamus. *Brain Res.*, **269**, 57–67

Araneda, S., Bobillier, P., Buda, M. and Pujol, J.-F. (1980). Retrograde axonal transport following injection of [^{3}H]serotonin in the olfactory bulb. I. Biochemical study. *Brain Res.*, **196**, 405–415

Awazi, N. and Guldberg, H. C. (1978). On the interaction of 5-hydroxytryptophan and 5-hydroxytryptamine with dopamine metabolism in the rat striatum. *Naunyn-Schmeidbergs Arch. Pathol. Exp. Pharmakol.*, **303**, 63–72

Azmitia, E. C. and Segal, M. (1978). An autographic analysis of the differential ascending projections of the dorsal and median raphe nuclei in the rat. *J. Comp. Neurol.*, **179**, 641–668

Barondes, S. H. (1974). Do tryptophan concentrations limit protein synthesis at specific sites in the brain? In *Aromatic Amino Acids in the Brain*. Elsevier, New York, pp. 265–274

Baumann, P. (1975). Metabolism of 5-hydroxytryptophan-^{14}C after intracisternal injection with and without the influence of drugs in the rat brain. *Psychopharmacologia (Berl.)*, **45**, 39–45

Beaudet, A. and Descarries, L. (1976). Quantitative data on serotonin nerve terminals in adult rat neocortex. *Brain Res.*, **111**, 301–309

Beaudet, A. and Descarries, L. (1979). Radioautographic characterization of a serotonin-accumulating nerve cell group in adult rat hypothalamus. *Brain Res.*, **160**, 231–243

Bevington, P. R. (1969). *Data Reduction and Error Analysis for the Physical Sciences*. McGraw-Hill, New York, pp. 92–118

Blundell, J. E. and Hill, A. J. (1987). Influence of tryptophan on appetite and food selection in man. In *Amino Acids in Health and Disease: New Prospectives* (ed. S. Kaufman). Alan R. Liss, New York, pp. 403–419

Bobillier, P., Petitjean, F., Salvert, D., Ligier, M. and Seguin, S. (1975). Differential projections of the nucleus raphe dorsalis and nucleus raphe centralis as revealed by autoradiography. *Brain Res.*, **85**, 205–210

Bobillier, P., Sequin, S., Petitjean, F., Salvert, D., Touret, M. and Michel, J. (1976). The raphe nuclei of the cat brain stem: a topographic atlas of their efferent projections as revealed by autoradiography. *Brain Res.*, **113**, 449–486

Bowsher, P. R. and Henry, D. P. (1986). Aromatic L-amino acid decarboxylase. In *Neuromethods; Neurotransmitter Enzymes*, Vol. 5 (ed. A. A. Boulton, G. B. Baker and P. H. Yu). Humana Press, Clifton, NJ, pp. 33–78

Bulat, M., Iskic, S., Stančic, L., Kveder, S. and Živkovic, B. (1970). Formation of 5-hydroxytryptophol from exogenous 5-hydroxytryptamine in cat spinal cord *in vivo*. *J. Pharm. Pharmacol.*, **22**, 67–68

Burton, A. C. (1936). The basis of the master reaction in biology. *J. Cell. Comp. Physiol.*, **9**, 1–14

Carlsson, A., Kehr, W. and Lindqvist, M. (1976). The role of intraneuronal amine levels in the feedback control of dopamine, noradrenaline and 5-hydroxytryptamine synthesis in rat brain. *J. Neur. Transmiss.*, **39**, 1–19

Chaly, T. and Diksic, M. (1988). Synthesis of 'no-carrier-added' α-[^{11}C]methyl-L-tryptophan. *J. Nucl. Med.*, **29**, 370–374

Christensen, H. N. and Handlogten, M. E. (1979). Interaction between parallel transport systems examined with tryptophan and related amino acids. *J. Neur. Transmiss. Suppl.*, **15**, 1–13

Coppen, A., Shaw, D. M. and Farrell, M. B. (1963). Potentiation of the antidepressive effect of a monoamine oxidase inhibitor by tryptophan. *Lancet*, **1**, 79–81

Čulman, J., Kiss, A. and Kvetnansky, R. (1984). Serotonin and tryptophan hydroxylase in isolated hypothalamic and brain stem nuclei of rats exposed to acute and repeated immobilization stress. *Exp. Clin. Endocrinol.*, **83**, 28–36

Curzon, G., Friedel, J. and Knott, P. J. (1973). The effects of fatty acids on the binding of tryptophan to plasma protein. *Nature*, **242**, 198–200

Curzon, G. and Green, A. R. (1969). Effects of immobilization on rat liver tryptophan pyrrolase and 5-hydroxytryptamine metabolism. *Br. J. Pharmacol.*, **37**, 689–697

Curzon, G., Joseph, M. H. and Knott, P. J. (1972). Effects of immobilization and food deprivation on rat brain tryptophan metabolism. *J. Neurochem.*, **19**, 1967–1974

Curzon, G. and Marsden, C. A. (1975). Metabolism of a tryptophan load in the hypothalamus and other brain regions. *J. Neurochem.*, **25**, 251–256

Dåhlström, A. and Häggendal, J. (1973). Localization and transport of serotonin. In *Serotonin and Behavior* (ed. J. Barchas and E. Usdin). Academic Press, New York, pp. 87–96

Davis, V. E., Cashaw, J. L., Huff, J. A. and Brown, H. (1966). Identification of 5-hydroxytryptophol as a serotonin metabolite in man. *Proc. Soc. Exp. Biol. Med.*, **122**, 890–893

Diksic, M., Nagahiro, S., Chaly, T., Sourkes, T. L., Yamamoto, Y. L. and Feindel, W. (1990a). The serotonin synthesis rate measured in living dog brain by PET. *J. Neurochem.* In press

Diksic, M., Nagahiro, S., Sourkes, T. L. and Yamamoto, Y. L. (1990b). A new method to measure brain serotonin synthesis *in vivo*. I. Theory and basic data for a biological model. *J. Cereb. Blood Flow Metab.*, **10**, 1–12

Diksic, M. and Sourkes, T. L. (1990). Autoradiographic measurement of the rate of serotonin synthesis in the rat brain. *Proceedings of ISTRY-89* (In press)

Diksic, M., Sourkes, T. L., Nagahiro, H., Chaly, T. and Missala, K. (1988). Influence of plasma tryptophan and $PaCO_2$ on brain serotonin synthesis in dog as measured with PET. *J. Nucl. Med.*, **29**, 784

Diksic, M., Sourkes, T. L., Nakai, H., Chaly, T., Missala, K. and Yamamoto, Y. L. (1987). *In vivo* rate of serotonin synthesis in the dog brain measured by positron emission tomography. *Proceedings of the 17th Annual Meeting of the Society for Neuroscience*, Abstract No. 224.5

Dodd, P. R., Hambley, J. W., Cowburn, R. F. and Hardy, J. A. (1988). A comparison of methodologies for the study of functional transmitter neurochemistry in human brain. *J. Neurochem.*, **50**, 1333–1345, and references therein

Doucet, G., Descarries, L., Audet, M. A., Garcia, S. and Berger, B. (1988). Radioautographic method for quantifying regional monoamine innervations in the rat brain. Application to the cerebral cortex. *Brain Res.*, **441**, 233–259

Duda, N. J. and Moore, K. E. (1985). Simultaneous determination of 5-hydroxytryptophan and 3,4-dihydroxyphenylalamine in rat brain by HPLC with electrochemical detection following electrical stimulation of the dorsal raphe nucleus. *J. Neurochem.*, **44**, 128–133

Ehret, M., Gobaille, S., Cash, C. D., Mandel P. and Maitre, M. (1987). Regional distribution in rat brain of tryptophan hydroxylase apoenzyme determined by enzyme-linked immunoassay. *Neurosci. Lett.*, **73**, (1), 71–76

Etienne, P., Young, S. N. and Sourkes, T. L. (1976). Inhibition by albumin of tryptophan uptake by rat brain. *Nature*, **262**, 144–145

Evans, A. C., Diksic, M., Yamamoto, Y. L., Kato, A., Dagher, A., Redies, C. and Hakim, A. (1986). Effect of vascular activity in the determination of rate constants for the uptake of ^{18}F-labelled 2-fluoro-2-deoxy-D-glucose: error analysis and normal values in older subjects. *J. Cereb. Blood Flow Metab.*, **6**, 724–738

Fernstrom, J. D. (1983). Role of precursor availability in control of monoamine biosynthesis in brain. *Physiol. Rev.*, **63**, 485–546

Fibiger, H. C., McGeer, E. G. and Atmadja, S. (1973). Axoplasmic transport of dopamine in nigrostriatal neurons. *J. Neurochem.*, **21**, 373–385

Finkelstein, L. and Carson, E. R. (1985). In *Mathematical Modelling of Dynamic Biological Systems*. Wiley, New York, pp. 51–58

Fowler, C. J. and Tipton, K. F. (1982). Deamination of 5-hydroxytryptamine by both forms of monoamine oxidase by the rat brain. *J. Neurochem.*, **38**, 733–736

Frankfurt, M. and Azmitia, E. (1984). Regeneration of serotonergic fibres in the rat hypo-thalamus following unilateral 5,7-dihydroxytryptamine injection. *Brain Res.*, **298**, 273–282

Friedlander, G., Kennedy, J. W. and Miller, J. M. (1955). *Nuclear and Radiochemistry*, pp. 69–85

Friedman, P. A., Kappelman, A. H. and Kaufman, S. (1972). Partial purification and characterization of tryptophan hydroxylase from rabbit hindbrain. *J. Biol. Chem.*, **247**, 4165–4173

Gal, E. M. and Christiansen, P. A. (1975). Alpha-methyltryptophan: Effects on cerebral monooxygenases *in vitro* and *in vivo*. *J. Neurochem.*, **24**, 89–95

Gal, E. M. and Sherman, A. D. (1978). Synthesis and metabolism of L-kynurenine in rat brain. *J. Neurochem.*, **30**, 607–613

Gess, G. L. and Tagliamonte, A. (1974). Serum free tryptophan: control of brain concentrations of tryptophan and of synthesis of 5-hydroxytryptamine. In: *Aromatic Amino Acids in the Brain*. Elsevier, New York, pp. 205–216

Ghadirian, A. M., Nair, N. P. V. and Schwartz, G. (1989). Effect of lithium and neuroleptic combination on lithium transport, blood pressure, and weight in bipolar patients. *Biol. Psychiat.*, **26**, 139–144

Goodnick, P. J. and Gershon, S. (1985). Lithium. In *Handbook of Neurochemistry*, 2nd edn, Vol. 9 (ed. A. Lajtha). Plenum Press, New York, pp. 103–149

Green, H., Greenberg, S. M., Erickson, R. W., Sawyer, J. L. and Ellison, T. (1962). Effect of dietary phenylalamine and tryptophan upon rat brain amine levels. *J. Pharmacol. Exp. Ther.*, **136**, 174–178

Green, A. R., Koslow, S. H. and Costa, E. (1973). Identification and quantitation of a new indolealkylamine in rat hypothalamus. *Brain Res.*, **51**, 371–374

Green, J. P. (1989). Histamine and serotonin. In *Basic Neurochemistry* (ed. G. Siegel, B. Agranoff, R. W. Albers and P. Molinoff). Raven Press, New York, pp. 253–269

Haggendal, C. J. and Dählström, A. B. (1969). The transport and life-span of amine storage granules in bulbospinal noradrenaline neurons of the rat. *J. Pharm. Pharmacol.*, 21, 55–57

Hamon, M., Bourgoin, S., Artaud, F. and Glowinski, J. (1979). The role of intraneuronal 5-HT and of tryptophan hydroxylase activation in the control of 5-HT synthesis in rat brain slices incubated in K⁺-enriched medium. *J. Neurochem.*, 33, 1031–1042.

Hamon, M., Bourgoin, S., and Glowinski, J. (1973). Feedback regulation of 5-HT synthesis in rat striatal slices. *J. Neurochem.*, 20, 1727–1745

Hoffman, E. J. and Phelps, M. E. (1986). Positron emission tomography: Principles and quantitation. In *Positron Emission Tomography and Autoradiography: Principles and Applications for the Brain and Health* (ed. M. E. Phelps, J. C. Mazziotta and H. R. Shelbert). Raven Press, New York, pp. 237–286

Johnston, J. P. (1968). Some observations upon a new inhibitor of monoamine oxidase in brain tissue. *Biochem. Pharmacol.*, 17, 1285–1297

Jones, B.E., Halaris, A. E., McIlhany, M. and Moore, R. Y. (1977). Ascending projections of the locus coeruleus in the rat. 1. Axonal transport in central noradrenaline neurons. *Brain Res.*, 127, 1–21

Jouvet, M. (1967). Neurophysiology of the states of sleep. *Physiol. Rev.*, 47, 117–177

Kato, A., Diksic, M., Yamamoto, Y. L., Strother, S. C. and Feindel, W. (1984a). An improved approach for measurement of regional cerebral rate constants in the deoxyglucose method. *J. Cereb. Blood Flow Metab.*, 4, 555–560

Kato, A., Menon, D., Diksic, M. and Yamamoto, Y. L. (1984b). Influence of the input function on the calculation of LCMRglu in the deoxyglucose model. *J. Cereb. Blood Flow Metab.*, 4, 41–46

Katz, I. R. (1980). Oxygen affinity of tyrosine and tryptophan hydroxylases in synaptosomes. *J. Neurochem.*, 35, 760–763

Kelder, D., Fagervall, I., Fowler, C. J. and Ross, S. B. (1989). Regulation of the monoamine concentrations in the rat brain by intraneuronal monoamine oxidase. *Biogenic Amines*, 6, 1–14

Kirchgessner, A. L., Gershon, M. D., Liu, K. P. and Tamir, H. (1988). Co-storage of serotonin binding protein with serotonin in the rat CNS. *J. Neurosci.*, 8, 3879–3890

Kirikae, M., Diksic, M. and Yamamoto, Y. L. (1989). Quantitative measurements of regional glucose utilization and rate of valine incorporation into proteins by double-tracer autoradiography in the rat brain tumor model. *J. Cereb. Blood Flow Metab.*, 9, 87–95

Kleven, M. S., Dwoskin, L. P. and Sparber, S. B. (1983). Pharmacological evidence for the existence of multiple functional pools of brain serotonin: analysis of brain perfusate from conscious rats. *J. Neurochem.*, 41, 1143–1149

Knapp, S. and Mandell, A. J. (1972). Narcotic drugs: effects on the serotonin biosynthetic systems of the brain. *Science, N.Y.*, 177, 1209–1211

Koe, B. K. and Weissmann, A. (1966). *p*-Chlorophenylalanine: a specific depleter of brain serotonin. *J. Pharmacol. Exp. Ther.*, 154, 499–516

Kopin, I. J. (1959). Tryptophan loading and excretion of 5-hydroxyindolacetic acid in normal and schizophrenic subjects. *Science, N.Y.*, 129, 835–836

Korf, J. (1985). Turnover rate assessments of cerebral neurotransmitter amines and acetylcholine. In *Neuromethods, Amines and their Metabolites* (ed. A. A. Boulton, G. B. Baker and J. M. Baker). Humana Press, Clifton, NJ, pp. 407–456

Kuhar, M. J., Aghajanian, G. H. and Roth, R. H. (1972). Tryptophan hydroxylase activity and synaptosomal uptake of serotonin in discrete brain regions after midbrain raphe lesions: correlations with serotonin levels and histochemical fluorescence. *Brain Res.*, 44, 165–176

Kuwabara, H., Evans, A. C. and Gjedde, A. (1990). Michaelis–Menten constraints improved cerebral glucose metabolism and regional lumped constant measurements with [¹⁸F]fluorodeoxyglucose. *J. Cereb. Blood Flow Metab.*, 10, 180–189

Lane, J. D. and Aprison, M. H. (1978). The flux of radioactive label through compartments of the serotonergic system following the injection of [³H]tryptophan: product-precursor anomalies providing evidence that serotonin exists in multiple pools. *J. Neurochem.*, 30, 671–678

McMillen, B. A., German, D. C. and Shore, P. A. (1980). Functional and pharmacological significance of brain dopamine and norepinephrine storage pools. *Biochem. Pharmacol.*, 29, 3045–3050

Macon, J. B., Sokoloff, L. and Glowinski, J. (1971). Feedback control of rat brain 5-hydroxytryptamine synthesis. *J. Neurochem.*, 18, 323–331

Madras, B. K. and Sourkes, T. L. (1965). Metabolism of α-methyl-tryptophan. *Biochem. Pharmacol.*, **14**, 1499–1506

Mandell, A. J. and Knapp, S. (1977). Regulation of serotonin biosynthesis in brain: role of the high affinity uptake of tryptophan into serotonergic neurons. *Fed. Proc.*, **36**, 2142–2148

Mandell, A. J. and Knapp, S. (1979). Asymmetry and mood, emergent properties of serotonin regulation. *Arch. Gen. Psychiat.*, **36**, 909–916

Michaelis, L. and Menten, M. L. (1913). Die Kinetik der Invertinwirkung. *Biochem. Z.*, **49**, 333–369

Miller, L. P., Pardridge, W. M., Braun, L. D. and Oldendorf, W. H. (1985). Kinetic constants for blood–brain barrier amino acid transport in conscious rats. *J. Neurochem.*, **45**, 1427–1432

Missala, K. and Sourkes, T. L. (1988). Functional cerebral activity of an analogue of serotonin formed *in situ*. *Neurochem. Int.*, **12**, 209–214

Miwa, S., Fujiwara, M., Lee, K. and Fujiwara, M. (1987). Determination of serotonin turnover in the rat brain using 6-fluorotryptophan. *J. Neurochem.*, **48**, 1577–1580

Moir, A. T. B. (1974). Tryptophan concentration in brain. In *Aromatic Amino Acids in the Brain* (Ciba Foundation Symposium 22). Elsevier, Amsterdam, pp. 195–206

Montine, T. J. and Sourkes, T. L. (1989). Behavior of alpha-methylserotonin in rat brain synaptosomes. *Neurochem. Int.*, **15**, 227–231

Moore, R. Y., Halaris, A. E. and Jones, B. E. (1987). Serotonin neurons of the midbrain raphe: ascending projections. *J. Comp. Neurol.*, **80**, 417–438

Nagahiro, S., Diksic, M., Yamamoto, Y. L. and Riml, H. (1990a). Non-invasive *in vivo* autoradiographic method to measure axonal transport in serotoninergic neurons in the rat brain. *Brain Res.*, **506**, 120–128

Nagahiro, S., Takada, A., Diksic, M., Sourkes, T. L., Missala, K. and Yamamoto, Y. L. (1990b). A new method to measure brain serotonin synthesis *in vivo*. II. A practical autoradiographic method tested in normal and lithium-treated rats. *J. Cereb. Blood Flow Metab.*, **10**, 13–21

Neckers, L. M. (1982). Serotonin turnover and regulation. In *Biology of Serotonergic Transmission* (ed. N. N. Osborne). Wiley, New York, pp. 139–158

Neff, N. H., Spano, P. F., Groppetti, A., Wang, C. T. and Costa, E. (1971). A simple procedure for calculating the synthesis rate of norepinephrine, dopamine and serotonin in rat brain. *J. Pharmacol. Exp. Ther.*, **176**, 701–710

Neff, N. H. and Tozer, T. N. (1968). *In vivo* measurement of brain serotonin turnover. *Adv. Pharmacol.*, **6A**, 97–109

Neff, N. H., Tozer, T. N. and Brodie, B. B. (1967). Application of steady-state kinetics to studies of the transfer of 5-hydroxyindolacetic acid from brain to plasma. *J. Pharmacol. Exp. Ther.*, **158**, 214–218

Nelson, T., Dienel, G. A., Mori, K., Cruz, N. F. and Sokoloff, L. (1987). Deoxyglucose-6-phosphate stability *in vivo* and deoxyglucose method: response to comments of Hawkins and Miller. *J. Neurochem.*, **49**, 1949–1960

Ng, L. K. Y., Chase, T. N. Colburn, R. W. and Kopin, I. J. (1972). Release of ^{3}H-dopamine by L-5-hydroxytryptophan. *Brain Res.*, **45**, 499–505

Oldendorf, W. H. (1971). Brain uptake of radiolabelled amino acids, amines, and hexoses after arterial injection. *Am. J. Physiol.*, **221**, 1629–1639

Oldendorf, W. H. and Szabo, J. (1976). Amino acid assignment to one of three blood–brain barrier acid carriers. *Am. J. Physiol.*, **230**, 94–98

Osborne, N. N. (ed.) (1982). *Biology of Serotonergic Transmission*. Wiley, New York

Palkovits, M., Brownstein, M., Kizer, J. S., Saavedra, J. M. and Kopin, I. J. (1976). Effect of stress on serotonin and tryptophan hydroxylase activity of brain nuclei. In *Catecholamines and Stress* (ed. E. Usdin *et al.*). Pergamon Press, Oxford, pp. 51–59

Pardridge, W. M. (1977). Kinetics of competitive inhibition of neutral amino acid transport across the blood–brain barrier. *J. Neurochem.*, **28**, 103–108

Pardridge, W. M. and Mietus, L. J. (1982). Kinetics of neutral amino acid transport through the blood–brain barrier of the newborn rabbit. *J. Neurochem.*, **38**, 955–962

Patlak, S. C., Blasberg, R.G. and Fenstermacher, J. D. (1983). Graphic evaluation of blood-to-brain transfer constants from multiple time uptake data. *J. Cereb. Blood Flow Metab.*, **3**, 1–9

Perez-Cruet, J., Tagliamonte, A., Tagliamonte, P. and Gessa G. L. (1971). Stimulation of serotonin synthesis by lithium. *J. Pharmacol. Exp. Ther.*, **178**, 325–330

Petersen, S. L., Hartman, R. D. and Barraclough, C. A. (1989). An analysis of serotonin secretion in hypothalamic regions based on 5-hydroxytryptophan accumulation or push–pull perfusion. Effects of mesencephalic raphe on locus coeruleus stimulation and correlated changes in plasma luteinizing hormone. *Brain Res.*, **495**, 9–19, and references therein

Phelps, M. E., Huang, S. C., Hoffman, E. J., Selin, M. S., Sokoloff, L. and Kuhl, D. E. (1979). Tomographic measurement of local cerebral glucose metabolic rate in humans with 2-[^{18}F]fluoro-2-deoxyglucose: validation of the method. *Ann. Neurol.*, **6**, 371–388

Philips, S. R., Durden, D. A. and Boulton, A. A. (1974). Identification and distribution of tryptamine in the rat. *Can. J. Biochem.*, **52**, 447–451

Redies, C. and Diksic, M. (1989). The deoxyglucose method in the ferret brain. I. Methodological considerations. *J. Cereb. Blood Flow Metab.*, **9**, 35–42

Redies, C., Diksic, M., Collier, B., Gjedde, A., Thompson, C. J., Gauthier, S. and Feindel, W. H. (1989). Influx of a choline analog to dog brain measured by positron emission tomography. *Synapse*, **2**, 406–411

Ritger, P. D. and Rose, N. J. (1968). In *Differential Equations with Applications*. McGraw-Hill, New York, pp. 224–307

Roberge, A. G., Missala, K. and Sourkes, T. L. (1972). Alpha-methyltryptophan: Effects on synthesis and degradation of serotonin in the brain. *Neuropharmacology*, **11**, 197–209

Sako, K., Diksic, M., Kato, A., Yamamoto, Y. L. and Feindel, W. (1984). Evaluation of [^{18}F]4-fluoroantipyrine as a new blood flow tracer for multinuclide autoradiography. *J. Cereb. Blood Flow Metab.*, **4**, 259–263

Sarna, G. S., Kantamaneni, B. D. and Curzon, G. (1985). Variables influencing the effect of a meal on brain tryptophan. *J. Neurochem.*, **44**, 1575–1580

Schirlin, D., Gerhart, F., Hornsperger, J. M., Hamon, M., Wagner, J. and Jung, M. J. (1988). Synthesis and biological properties of α-mono- and α-difluoromethyl derivatives of tryptophan and 5-hydroxytryptophan. *J. Med. Chem.*, **31**, 30–36

Schubert, J. (1974). Labelled 5-hydroxytryptamine and 5-hydroxyindolacetic acid formed *in vivo* from ^{3}H-tryptophan in rat brain: effect of probenecid. *Acta Physiol. Scand.*, **9**, 401–408

Schute, H. H. (1976). Het Metabolisme van Serotonine in Rattehersenen. Thesis, University of Groningen

Sedvall, G. (1981). Serotonin metabolite concentrations in cerebrospinal fluid from schizophrenic patients—relationships to family history. In *Serotonin Current Aspects and Neurochemistry and Function* (ed. B. Haber, S. Gabay, M. R. Issidorides and S. G. A. Alivisatos). Plenum Press, New York, pp. 719–725, and references therein

Sharp, T., Bramwell, S. R., Clark, D. and Grahame-Smith, D. G. (1989). *In vivo* measurement of extracellular 5-hydroxytryptamine in hippocampus of the anesthetized rat using microdialysis: changes in relation to 5-hydroxytryptaminergic neuronal activity. *J. Neurochem.*, **53**, 234–240, and references therein

Sheppard, C. W. (1948). The theory of the study of transfers within a multicompartment system using isotopic tracers. *J. Appl. Phys.*, **19**, 70–76

Shields, P. J. and Eccleston, D. (1972). Effects of electrical stimulation of rat midbrain on 5-hydroxytryptamine synthesis as determined by a sensitive radioisotope method. *J. Neurochem.*, **19**, 265–272

Smith, Q. R., Momma, S., Aoyagi, M. and Rappaport, Sl. (1987). Kinetics of neutral amino acid transport across the blood–brain barrier. *J. Neurochem.*, **49**, 1651–1658

Sokoloff, L., Reivich, M., Kennedy, C., Des Rosiers, M. H., Patlak, C. S., Pettigrew, K. D., Sakurada, O. and Shinohard, M. (1977). The ^{14}C-deoxyglucose method for the measurement of local glucose utilization: theory, procedure, and normal values in the conscious and anesthetized albino rat. *J. Neurochem.*, **28**, 897–916.

Sourkes, T. L. (1971). Alpha-methyltryptophan and its action on tryptophan metabolism. *Fed. Proc.*, **30**, 897–903

Steinbush, H. W. M., Verhofstad, A. A. J. and Joosten, W. J. (1978). Localization of serotonin in the central nervous system by immunohistochemistry: description of a specific and sensitive technique and some applications. *Neuroscience*, **3**, 811–819

Stewart, P. M., Atherdel, S. M., Stewart, S. E., Whalley, L., Edwards, C. R. W. and Padfield, P. L. (1988). Lithium carbonate—a competitive aldosterone antagonist? *Br. J. Psychiat.*, **153**, 205–207

Susilo, R., Rommelspacher, H. and Höfle, G. (1989). Formation of thiazolidine-4-carboxylic acid represents a main metabolic pathway of 5-hydroxytryptamine in rat brain. *J. Neurochem.*, **52**, 1793–1800

Sze, P. Y. (1981). Developmental-regulatory aspects of brain tryptophan hydroxylase. In *Serotonin Current Aspects and Neurochemistry and Function* (ed. B. Haber, S. Gabay, M. R. Issidorides and S. G. A. Alivisatos). Plenum Press, New York, pp. 507–523

Tagaki, H., Shiosaka, S., Tohyama, M., Senba, E. and Sakanaka, M. (1980). Ascending components of the medial forebrain bundle from the lower brain stem in the rat, with special reference to raphe and catecholamine cell groups. *Brain Res.*, **193**, 315–337

Tamir, H., Klein, A. and Rapport, M. M. (1976). Serotonin binding protein: Enhancement of binding by Fe^{2+} and inhibition of binding by drugs. *J. Neurochem.*, **26**, 871–878

Tappaz, M. and Pujol, J.-F. (1980). Estimation of the rate of tryptophan hydroxylation *in vivo*: A sensitive microassay in discrete rat brain nuclei. *J. Neurochem.*, **34**, 933–940

Teorell, T. (1937). Kinetics of distribution of substances administered to the body. I. Extravascular modes of administration. *Arch. Int. Pharmacodyn.*, **57**, 205–240

Tozer, T. N., Neff, N. H. and Brodie, B. B. (1966). Application of steady-state kinetics to the synthesis rate and turnover time of serotonin in the brain of normal and reserpine-treated rats. *J. Pharmacol. Exp. Ther.*, **153**, 177–182

Tracqui, P., Brézillon, P., Staub, J. F., Morot-Gaudry, Y., Hamon, M. and Perault-Staub, A. M. (1983a). Model of brain serotonin metabolism. I. Structure determination–parameter estimation. *Am. J. Physiol.*, **244**, R193–R205

Tracqui, P., Morot-Gaudry, Y., Staub, J. F., Brézillon, P., Perault-Staub, A. M., Burgoin, S. and Hamon, M. (1983b). Model of brain serotonin metabolism. II. Physiological interpretation. *Am. J. Physiol.*, **244**, R206–R215

van Wijk, M. and Korf, J. (1981). Postmortem changes of 5-hydroxytryptamine and 5-hydroxyindoleacetic acid in mouse brain and their prevention by pargyline and microwave irradiation. *Neurochem. Res.*, **6**, 425–430

van Wijk, M., Sebens, J. B. and Korf, J. (1979). Probenecid-induced increase of 5-hydroxytryptamine synthesis in rat brain as measured by formation of 5-hydroxytryptophan. *Psychopharmacology*, **60**, 229–235

Weissman, D., Belin, M. F., Aguera, M., Meuniere, C., Maitre, M., Cash, C. D., Ehret, M., Pandel, P. and Pujol, J. F. (1987). Immunohistochemistry of tryptophan hydroxylase in the rat brain. *Neuroscience*, **23**, 291–304

Yamamoto, Y. L., Thompson, C. J., Meyer, E., Robertson, J. and Feindel, W. L. (1977). Dynamic positron emission tomography for study of cerebral haemodynamics in a cross-section of the head using positron emitting ^{68}Ga-EDTA and Kr^{77}. *J. Comp. Assist. Tomogr.*, **1**, 43–56

Young, S. N., Chouinard, G. and Annable, A. (1981). Tryptophan in treatment of depression. In *Serotonin Current Aspects and Neurochemistry and Function* (ed. B. Haber, S. Gabay, M. R. Issidorides and S. G. A. Alivisatos). Plenum Press, New York, pp. 727–737, and references therein

Young, S. N. and Sourkes, T. L. (1977). Tryptophan in the central nervous system: regulation and significance. *Adv. Neurochem.*, **2**, 133–191

Young, S. N. and Teff, K. L. (1989). Tryptophan availability, 5HT synthesis and 5HT function. *Progr. Neuro-Psychopharmacol. Biol. Psychiat.*, **13**, 373–379

Yudilevich, D. L., DeRose, N. and Sepulveda, F. V. (1972). Facilitated transport of amino acids through the blood–brain barrier of the dog studied in a single capillary circulation. *Brain Res.*, **44**, 569–578

3

The Area Postrema and Vomiting: How Important is Serotonin?

R. A. LESLIE[1] and D. J. M. REYNOLDS[2]

[1]*Oxford University—Beecham Centre for Applied Neuropsychobiology*
[2]*MRC Unit and University Department of Clinical Pharmacology, Radcliffe Infirmary, Woodstock Road, Oxford OX2 6HE, UK*

Contents

Current Aspects of the Neurosciences, Vol. 3. Edited by N. N. Osborne. © The Macmillan Press Ltd 1991

1. Introduction

In the last few years there has been a marked upsurge of interest in research regarding the neural mechanisms of control of nausea and vomiting, following the recent recognition (Miner and Sanger, 1986) that a poorly understood class of drugs has potent antiemetic properties for some forms of emesis. In particular, these drugs appear to be selective for emesis that is experienced by most cancer patients when they receive chemotherapy or radiotherapy for their condition. The drugs are 'blockers' of the 'M' type of serotonin (5-HT) receptor of Gaddum and Picarelli (1957), which is now classified as the 5-HT$_3$ receptor (Bradley *et al.*, 1986). Since the somewhat startling discovery that 5-HT$_3$ receptor antagonists can be so potent and selective in this regard, a host of new drugs has been developed by several pharmaceutical companies to introduce even more potent and more selective drugs of this type.

The neural mechanisms controlling the related syndromes of nausea and vomiting are still very poorly understood, despite the large amount of work that has been devoted to this subject—especially since the pioneering work of Wang, Borison, Brizzee and their colleagues, dating from the late 1940s and the 1950s. The standard textbook description of the chemoreceptive trigger zone for vomiting and the vomiting centre, both located in the caudal rhomencephalon, is derived from their work. None the less, there is still much uncertainty about the actual morphological structures, and certainly the neurochemical mechanisms, involved in these processes. It is clear that ablation of the area postrema, a circumventricular organ located at or near the obex of the fourth ventricle, disrupts certain forms of chemoreception that trigger the vomiting response (Borison, 1974). Similarly, a region in or near the parvicellular reticular formation of the caudal medulla oblongata has been described as a 'centre' for the initiation of vomiting (Brizzee and Mehler, 1986) or as a 'pattern generator' (Carpenter, 1988) which plays a role in co-ordinating the vomiting response.

However, recent experimental evidence has questioned the physiological significance of these sites *vis-à-vis* the vomiting response (Miller and Wilson, 1983). Rather than a discrete vomiting centre in the hindbrain, there may, in fact, be a series of scattered neuronal cell bodies throughout the neuraxis which co-ordinate the vomiting response (Carpenter, 1988). The 'chemoreceptive trigger zone', likewise, may not be a discrete entity in the caudal brainstem; vagal sensory nerve fibres themselves might be chemoreceptive.

The present chapter, then, may just as well have been entitled 'Serotonin and vomiting—how important is the area postrema?' The questions address the interrelationship between structure and function of different specific elements involved in the vomiting response, in both, as we shall see, the peripheral and central nervous systems. The fundamental importance of the area postrema and the so-called vomiting centre, as well as the significance of 5-HT as a neuromediator of the vomiting response, will be addressed here. We shall try to put these questions into the context of modern neurobiological research on a most fascinating and clinically vexing problem—why and how do we vomit, and what can we do about it?

2. *The Disparate Nature of Emetic Stimuli*

A large number of drugs and other stimuli can cause nausea and vomiting (for recent reviews see Barnes, 1984; Grahame-Smith, 1986). The vomiting response appears to have developed for the purpose of ridding the gastrointestinal tract of toxic ingested items, and thus it is reasonable that so many different substances should result in expulsion of stomach contents by this mechanism. Nevertheless, there are puzzling phenomena which do not fit with such an explanation. For example, it has never been satisfactorily explained why unnatural motion should result in nausea and vomiting for susceptible people or animals. An interesting hypothesis suggests that the vestibular mechanism was recruited to the purpose of vomiting because of its exquisite sensitivity to certain stimuli (Treisman, 1977), but it is difficult to imagine how to prove or disprove this. Morning sickness of pregnancy is another type of vomiting which seems to have no evolutionary explanation— it would, in fact, appear to be counterproductive rather than protective for the suffering mother. Regardless of why these other forms of emesis developed, it is certainly true that a large number of chemicals that find their way into the systemic circulation can have the effect of stimulating nausea or emesis. Is there any evidence that receptors for such a large variety of substances exist somewhere in the brain circuitry implicated in the vomiting response? In fact, there is good evidence that several different kinds of receptor may occur on the plasma membranes of single neuronal somata within the area postrema (Carpenter *et al.*, 1983). Of interest to our present discussion is the question of how 5-HT might be involved in the initiation of emesis. As discussed below, it seems likely that irritation of the epithelium lining the gut releases 5-HT from enterochromaffin cells and stimulates 5-HT$_3$ receptors either on enteric neurons or on the distal, receptive terminals of vagal afferent fibres in the vicinity. In addition, serotonergic mechanisms within the dorsal vagal complex of the caudal brainstem are most probably involved in modulation of the emetic response. This complex incorporates vagal sensory and motor nuclei, and includes the nucleus of the solitary tract, the area postrema and the dorsal motor nucleus of the vagus nerve.

3. *The Area Postrema as a Chemoreceptor Trigger Zone for Vomiting*

Morphology of the Area Postrema

The area postrema is one of the so-called circumventricular organs which occur around the circumference of the brain ventricles. These organs, which are, in fact, brainstem nuclei, are known to be involved in the control of some autonomic functions. For example, the subfornical organ, located at the rostral tip of the third ventricle, is involved in the control of thirst and ingestion of liquids, while the area postrema, as well as being implicated in initiating the vomiting response, may well be involved in control of satiety (Edwards and Ritter, 1981). Indeed, many disparate functions have been ascribed to the area postrema over the years (see Leslie, 1986, for a recent review).

The structure of the area postrema makes it particularly suited for receiving information about the chemical environment of the brain, and even structures further afield, such as the thoracic and abdominal viscera. The morphology has been discussed in detail elsewhere (Leslie, 1986), but a brief description will be given here. The organ is situated at the caudal end of the fourth ventricle, and, depending upon the species, forms either a midline structure or twin spindle-shaped structures which make up part of the roof, sides or floor of the ventricle at or near the obex. It consists of a scattered collection of small neuronal cell bodies embedded in a matrix of astrocyte-like glial cells and bundles of largely unmyelinated axons which convey information to the nucleus from thoracic and abdominal viscera via the vagus nerve (Gwyn and Leslie, 1979; Gwyn et al., 1979; Kalia and Mesulam, 1979), or from the nucleus to various sites (Leslie and Gwyn, 1984). A rich plexus of small blood vessels with peculiarly large perivascular spaces surrounding their walls courses throughout the parenchyma of the nucleus (Figure 1). The large dilated perivascular spaces are not simply artefacts of tissue preparation, as they are never seen, in the same sections, in the immediately underlying nucleus of the solitary tract. This fact provides a means of detecting, in histological sections, the otherwise indistinct boundary between the area postrema and adjacent brainstem structures. These blood vessels, like those of most of the other circumventricular organs, are unique in the brain in that their endothelial cells are not linked to each other with zonulae occludentes, or tight junctions that would restrict the passage of macromolecules across this epithelium. Thus, the area postrema is often said to 'lie outside the blood–brain barrier', by which is meant that it has a deficient blood–brain diffusion barrier to lipophobic molecules.

The ependyma overlying the organ, also in common with that of other circumventricular organs, consists of a monolayer of distinctive, rather squamous, modified ependymal cells that bear prominent tufts of branched microvilli (Leslie et al., 1978) and there are no traces of the kinocilia which decorate normal ependymal cells. The epithelial cells are linked with specialized cell junctions, similar to but 'leakier' than tight junctions, which form a partial barrier to the possible entrance into the parenchyma of macromolecules from the cerebrospinal fluid which bathes the surface of the organ. Furthermore, cytoplasmic flanges of tanycyte-like cells extend from the

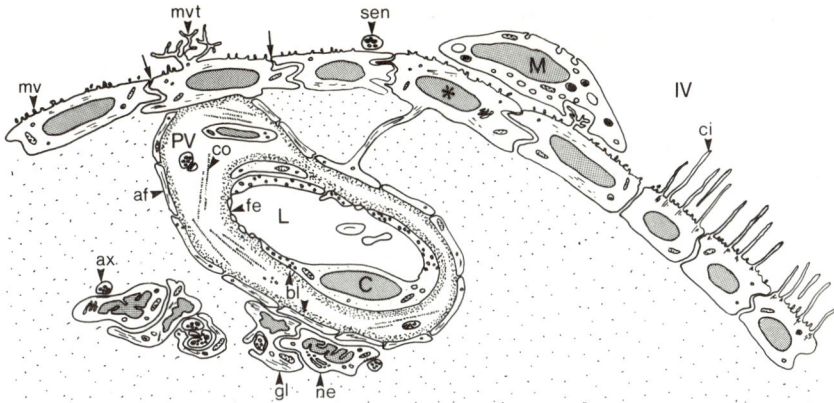

Figure 1 Diagrammatic representation of a cross-section of the cat area postrema. The transition between normal ciliated ependyma (ci) and non-ciliated but microvillus-bearing (mv) ependyma overlying the area postrema is indicated. Microvillous tufts (mvt) occur frequently on the apical surfaces of these cells. These are sometimes enveloped by supraependymal macrophages (M). Occasionally, supraependymal cell profiles, resembling axons in section (sen), are seen. Arrows indicate the sites of poorly defined specialized cell junctions at the apices of ependymal cells which have been shown to be leaky to large tracer molecules. One ependymal cell (⋆) is shown with a basal process forming part of the wall of a much-distended perivascular space (PV) which encloses a fenestrated (fe) capillary (C). This basal process forms one of the astrocyte-like endfeet (af) delimiting the wall of the perivascular space. The capillary is associated with a dorsally positioned pericyte which is enclosed within the continuous basal lamina (bl) of the endothelium. A second continuous basal lamina lines the wall of the perivascular space. The space itself contains abundant collagen fibres (co) as well as fibroblasts and profiles of vesiculated axonal varicosities. Several small neuronal somata (ne) are represented within the parenchyma of the area postrema and these are closely associated with astrocyte-like glial elements (gl). Several axosomatic synapses are illustrated here (ax), although, more commonly, axo-dendritic synapses (double arrowheads) are seen. (Figure previously published in Davis *et al.*, 1986)

ependymal surface to surround the outer basement membrane of the perivascular spaces surrounding the blood vascular elements of the organ. The area postrema, then, can be seen to be particularly suited for receiving and relaying neuronal or hormonal information from a wide variety of sources, including the blood, meningeal or ventricular cerebrospinal fluid, or any of the sources of afferent neuronal fibres that terminate here. This information can be carefully modulated by means of the specialized cell junctions at the ependymal surface, the palisades of glial (tanycyte) endfeet surrounding the blood vessels and the probable neuroendocrine elements that terminate near the blood vessel walls (Figure 1).

The Neurochemistry of the Area Postrema

A large number of neurotransmitters, neuromodulators and their receptors have been demonstrated in the area postrema (see Leslie, 1985; Palkovits, 1985). Many techniques have been used to demonstrate these, ranging from biochemical assays for the determination of neurochemicals to physiological ablation studies in concert with drug administration and behavioural experiments to determine which receptors occur here. More recently, immunocytochemistry and receptor radioligand binding assays have been used to extend the list. As well as a host of peptide neuromodulators, most of the classical neurotransmitters are thought to be present, along with some of their receptor subtypes. 5-HT-containing neuronal cell bodies have been shown to be present in the area postrema in early fluorescent histochemical studies (Dahlstrom and Fuxe, 1964; Fuxe and Owman, 1965). All the immunocytochemical studies of various species that have been undertaken more recently (e.g. Newton *et al.*, 1985) have demonstrated 5-HT immunoreactivity in axon varicosities in the nucleus, and often in punctate structures surrounding blood vascular elements (Leslie and Osborne, 1984). Curiously, although 5-HT-immunoreactive cell bodies are readily and consistently demonstrated in the rodent and lagomorph area postrema (Howe *et al.*, 1983; Newton *et al.*, 1985), no similar findings have ever been reported in any other mammals. It seems likely that this does not represent an 'absolute' difference in species, but rather that 5-HT occurs in area postrema neurons of other species, but at levels below the threshold of detection with current immunocytochemical techniques.

The origin of the 5-HT found in the area postrema is still poorly understood. At least some of the vagal afferent fibres which project to the area postrema have been shown to be serotonergic (Gaudin-Chazal *et al.*, 1982). It is possible that some of the 5-HT-immunoreactive terminals found here arise from intrinsic cell bodies within the nucleus, although, as stated above, it appears that only in the rat does 5-HT occur in large amounts in area postrema cell bodies. However, it is equally possible that these terminals could be on axons arising from 5-HT cells in the raphe nuclei in the adjacent reticular formation. Mast cells occur with some frequency in the area postrema (Leslie, 1986), and these might provide a certain amount of 5-HT which might be released upon suitable stimulation. Finally, circulating platelets could conceivably release 5-HT in the area postrema in response to certain stimuli. As we shall see below, there is convincing, albeit as yet circumstantial, evidence that 5-HT$_3$ receptors occur in the nucleus of the solitary tract in large numbers on vagal afferent terminals arising from abdominal viscera.

Evidence for the Area Postrema as a Chemoreceptive Trigger Zone

Studies undertaken by Wang and Borison (1952) have shown that removal of the area postrema renders the experimental animal (or human: see Lindstrom and Brizzee, 1962) refractory to vomiting in response to certain drug challenges. For example, apomorphine, when given to dogs with surgical ablations of the area postrema, will not cause emesis in the animals. Thus, the area postrema has come to be known as a 'chemoreceptive trigger zone' for the emetic response (Borison, 1974). The hypothesis is an attractive one, especially as it is clear that drugs which do not penetrate ordinary brain parenchyma easily can be potent emetics, and the area postrema would provide a 'window' into the brain for these agents by virtue of its deficient blood–brain barrier. However, it has never been clear which cellular elements within the area postrema might be chemosensitive. Recent studies have indicated that stimulation of the vagal afferent fibres arising in the abdominal viscera can evoke emesis in the ferret (Andrews *et al.*, 1986). Ablation of the area postrema will, of necessity, remove the axon terminals of vagal afferent fibres which terminate there, so it is tempting to speculate that it is the membranes of these terminals which bear the chemosensitive elements. There is evidence from several laboratories that ligand binding sites for muscarinic cholinergic, delta opioid, angiotensin II, neurotensin, cholecysto-kinin and $5-HT_3$ receptors are located on some of these terminals (Diz *et al.*, 1986; Ladenheim *et al.*, 1988; Leslie *et al.*, 1989a, 1990). Area postrema ablation, then, would be simply a (partial) 'high-level vagotomy' which would have the effect of abolishing the emetic response to drugs which affected these receptors.

4. *The Role of the Gut in the Vomiting Response*

Vomiting has evolved as a protective reflex to enable the rapid expulsion of potentially harmful ingested material before significant amounts are absorbed into the bloodstream. It is, therefore, particularly important that the luminal contents of the proximal gut be monitored for the presence of toxins and that the emetic response can be triggered with the minimum of delay. Far from playing a passive role in vomiting, orchestrated by medullary brainstem nuclei, the proximal gut fulfils a vital sensory role in the detection of ingested toxins (see Andrews and Davis, 1990, for a recent review). The organization of the emetic reflex has been viewed as a hierarchical system with taste and smell providing the first line of defence, sensory mechanisms in the proximal gut providing a major second line and the chemoreceptor trigger zone in the brain acting as a final back-up to detect toxins which have been absorbed (Davis *et al.*, 1986).

In disease states a wide variety of pathological stimuli may activate this protective system, resulting in seemingly purposeless and often counterproductive nausea and vomiting (Grahame-Smith, 1986). Cancer patients receiving radiotherapy or antineoplastic drugs frequently suffer severe and protracted nausea and vomiting which is both distressing and debilitating and can force the withdrawal of treatment. The neuropharmacology of vomiting induced by radiotherapy and chemotherapy has been the subject of much research in recent years (Andrews *et al.*, 1988), but it remains unclear at what level these agents stimulate the emetic reflex.

Gastrointestinal Chemoreceptors

Visceral afferent fibres convey sensory information from the proximal gut via sympathetic (splanchnic nerves) and parasympathetic (vagus nerves) pathways (Andrews, 1986). They are largely unmyelinated and convey information relating to gut motility, temperature, pain, and the osmolarity and the chemical nature of the luminal contents (Mei, 1985). The sensory terminals within the gut are relatively poorly described in the literature, but there is evidence to support the existence of chemoreceptors and mechanoreceptors associated with both sympathetic and parasympathetic fibres (Mei, 1985). Vagal afferent nerve endings can function as mechanoreceptors and chemoreceptors (Clarke and Davison, 1978), but it is not known whether the free endings themselves possess chemosensitivity. It is possible that mechanoreceptors could evoke emesis by detecting the motility changes associated with chemoreceptor-initiated vago-vagal reflexes (Andrews and Wood, 1988). However, it seems more probable that the emetic reflex is triggered directly by chemoreceptors situated in visceral afferent fibres. Alternatively, the trigger may be the release of emetic neurohumoral agents which act at the 'chemoreceptor trigger zone'.

There are epithelial cells within the gut mucosa which could function as chemosensors. These include endocrine cells which release neuroactive peptide hormones (such as vasoactive intestinal peptide, cholecytoskinin, secretin, gastrin, bombesin, somatostatin) in response to luminal chemical stimuli. These gut hormones could act at the level of the area postrema (Carpenter *et al.*, 1983) or the liver (Andrews *et al.*, 1988), or locally on visceral afferent fibres. Cells with morphological similarities to the taste cells of the gustatory epithelium have also been described in the gut mucosa (Newson *et al.*, 1982) and these might play a role analogous to that of taste cells in the detection of toxins in the gut lumen. Enterochromaffin cells have numerous microvilli on their mucosal surface and are good candidates for structures involved in the preabsorption detection of toxins. They contain abundant stores of 5-HT (Erpsamer, 1954) which can be released in response to a variety of physiological stimuli (Verbeuren, 1989). Electron microscopy and axon tract tracing studies (Newson *et al.*, 1982) have revealed distal vagal afferent endings adjacent to enterochromaffin cells. It is conceivable, therefore, that emetic substances are detected by chemoreceptors on the luminal surface of enterochromaffin cells, which causes them to release 5-HT from their basal surface which then evokes depolarization of nearby vagal sensory terminals.

Evidence for the Role of Vagal Afferents in the Emetic Reflex

The contribution of gut vagal afferent fibres to the emetic reflex has been investigated with electrophysiological recording, and stimulation and lesioning experiments. Rodents and lagomorphs do not vomit, and care is needed in interpreting work which has been performed in these species. The ferret has emerged in recent years as a good animal model for emesis research (Florczyk *et al.*, 1982; Davis, 1989), largely replacing cats, dogs and monkeys, which were used in many of the earlier studies. Marked interspecies differences occur in the sensitivities of experimental animals to emetic stimuli: for example, cats appear to be relatively insensitive to radiation compared with ferrets or humans (cf. Borison, 1957). However, it is unclear how useful the ferret model may prove to be in cases of emesis evoked by stimuli other than radiation or cytostatic drugs; they may be unsuitable for motion sickness studies, for example.

At the end of the last century, Openchowski induced vomiting in dogs, using intragastric copper sulphate, and observed that the effect could be blocked by prior bilateral vagotomy (quoted in Hatcher, 1924). It is now apparent that vomiting due to a large variety of stimuli can be blocked or significantly modified by vagotomy or the combination of vagotomy and splanchnectomy. Vagotomy, of course, does not simply remove the afferent fibres: the vagus is a mixed sensory and motor nerve and the efferent pathways will be destroyed as well. In addition, the subdiaphragmatic vagus nerves are situated in close proximity to sympathetic fibres, some of which are almost certainly destroyed by a 'vagal' lesion. Vagal efferents play an important role in the control of gut motility, blood flow and secretion, as well as innervating some of the epithelial cells which may be involved in chemoreception. The combined effects of such efferent denervation may well be significant, but little published work exists which addresses the contribution of vagal efferent pathways to the vomiting response.

One of the first signs of radiation toxicity is nausea and vomiting (Young, 1986), and, in the clinical context, radiotherapy-induced emesis is a common and troublesome complication. In 1957 Borison observed that postirradiation vomiting in cats could be prevented by shielding the abdomen from the source of radiation or by abdominal denervation, and he concluded that radiation-induced vomiting in the cat is initiated in the abdomen, with the afferent impulses passing in the vagus and dorsal spinal roots. In man as well, irradiation of the upper abdoman is a particularly potent stimulus for vomiting (Gerstner, 1960). In a study by Andrews and Hawthorn (1987) total body irradiation of the ferret resulted in vomiting after a latency of about 17

min, which had peaked by 60 min and thereafter declined. Bilateral abdominal vagotomy 7 days before irradiation virtually abolished retching and
vomiting in the first 30 min but the later phases of the emetic response were
unaffected. The authors concluded that radiation-induced emesis may be
divided into an early, vagally dependent phase and a later phase which is
independent of vagal afferent innervation, perhaps mediated by a humoral
emetic substance acting at the chemoreceptor trigger zone.

A large number of cytotoxic drugs and inhibitors of protein synthesis are
potent emetics (Harris and Cantwell, 1986), which gives rise to considerable
problems in treating cancer patients. The time-course of vomiting due to
these agents is very variable, even within a single species (see Andrews *et al.*,
1988). None of them acts as rapidly as apomorphine, and the latencies suggest
that a direct action on afferent neuronal pathways or the chemoreceptor
trigger zone is unlikely. In the cat the cytotoxic antineoplastic drug cisplatin
causes vomiting with a latency of approximately 100 min, but its emetic action
is not seen in postremectomized animals (McCarthy and Borison, 1984).
Using the ferret as their model, Hawthorn *et al.* (1988) found that the
abdominal innervation played a crucial role in cyclophosphamide- and
cisplatin-induced vomiting. Since some elements of the central nervous
system that are involved with the vomiting response have a poor blood–brain
diffusion barrier, as described above, it seems likely that cytotoxic drugs
(which tend to be administered by the intravenous route) activate both gut
sensory mechanisms and central ones. Administration of reserpine, para-
chlorophenylalanine or fenfluramine in the ferret antagonizes cisplatin-
induced emesis (Barnes *et al.*, 1988b), which suggests the involvement of
5-HT in the emetic response, although it is not possible to distinguish between
the contribution of central and peripheral 5-HT with these agents.

More direct evidence for the role of abdominal vagal and splanchnic
innervation in the emetic reflex comes from electrical stimulation experiments. Stimulation of the central end of the subdiaphragmatic vagus (i.e.
afferent stimulation) in the conscious ferret elicits the prodromata of vomiting
within a few seconds, and retching and vomiting occur within 1–2 min
(Andrews and Davidson, 1990). In the anaesthetized animal similar responses
are observed. Efferent stimulation does not elicit retching or any of the
emetic epiphenomena (P. L. R. Andrews, personal communication). Stimulation of the splanchnic afferents or efferents also fails to evoke retching or
prodromic behaviour. Although electrical stimulation does not reproduce the
'physiological' pattern of afferent impulses, this work emphasizes further the
potential for vagal sensory information to trigger the emetic reflex.

Evidence for Gut-derived Humoral Emetic Mediators

In the dog it has been shown that radiation elicits vomiting which is
dependent on the integrity of the area postrema but not the vagal afferent

pathways (Wang *et al.*, 1958; Carpenter *et al.*, 1986). Carpenter and co-workers (1986) further demonstrated that, following abdominal irradiation, neurons within the area postrema become spontaneously electrically active but fire at a relatively slow rate, which suggests that radiation-induced vomiting in dogs may be humorally mediated. A number of candidate substances for such a humoral endogenous emetic have been proposed. Ileal 5-HT is released by irradiation (Matsuoka *et al.*, 1962) and cytotoxic drugs produce marked histological changes in the ileum associated with increased mucosal levels of 5-HT (Gunning *et al.*, 1987). 5-HT released into the portal vein in response to noxious stimuli could exert a significant effect in the liver, perhaps acting on hepatic vagal afferents (Andrews *et al.*, 1988). However, it is unclear whether significant levels of 5-HT spill over into the systemic circulation to act at a central site such as the chemoreceptor trigger zone, because of the highly efficient uptake of 5-HT by platelets (Born and Gillson, 1959) and probable degradation in liver and lung (Ahlman and Dahlstrom, 1982). Furthermore, it is interesting to note that vomiting is not a prominent feature of the carcinoid syndrome where circulating levels of 5-HT are pathologically high (Grahame-Smith, 1972).

Using electrophysiological techniques, Carpenter and colleagues (1983, 1988) have found that, in anaesthetized dogs, the normally silent area postrema neurons could be excited by iontophoretic application of neuro-transmitters (including glutamate, dopamine, 5-HT and noradrenaline), peptides (gastrin, angiotensin II, thyrotropin-releasing hormone, vasoactive intestinal peptide, vasopressin, substance P, neuropeptide Y and leu-enkephalin, but not cholecystokinin or somatostatin) and cyclic nucleotides.

Some evidence exists to support the role of peptide YY (PYY) as a humoral emetic agent released from the gut. Harding *et al.* (1985) identified a peptide fraction in porcine intestinal extract which coeluted with PYY on reverse phase HPLC and which was emetic when injected into dogs. PYY is present in gut epithelial cells (Lundberg *et al.*, 1982), and receptor binding sites for PYY have been demonstrated autoradiographically in the dog area postrema and nucleus of the solitary tract (Leslie *et al.*, 1988). A report has suggested that the postprandial release of PYY can be decreased by the 5-HT$_3$ receptor antagonist GR 38032F (Talley *et al.*, 1989). This raises the possibility that 5-HT$_3$ receptor antagonists might also influence PYY release in patholo-gical situations. In man, however, infusion of PYY at a dose sufficient to inhibit gastric emptying was not associated with nausea or vomiting (Allen *et al.*, 1984).

There is, therefore, much circumstantial evidence to link gut 5-HT with the emetic reflex, and the presence of very large numbers of 5-HT$_3$ receptor binding sites in the dorsal vagal complex of the brain suggests that there might also be a central effect of 5-HT in this response. The 5-HT$_3$ receptor antagonist drugs have emerged over the last few years as potent antiemetics for the treatment of cytotoxic- and radiation-induced nausea and vomiting. The site of action of these exciting new agents is discussed below.

5. 5-HT₃ Receptor Antagonists as Antiemetics

Clinically useful antiemetic activity has been ascribed to many classes of drugs, including dopamine D2 receptor antagonists, histamine H1 blockers, antimuscarinics, cannabinoids, benzodiazepines, steroids, tricyclic antidepressants (reviewed in Barnes, 1984) and, more recently, 5-HT$_3$ receptor antagonists (Miner and Sanger, 1986). The lack of a unified therapeutic approach is perhaps a reflection of the diversity of biological mechanisms underlying the different causes of nausea and vomiting, and clearly, if a 'final common pathway' is involved, it has so far eluded pharmacological characterization. The use of radiotherapy and antineoplastic drugs as anticancer treatments has brought with it the therapeutic challenge of producing drugs to ameliorate the severe nausea and vomiting which affect the majority of cancer patients undergoing therapy.

The development of specific 5-HT$_3$ receptor antagonist drugs has been well discussed in the literature (Richardson and Engel, 1986; Sanger and King, 1988). These drugs have emerged as powerful pharmacological tools and as promising therapeutic agents. In man the antiemetic effect of 5-HT$_3$ receptor antagonists has been the first of their properties to be exploited, and one of these drugs is now available commercially for this use. Even allowing for the initial enthusiasm which accompanies the introduction of many new drugs, 5-HT$_3$ receptor antagonists do appear to represent a major advance in emetic control in patients receiving cytotoxic therapy and radiotherapy, with efficacy rates at least as good as those of current combination therapy and with apparently significantly fewer side-effects.

5-HT$_3$ receptor antagonists are not effective in blocking emesis from all causes. They appear to have no activity against vomiting due to apomorphine (Miner *et al.*, 1987; Bermudez *et al.*, 1988; Davis, 1989), motion sickness, xylazine (Lucot, 1989b) or intragastric irritants such as copper sulphate or sodium chloride (Davis, 1989). Apomorphine-induced vomiting is antagonized by dopamine D2 receptor blockers such as domperidone, and lesioning work would suggest that the emetic action of apomorphine is exerted in the region of the area postrema (Borison *et al.*, 1984). Vomiting elicited by intragastric irritants is largely dependent on the integrity of visceral afferent fibres. However, the observation that 5-HT$_3$ receptor antagonists have no activity against vomiting due to these agents raises the possibility that some toxins are capable of activating gastrointestinal afferent pathways independent of 5-HT. It may be that stimulation of such gut chemoreceptors which do not require 5-HT as an intermediary may produce vagal depolarization and result in emesis.

5-HT$_3$ receptor antagonists have been shown to inhibit vomiting evoked by a range of cytotoxic drugs (Leibundgut and Lancranjan, 1987), protein synthesis inhibitors (Davis, 1989), radiation (Andrews and Hawthorn, 1987) and PYY (R. K. Harding, personal communication). The possible sites of action of 5-HT$_3$ receptor antagonists are discussed below.

Peripheral 5-HT$_3$-mediated Antiemetic Action

It is from work in animal models that the use of 5-HT$_3$ receptor antagonists has provided further evidence to support the role of 5-HT in the emetic response. 5-HT$_3$ receptors in both peripheral and central sites may be important in processing emetic information. 5-HT$_3$ receptor-mediated effects in peripheral nervous tissue have been investigated, using a number of bioassay systems (Richardson and Buchheit, 1988). 5-HT$_3$ receptors located on peripheral sensory, autonomic or enteric nerve fibres mediate the excitatory response to 5-HT (Richardson and Engel, 1986; Round and Wallis, 1987; Ireland and Tyers, 1987). 5-HT causes depolarization of vagal fibres which can be blocked by 5-HT$_3$ receptor antagonists (Richardson *et al.*, 1985; Ireland and Tyers, 1987). It is, therefore, plausible that some emetic agents could activate the release of 5-HT in the gut (perhaps from enterochromaffin cells), which binds to 5-HT$_3$ receptors in vagal sensory fibres in the gut, resulting in depolarization and stimulation of emetic pathways in the brainstem. The substituted benzamide BRL 24924 (renzapride) has 5-HT$_3$ receptor antagonist activity and in low dose it has been shown to mimic the effect of abdominal vagotomy in inhibiting the 'vagally dependent' phase of radiation-induced vomiting in the ferret (Andrews and Hawthorn, 1987). In higher doses it almost totally antagonizes the later (vagally independent) phase of the response as well. Therefore, an additional extra-abdominal site of action of 5-HT$_3$ receptor antagonism was suggested (Andrews and Hawthorn, 1987).

The Involvement of Central 5-HT$_3$ Receptors in Emesis

5-HT$_3$ receptor binding in the brain was first demonstrated by use of the radiolabelled antagonist [^{3}H]GR65630 in homogenates of rat brain (Kilpatrick *et al.*, 1987). Subsequent membrane binding studies have been performed using other radiolabelled antagonists such as [^{3}H]quaternized ICS 205-930 (Watling *et al.*, 1988), [^{3}H]zacopride (Barnes *et al.*, 1988a), [^{3}H]BRL 43694 (Nelson and Thomas, 1989) and [^{3}H]quipazine (Peroutka and Hamik, 1988). A number of autoradiographic studies have also demonstrated central binding sites for radiolabelled 5-HT$_3$ receptor antagonists with particularly high density of binding in the dorsal vagal complex of the medulla oblongata (Kilpatrick *et al.*, 1988; Pratt and Bowery, 1989; Reynolds *et al.*, 1989a,b; Waeber *et al.*, 1988, 1989; Leslie *et al.*, 1990).

Different authors have used a number of 5-HT$_3$ receptor radioligands in a variety of species, and their reports indicated some variation in the exact distribution of binding within the dorsal vagal complex. This led to speculation about the existence of more than one 5-HT$_3$ receptor subtype in the brainstem. However, it is now clear that the apparent differences were due to problems in defining the boundaries between the brainstem nuclei which constitute the dorsal vagal complex. A consensus has now been reached that the binding is principally within the dorsomedial part of the nucleus of the solitary tract, with lesser levels of binding in the area postrema and dorsal motor nucleus of the vagus (Pratt *et al.*, 1990). Nevertheless, interspecies variations do exist (see Figure 2). For example, in the rat, cat and man there is a high denisty of 5-HT$_3$ receptor radioligand binding in the nucleus of the solitary tract, with very low levels in the area postrema. In contrast, in the

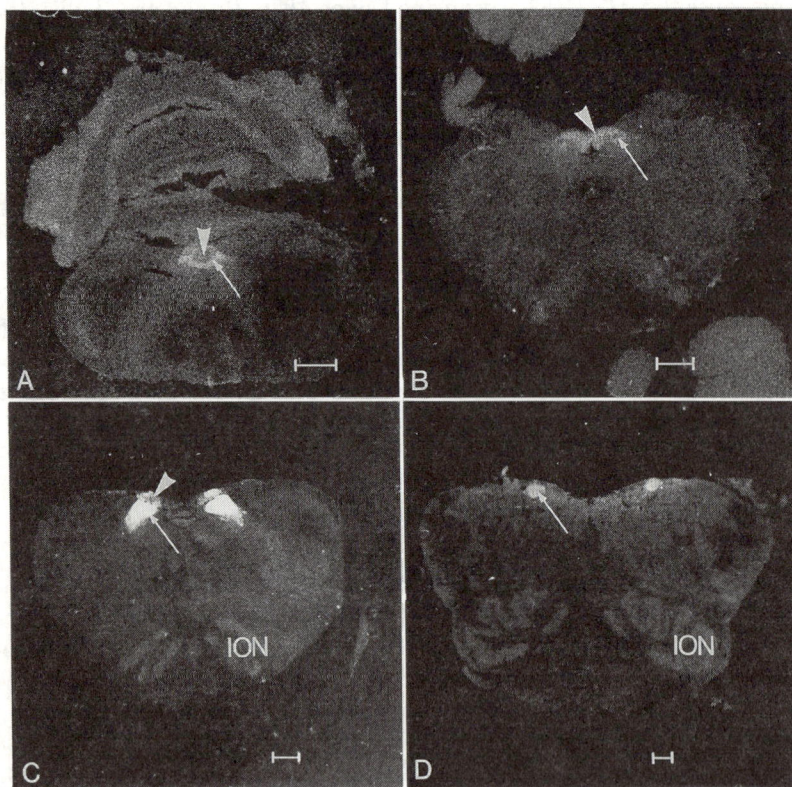

Figure 2   Negative images of autoradiograms generated over 12 μm frozen sections of rat (A), ferret (B), cat (C) and human (D) caudal brainstem, showing total binding of 1 nM [^{3}H]GR 65630. The sections were incubated with 1 nM [^{3}H]GR 65630 (specific activity 87 Ci/mmol) in 50 mM HEPES buffer, pH 7.4 at room temperature for 45 min. Dense binding is seen within the dorsal vagal complex of each species. In the ferret (B) binding is similar in the area postrema (AP, arrowhead) and the subjacent nucleus of the solitary tract (NTS, arrow). In contrast, the binding in the AP (arrowheads) is much less than that in the NTS (arrows) in the rat (A) and cat (C). In man (D) there is little evidence of any binding in the AP. The binding visible in the inferior olivary nucleus (ION, in sections B–D) is not displaced by 10 μM zacopride or 10 μM BRL 43694. Bars = 1 mm

ferret, although the binding is still higher in the nucleus of the solitary tract, there is proportionally much more binding in the area postrema (Figure 2).

From the autoradiographic appearance of the distribution of binding of [^{3}H]ICS205-930, Waeber *et al.* (1988) postulated that, as in the periphery, 5-HT$_3$ receptors might be located on sensory afferent terminals, Lesions of the nodose ganglion in rats (Pratt and Bowery, 1989) and in ferrets (Leslie *et al.*, 1989b, 1990) result in a marked reduction of the binding of [^{3}H]BRL 43694 in the nucleus of the solitary tract ipsilateral to the lesion, suggesting that 5-HT$_3$ receptors are located on vagal afferent terminals. Bilateral subdiaphragmatic vagotomy in the ferret abolishes 5-HT$_3$ receptor binding in the dorsal vagal complex (Reynolds *et al.*, 1989b; Leslie *et al.*, 1990). Cervical vagal lesions do not discriminate between vagal afferents from any particular source, whereas subdiaphragmatic lesions selectively remove abdominal visceral afferents which are known from studies in cat (Gwyn *et al.*, 1979) and rat (Leslie *et al.*, 1982) to be very largely gastric in origin. Abolition of 5-HT$_3$ receptor binding sites after subdiaphragmatic vagotomy provides strong circumstantial evidence that these receptors are located primarily on the vagal afferents which emanate from the upper gastrointestinal tract. The central projections of vagal afferents in the cat are well documented and correlate very well with the distribution of 5-HT$_3$ receptor binding sites in the brainstem of this animal (Figure 3; Reynolds *et al.*, 1990).

Intravenous or intraperitoneal injections of cisplatin induce retching and vomiting with a latency of about 60 min in the ferret (Davis, 1989) and 100 min in the cat (Smith *et al.*, 1988). If the cytotoxic drug is injected directly into the fourth ventricle, vomiting in the cat occurs within 4 min, and this can be prevented by intracerebroventricular (i.c.v.) injection of zacopride 15 min before the cytotoxic drug (Smith *et al.*, 1988). These authors also found that once cisplatin-induced emesis was established, i.c.v. injection of zacopride would inhibit further episodes of vomiting. Higgins *et al.* (1989) observed that injections of 5-HT$_3$ receptor antagonists into the region of the dorsal medulla in the ferret inhibited vomiting due to intraperitoneal cisplatin. This provides evidence to argue for a central site of action of 5-HT$_3$ receptor antagonists in blocking cisplatin-evoked emesis. The presence of 5-HT$_3$ receptors on vagal afferent terminals in the dorsal vagal complex would support such an argument. In the gut 5-HT$_3$ receptor antagonists block the excitatory effect of 5-HT on myenteric GABAergic neurones (Shirakawa *et al.*, 1989). There is evidence in the central nervous system that 5-HT, acting via 5-HT$_3$ receptors, may modulate the release of dopamine (Blandina *et al.*, 1988) and acetylcholine (Barnes *et al.*, 1989). How 5-HT$_3$ receptors, located on central vagal afferent terminals in the dorsal vagal complex, may modulate the emetic response is unknown. As discussed above, firing of vagal afferents is associated with emesis, and blockade of 5-HT$_3$ receptors is antiemetic. If it is postulated that toxins within the gut cause 5-HT release which, in turn, activates distal vagal sensory endings in the gut, then a similar situation may

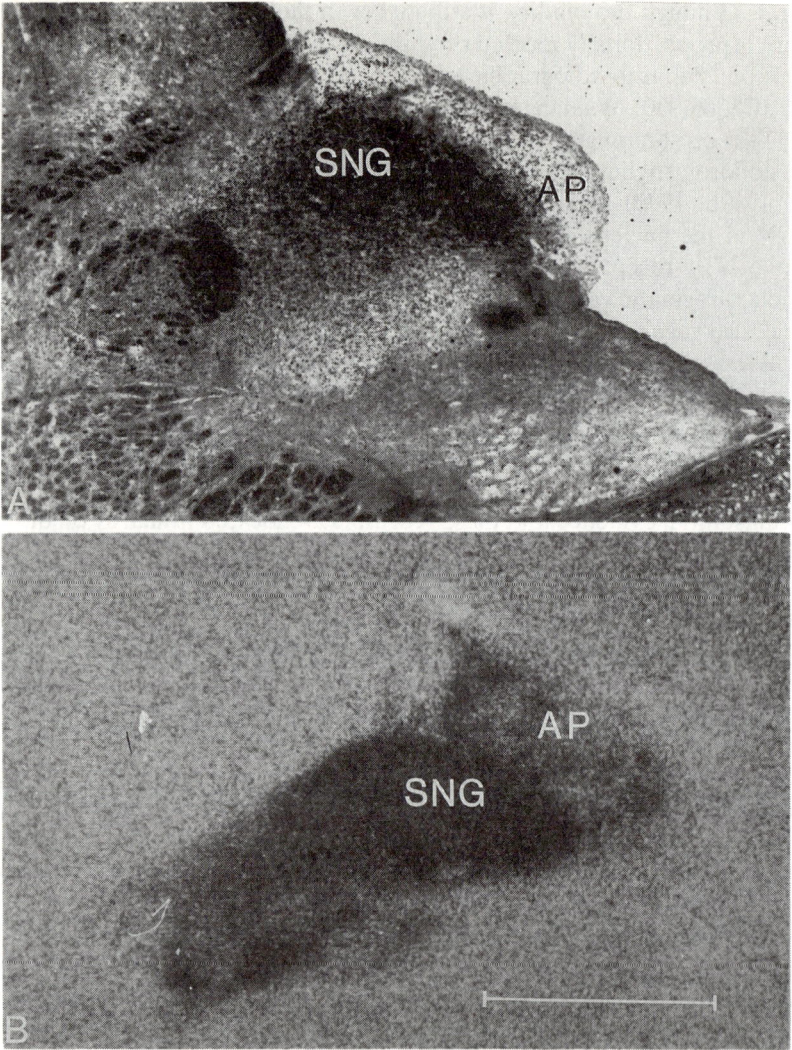

Figure 3   A: Autoradiograph generated over a transverse section through the cat caudal brainstem at the level of the area postrema (AP) 4 days following an injection of 25 μCi of [³H]leucine into the nodose ganglion (material taken from Gwyn *et al.*, 1979). Note the heavy labelling in the subnucleus gelatinosus (SNG), with much lower levels in the AP. The distribution of silver grains representing the labelled vagus nerve fibres and terminals is very similar to that seen in Figure 2(B), which illustrates the binding of [³H]GR 65630 to the cat brainstem. B: Positive image, at higher power, of an autoradiograph similar to that in Figure 2(C). Bar = 100 μm; magnification is the same in Figures 3(A) and 3(B)

exist for blood- or CSF-borne toxins acting on chemoreceptors in the area postrema. 5-HT, released in the gut or the area postrema, acting on 5-HT_3 receptors, would have the same effect—i.e. to cause depolarization of vagal afferent terminals and result in activation of emetic pathways.

6. *The Importance of Other 5-Hydroxytryptamine Receptors*

So far we have discussed only the involvement of 5-HT_3 receptors in the emetic response, but other 5-HT receptor subtypes might also be important. Autoradiographic radioligand binding studies have revealed 5-HT_{1A} receptor recognition sites in the nucleus of the solitary tract in man, as defined by binding of [^{3}H]8-OH-DPAT ([^{3}H]8-hydroxy-2-[di-n-propylamino] tetralin) and lower levels of 5-HT_{1C} and 5-HT_2 receptors (Pazos *et al.*, 1987a,b). There is some evidence to suggest that 5-HT_{1A} receptors might be involved in the control of emesis. Lucot and Crampton (1987) have shown in cats that the 5-HT_{1A} receptor agonist busiprone at a dose of 4 mg/kg blocks the retching and vomiting evoked by cisplatin. However, buspirone possesses dopamine blocking activity (McMillen and Mattiace, 1983) and its principal metabolite is a potent adrenergic alpha$_2$ antagonist (Caccia *et al.*, 1986). Its antiemetic effect, therefore, cannot at this stage be attributed to 5-HT_{1A} receptor agonist activity. More recently there has been a preliminary report that the prototypic 5-HT_{1A} agonist 8-OH-DPAT is also antiemetic in cats, but no details were given (Lucot, 1989a). An antiemetic effect of 5-HT_{1A} agonists could be related to activation of 5-HT_{1A} autoreceptors resulting in decreased 5-HT release (Sharp *et al.*, 1989) or to a postsynaptic 5-HT_{1A} receptor effect, but this remains speculative at this stage.

In 1988 Dumuis and colleagues described a 5-HT receptor coupled to adenylyl cyclase in mouse embryo colliculi neurons which did not fit into the 5-HT_1, 5-HT_2 or 5-HT_3 classification and which they designated the 5-HT_4 receptor. Subsequently it has been shown that the 5-HT_3 receptor antagonist ICS 205-930 also acts as an antagonist at the 5-HT_4 receptor and that some substituted benzamides (e.g. metoclopramide, zacopride, cisapride and renzapride) act as 5-HT_4 receptor agonists (Dumuis *et al.*, 1988, 1989). It seems probable that the gastrokinetic actions of the substituted benzamides discussed here arise through activation of 5-HT_4 receptors in the enteric nervous system (Clark *et al.*, 1989). These substituted benzamide drugs are also 5-HT_3 receptor antagonists and potent inhibitors of radiation- and cytotoxic-drug-induced vomiting. It remains to be seen whether or not 5-HT_4 receptors are involved in the emetic reflex as well as in the control of gut motility.

7. Prospects for the Future: A Better Understanding of the Mechanisms of and New Treatments for Nausea and Vomiting

From the discussion above, it is clear that a large number of important questions about the mechanisms of nausea and vomiting are still unanswered. In fact, recent investigations have posed new, intriguing questions such as: What role (if any) do the 5-HT$_3$ receptor binding sites in the dorsal vagal complex play in the emetic reflex? The extremely dense and highly localized nature of these binding sites in this tiny region of the brain is remarkable; nowhere else in the entire central nervous system has such a dense accumulation of these sites. Other questions include: How do these binding sites interact with all the others that are found in this region of the brain and that are known to be involved in the emetic reflex? Where does the endogenous ligand for these receptors arise?

There are a number of approaches that may be taken to attempt to answer some of these questions. Obviously, further studies aimed at elucidating the anatomy and neurochemistry of the relevant neuronal circuits would go a long way to helping with these investigations. Modern methods of immunocytochemical identification of neuromodulatory substances, and now even receptor sites, can be combined with electron microscopy to give details of the exact interconnections between neuronal elements within the brain. Thus, it should be possible eventually to determine which cells and which parts of cells bear the 5-HT$_3$ receptors in the dorsal vagal complex, and which cells provide the endogenous ligand for these receptors. Furthermore, it should be possible to determine the anatomical nature of the connections between cholinergic, adrenergic and peptidergic components with the serotonergic elements in this brain region.

New methods of determining which neurons are metabolically active at any given time following peripheral stimuli should prove of importance in such investigations. For example, 2-deoxyglucose uptake studies (Sokoloff *et al.*, 1977) or mapping of active neuronal pathways by localization of immediate-early gene expression (Robertson and Dragunow, 1990) should enable investigators to detect how identified neuronal elements interact during nausea or vomiting episodes.

It will prove interesting to investigate the pharmacology of these processes by means of further electrophysiological recording studies, either *in situ* or in brain slice preparations of the relevant brain regions. Another way of approaching these questions is to use brain microdialysis techniques to study the pharmacological mechanisms of neurotransmitter release in the dorsal vagal complex. These studies can be pursued at the distal end of some of the pathways involved as well. For example, *in vivo* or *in vitro* gut preparations can be investigated for their ability to respond to known emetogenic stimuli by releasing substances which are candidates for the 'endogenous emetic'. An obvious material to search for in such preparations is 5-HT itself, but other suggested candidates for this role include prostaglandins and various peptides such as PYY.

Once we arrive at a better understanding of the anatomical, pharmacological and physiological elements involved in the vomiting response, it should be possible to design better drugs to deal with the outstanding problems involving unwanted nausea and emesis. It may be that 5-HT$_3$ receptor antagonist compounds are just the start of such targeted therapies. One hopes that safe and more effective drugs will become available to treat such diverse problems as motion (and space) sickness, morning sickness and sickness induced by pathological toxins released by viral or bacterial infections.

Acknowledgements

We wish to thank J. M. Harvey and C. M. Allen for expert technical assistance, and Professor D. G. Grahame-Smith and Drs P. L. R. Andrews, G. F. Sanger and T. P. Flanigan for helpful discussions.

References

Ahlman, H. and Dahlstrom, A. (1982). Storage and release of 5-hydroxytryptamine in enterochromaffin cells of the small intestine. In *5-Hydroxytryptamine in Peripheral Reactions* (ed. F. De Clerck and P. M. Vanhoutte). Raven Press, New York, pp. 1–21

Allen, J. M., Fitzpatrick, M. L., Yeats, J. C., Darcy, K., Adrian, T. E. and Bloom, S. R. (1984). Effects of peptide YY and neuropeptide Y on gastric emptying in man. *Digestion*, **30**, 255–262

Andrews, P. L. R. (1986). Vagal afferent innervation of the gastrointestinal tract. *Prog. Brain Res.*, **67**, 65–85

Andrews, P. L. R. and Davidson, H. I. M. (1990). A method for the induction of emesis in the conscious ferret by abdominal vagal stimulation. *J. Physiol.* (in press)

Andrews, P. L. R. and Davis, C. J. (1990). The role of the gastrointestinal tract in nausea and vomiting. In *Nausea and Vomiting* (ed. R. K. Harding). CRC Press, Cleveland

Andrews, P. L. R., Davis, C. J., Grahame-Smith, D. G. and Leslie, R. A. (1986). Increase in [^{3}H]-2-deoxyglucose uptake in the ferret area postrema produced by apomorphine administration or electrical stimulation of the abdominal vagus. *J. Physiol.*, **383**, 187P

Andrews, P. L. R. and Hawthorn, J. (1987). Evidence for an extra-abdominal site of action for the 5-HT$_3$ receptor antagonist BRL 24924 in the inhibition of radiation-evoked emesis in the ferret. *Neuropharmacology*, **26**, 1367–1370

Andrews, P. L. R., Rapeport, W. G. and Sanger, G. J. (1988). Neuropharmacology of emesis induced by anti-cancer therapy. *Trends Pharm. Sci.*, **9**, 334–341

Andrews, P. L. R. and Wood, K. L. (1988). Vagally mediated gastric motor and emetic reflexes evoked by stimulation of the antral mucosa in anaesthetized ferrets. *J. Physiol.*, **395**, 1–16

Barnes, J. H. (1984). The physiology and pharmacology of emesis. *Molec. Aspects Med.*, **7**, 397–508

Barnes, J. M., Barnes, N. M., Costall, B., Naylor, R. J. and Tyers, M. B. (1989). 5-HT$_3$ receptors mediate inhibition of acetylcholine release in cortical tissue. *Nature*, **338**, 762–763

Barnes, N. M., Costall, B. and Naylor, R. J. (1988a). [^{3}H]Zacopride: ligand for the identification of 5-HT$_3$ recognition sites. *J. Pharm. Pharmcol.*, **40**, 548–551

Barnes, N. M., Costall, B., Naylor, R. J. and Tattersall, F. D. (1988b). Reserpine, para-chlorophenylalanine and fenfluramine antagonise cisplatin-induced emesis in the ferret. *Neuropharmacology*, **27**, 783–790

Bermudez, J., Boyle, E. A., Miner, W. D. and Sanger, G. J. (1988). The anti-emetic and anti-nauseant potential of the 5-hydroxytryptamine3 receptor antagonist BRL 43694. *Br. J. Cancer*, **58**, 644–650

Blandina, P., Goldfarb, J. and Green, J. P. (1988). Activation of a 5-HT$_3$ receptor releases dopamine from rat striatal slices. *Eur. J. Pharmacol.*, **155**, 349–350

Borison, H. L. (1957). Site of emetic action of X-irradiation in the cat. *J. Comp. Neurol.*, **107**, 439–453

Borison, H. L. (1974). Area postrema: chemoreceptive trigger zone for vomiting—is that all? *Life Sci.*, **14**, 1807–1817

Borison, H. L., Borison, R. and McCarthy, L. E. (1984). Role of the area postrema in vomiting and related functions. *Fed. Proc.*, **43**, 2955–2958

Born, G. V. R. and Gillson, R. E. (1959). Studies on the uptake of 5-HT by blood platelets. *J. Physiol.*, **146**, 472–491

Bradley, P. B., Engel, G., Feniuk, W., Fozard, J. R., Humphrey, P. P. A., Middlemiss, D. N., Mylecharane, E. J., Richardson, B. P. and Saxena, P. R. (1986). Proposals for the classification and nomenclature of functional receptors for 5-hydroxytryptamine. *Neuropharmacology*, **25**, 563–576

Brizzee, K. R. and Mehler, W. R. (1986). The central nervous connections involved in the vomiting reflex. In *Nausea and Vomiting: Mechanisms and Treatment* (ed. C. J. Davis, G. V. Lake-Bakaar and D. G. Grahame-Smith). Springer-Verlag, Berlin, pp. 31–55

Caccia, S., Conti, I., Vigano, G. and Garattini, S. (1986). 1-(2-Pyrimidinyl)-piperazine as active metabolite of buspirone in man and rat. *Pharmacology*, **33**, 46–51

Carpenter, D. O. (1988). Central nervous system mechanisms in deglutition and emesis. In *Handbook of Physiology*, Vol. IV: *Motility and Circulation* (ed. J. W. Wood). American Physiological Society, Bethesda

Carpenter, D. O., Briggs, D. B., Knox, A. P. and Strominger, N. (1986). Radiation-induced emesis in the dog: effects of lesions and drugs. *Radiat. Res.*, **108**, 307–316

Carpenter, D. O., Briggs, D. B., Knox, A. P. and Strominger, N. (1988). Excitation of area postrema neurons by transmitters, peptides and cyclic nucleotides. *J. Neurophysiol.*, **59**, 358–369

Carpenter, D. O., Briggs, D. B. and Strominger, N. (1983). Responses of neurons of canine area postrema to neurotransmitters and peptides. *Cell. Molec. Neurol.*, **3**, 113–126

Clarke, D. E., Craig, D. A. and Fozard, J. R. (1989). The 5-HT$_4$ receptor: naughty, but nice. *Trends Pharmacol. Sci.*, **10**, 385–386

Clarke, G. D. and Davison, J. S. (1978). Mucosal receptors in the gastric antrum and small intestine of the rat with afferent fibres in the cervical vagus. *J. Physiol.*, **284**, 55–67

Dahlstrom, A. and Fuxe, K. (1964). Evidence for the existence of monoamine-containing neurons in the central nervous system. *Acta Physiol. Scand.*, **62**, Suppl. 232, 1–55

Davis, C. J. (1989). Neuropharmacological Investigations into the Mechanisms of Emesis Caused by Cytotoxic Drugs and Radiation. D. Phil. Thesis, University of Oxford

Davis, C. J., Harding, R. K., Leslie, R. A. and Andrews, P. L. R. (1986). The organisation of vomiting as a protective reflex. In *Nausea and Vomiting: Mechanisms and Treatment* (ed. C. J. Davis, G. V. Lake-Bakaar and D. G. Grahame-Smith). Springer-Verlag, Berlin, pp. 65–75

Diz, D. I., Barnes, D. L. and Ferrario, C. M. (1986). Contribution of the vagus nerve to angiotensin II binding sites in the canine medulla. *Brain Res. Bull.*, **17**, 497–505

Dumuis, A., Bouhelal, R., Sebben, M. and Bockaert, J. (1988). A 5-HT receptor in the central nervous system, positively coupled with adenylate cyclase, is antagonized by ICS 205 930. *Eur. J. Pharmacol.*, **146**, 187–188

Dumuis, A., Sebben, M. and Bockaert, J. (1989). The gastrointestinal prokinetic benzamide derivatives are agonists at the non-classical 5-HT receptor (5-HT$_4$) positively coupled to adenylate cyclase in neurons. *Naunyn-Schmiedebergs Arch. Pathol. Exp. Pharmakol.*, **340**, 403–410

Edwards, G. L. and Ritter, R. C. (1981). Ablation of the area postrema causes exaggerated consumption of preferred foods in the rat. *Brain Res.*, **216**, 265–276

Erpsamer, V. (1954). Pharmacology of indole alkylamines. *Pharmacol. Rev.*, **6**, 425–487

Florczyk, A. P., Schurig, J. E. and Bradner, W. T. (1982). Cisplatin-induced emesis in the ferret: a new animal model. *Cancer Treat. Rep.*, **66**, 187–189

Fuxe, K. and Owman, C. (1965). Cellular localization of monoamines in the area postrema of certain mammals. *J. Comp. Neurol.*, **125**, 337–354

Gaddum, J. H. and Picarelli, Z. P. (1957). Two kinds of tryptamine receptor. *Br. J. Pharmacol.*, **12**, 323–328

Gaudin-Chazal, G., Seyfritz, N., Araneda, S., Vigier, D. and Puizillout, J. J. (1982). Selective retrograde transport of [^{3}H]serotonin in vagal afferents. *Brain Res. Bull.*, **8**, 503–509

Gerstner, H. B. (1960). Reaction to short term radiation in man. *Ann. Rev. Med.*, **11**, 389–402

Grahame-Smith, D. G. (1972). *The Carcinoid Syndrome*. Heinemann, London

Grahame-Smith, D. G. (1986). The multiple causes of vomiting: is there a common mechanism? In *Nausea and Vomiting: Mechanisms and Treatment* (ed. C. J. Davis, G. V. Lake-Bakaar and D. G. Grahame-Smith). Springer-Verlag, Berlin, pp. 1–8

Gunning, S. J., Hagan, R. M. and Tyers, M. B. (1987). Cisplatin induces biochemical and histological changes in the small intestine of the ferret. *Br. J. Pharmacol.*, **90**, 135P

Gwyn, D. G. and Leslie, R. A. (1979). Retrograde degeneration studies on the afferents of the vagus nerve to the area subpostrema of the cat. *Brain Res.*, **161**, 335–341

Gwyn, D. G., Leslie, R. A. and Hopkins, D. A. (1979). Gastric afferents in the nucleus of the solitary tract in the cat. *Neurosci. Lett.*, **14**, 13–17

Harding, R. K., McDonald, T. J., Hugenholtz, H., Kucharczyk, J. and Leach, K. E. (1985). PYY: a relevant emetic peptide? *Gastroenterology*, **88**, 1413

Harris, A. L. and Cantwell, B. M. J. (1986). Mechanisms and treatment of cytotoxic-induced nausea and vomiting. In *Nausea and Vomiting: Mechanisms and Treatment* (ed. C. J. Davis, G. V. Lake-Bakaar and D. G. Grahame-Smith). Springer-Verlag, Berlin, pp. 78–93

Hatcher, R. A. (1924). The mechanisms of vomiting. *Physiol. Rev.*, **4**, 479–504

Hawthorn, J., Ostler, K. J. and Andrews, P. L. R. (1988). The role of the abdominal visceral innervation and 5-hydroxytryptamine M-receptors in vomiting induced by the cytotoxic drugs cyclophosphamide and cisplatin in the ferret. *J. Exp. Physiol.*, **73**, 7–21

Higgins, G. A., Kilpatrick, G. J., Bunce, K. T., Jones, B. J. and Tyers, M. B. (1989). 5-HT$_3$ receptor antagonists injected into the area postrema inhibit cisplatin-induced emesis in the ferret. *Br. J. Pharmacol.*, **97**, 247–255

Howe, P. R. C., Moon, E. and Dampney, R. A. L. (1983). Distribution of serotonin nerve cells in the rabbit brainstem. *Neurosci. Lett.*, **38**, 125–130

Ireland, S. J. and Tyers, M. B. (1987). Pharmacological characterization of 5-hydroxytryptamine-induced depolarization of the rat isolated vagus nerve. *Br. J. Pharmacol.*, **90**, 229–238

Kalia, M. and Mesulam, M.-M. (1979). Brain stem projections of sensory and motor components of the vagus complex in the cat. II. Laryngeal, tracheo-bronchial, pulmonary, cardiac and gastrointestinal branches. *J. Comp. Neurol.*, **193**, 467–508

Kilpatrick, G. J., Jones, B. J. and Tyers, M. B. (1987). Identification and distribution of 5-HT$_3$ receptors in rat brain using radioligand binding. *Nature*, **330**, 746–748

Kilpatrick, G. J., Jones, B. J. and Tyers, M. B. (1988). The distribution of specific binding of the 5-HT$_3$ receptor ligand [^{3}H]GR65630 in rat brain using quantitative autoradiography. *Neurosci. Lett.*, **94**, 156–160

Ladenheim, E. E., Speth, R. C. and Ritter, R. C. (1988). Reduction of CCK-8 binding in the nucleus of the solitary tract in unilaterally nodosectomized rats. *Brain Res.*, **474**, 125–129

Leibundgut, U. and Lancranjan, I. (1987). First results with ICS 205-930 (5-HT$_3$ receptor antagonist) in prevention of chemotherapy-induced emesis. *Lancet*, **1**, 1198

Leslie, R. A. (1985). Neuroactive substances in the dorsal vagal complex of the medulla oblongata: nucleus tractus solitarius, area postrema and dorsal motor nucleus of the vagus. *Neurochem. Int.*, **7**, 191–121

Leslie, R. A. (1986). Comparative aspects of the area postrema: fine structural considerations help to determine its function. *Cell. Molec. Neurobiol.*, **6**, 95–120

Leslie R. A. and Gwyn, D. G. (1984). Neuronal connections of the area postrema. *Fed. Proc.*, **43**, 2941–2943

Leslie R. A., Gwyn, D. G. and Hopkins, D. A. (1982). The central distribution of the cervical vagus nerve and gastric afferent and efferent projections in the rat. *Brain Res. Bull.*, **8**, 37–43

Leslie, R. A., Gwyn, D. G. and Morrison, C. M. (1978). The fine structure of the ventricular surface of the area postrema of the cat, with particular reference to supraependymal structures. *Am. J. Anat.*, **153**, 273–290

Leslie, R. A., MacDonald, T. J. and Robertson, H. A. (1988). Autoradiographic localization of Peptide YY and Neuropeptide Y binding sites in the medulla oblongata. *Peptides*, **9**, 1071–1076

Leslie, R. A., Murphy, K. M. and Robertson, H. A. (1989a). Nodose ganglionectomy selectively reduces muscarinic cholinergic and delta opioid binding sites in the dorsal vagal complex of the cat. *Neuroscience*, **32**, 481–492

Leslie, R. A. and Osborne, N. N. (1984). Amines and other transmitter-like compounds in the bovine area postrema. *Brain Res. Bull.*, **13**, 357–362

Leslie, R. A., Reynolds, D. J. M., Andrews, P. L. R., Grahame-Smith, D. G., Davis, C. J. and Harvey, J. M. (1990). Evidence for presynaptic 5-HT$_3$ recognition sites on vagal afferent terminals in the brainstem of the ferret. *Neuroscience* (in press)

Leslie, R. A., Reynolds, D. J. M., Grasby, P. M. and Grahame-Smith, D. G. (1989b). Autoradiographic localisation of the 5-HT$_3$ antagonist [^{3}H]BRL 43694 in the dorsal vagal complex of the ferret. *Proc. Soc. Neurosci.*, **15**, 586

Lindstrom, P. A. and Brizzee, K. R. (1962). Relief of intractable vomiting from surgical lesions in the area postrema. *J. Neurosurg.*, **19**, 228–236

Lucot, J. B. (1989a). RU 24969-induced emesis in the cat: serotonin-1$_D$ sites implicated. *Proc. Soc. Neurosci.*, **15**, 220

Lucot, J. B. (1989b). Blockade of 5-hydroxytryptamine$_3$ receptors prevents cisplatin-induced but not motion- or xylazine-induced emesis in the cat. *Pharmacol. Biochem. Behav.*, **32**, 207–210

Lucot, J. B. and Crampton, G. H. (1987). Buspirone blocks cisplatin-induced emesis in cats. *J. Clin. Pharmacol.*, **27**, 817–818

Lundberg, J. M., Tatemoto, K., Terenius, L., Hellstrom, P. M., Mutt, V., Hokfelt, T. and Hamberger, B. (1982). Localisation of peptide YY (PYY) in gastrointestinal endocrine cells and effects on intestinal blood flow and motility. *Proc. Natl Acad. Sci. USA*, **79**, 4471–4475

McCarthy, L. E. and Borison, H. L. (1984). Cisplatin-induced vomiting eliminated by ablation of the area postrema in cats. *Cancer Treat. Rep.*, **68**, 401–404

McMillen, B. A. and Mattiace, L. A. (1983). Comparative neuropharmacology of buspirone and MJ-13805, a potential anti-anxiety drug. *J. Neural. Trans.*, **57**, 255–265

Matsuoka, O., Tsuchiya, T. and Furukawa, Y. (1962). The effect of X-irradiation on 5-hydroxytryptamine (serotonin) contents in the small intestines of experimental animals. *J. Radiat. Res.*, **3**, 104–108

Mei, N. (1985). Intestinal chemosensitivity. *Physiol. Rev.*, **65**, 211–237

Miller, A. D. and Wilson, V. J. (1983). 'Vomiting center' reanalyzed: an electrical stimulation study. *Brain Res.*, **270**, 154–158

Miner, W. D. and Sanger, G. J. (1986). Inhibition of cisplatin-induced vomiting by selective 5-hydroxytryptamine M receptor antagonism. *Br. J. Pharmacol.*, **88**, 497–499

Miner, W. D., Sanger, G. J. and Turner, D. H. (1987). Evidence that 5-hydroxytryptamine$_3$ receptors mediate cytotoxic drug and radiation-evoked emesis. *Br. J. Cancer*, **56**, 159–162

Nelson, D. R. and Thomas, D. R. (1989). [^{3}H]-BRL 43694 (Granisetron), a specific ligand for 5-HT$_3$ binding sites in rat brain cortical membranes. *Biochem. Pharmacol.*, **38**, 1693–1695

Newson, B., Ahlman, H., Dahlstrom, A. and Nyhus, L. M. (1982). Ultrastructural observations in the rat ileal mucosa of possible epithelial 'taste cells' and submucosal sensory neurons. *Acta Physiol. Scand.*, **114**, 161–164

Newton, B. W., Maley, B. and Traurig, H. (1985). The distribution of substance P, enkephalin, and serotinin immunoreactivities in the area postrema of the rat and cat. *J. Comp. Neurol.*, **234**, 87–104

Palkovits, M. (1985). Distribution of neuroactive substances in the dorsal vagal complex of the medulla oblongata. *Neurochem. Int.*, **7**, 213–219

Pazos, A., Probst, A. and Palacios, J. M. (1987a). Serotonin receptors in the human brain. III. Autoradiographic mapping of serotonin-1 receptors. *Neuroscience*, **21**, 97–122

Pazos, A., Probst, A. and Palacios, J. M. (1987b). Serotonin receptors in the human brain. IV. Autoradiographic mapping of serotonin-2 receptors. *Neuroscience*, **21**, 123–139

Peroutka, S. J. and Hamik, A. (1988). [^{3}H]quipazine labels 5-HT$_3$ recognition sites in rat cortical membranes. *Eur. J. Pharmacol.*, **148**, 297–299

Pratt, G. D. and Bowery, N. G. (1989). The 5-HT$_3$ receptor ligand [^{3}H]-BRL 43694 binds to presynaptic sites in the nucleus tractus solitarius of the rat. *Neuropharmacology*, **28**, 1367–1376

Pratt, G. D., Bowery, N. G., Kilpatrick, G. J., Leslie, R. A., Barnes, N. M., Naylor, R. J., Jones, B. J., Nelson, D. R., Palacios, J. M., Slater, P. and Reynolds, D. J. M. (1990). Consensus meeting agrees distribution of 5-HT$_3$ receptors in mammalian hindbrain. *Trends Pharm. Sci.*, **11**, 135–137

Reynolds, D. J. M., Andrews, P. L. R., Leslie, R. A., Harvey, J. M., Grasby, P. M. and Grahame-Smith, D. G. (1989b). Bilateral abdominal vagotomy abolishes binding of [^{3}H]BRL 43694 in ferret dorsovagal complex. *Br. J. Pharmacol.*, **98**, 692P

Reynolds, D. J. M., Leslie, R. A., Grahame-Smith, D. G. and Harvey, J. M. (1989a). Localization of 5-HT$_3$ receptor binding sites in human dorsal vagal complex. *Eur. J. Pharmacol.*, **174**, 127–130

Reynolds, D. J. M., Leslie, R. A., Grahame-Smith, D. G. and Harvey, J. M. (1990). Autoradiographic localization of 5-HT$_3$ receptor ligand binding in the cat brainstem. *Neurochem. Int..*, in press

Richardson, B. P. and Buchheit, K. H. (1988). The pharmacology, distribution and function of 5-HT$_3$ receptors. In *Neuronal Serotonin* (ed. N. N. Osborne and M. Hamon). Wiley, Chichester, pp. 465–506

Richardson, B. P. and Engel, G. (1986). The pharmacology and function of 5-HT$_3$ receptors. *Trends Neurosci.*, **9**, 424–428

Richardson, B. P., Engel, G., Donatsch, P. and Stadler, P. A. (1985). Identification of serotonin M-receptor subtypes and their specific blockade by a new class of drugs. *Nature*, **316**, 126–131

Robertson, H. A. and Dragunow, M. (1990). From synapse to genome: the role of immediate-early genes in permanent alterations in the central nervous system. In *Current Aspects of the Neurosciences*, Vol. 2 (ed. N. N. Osborne). Macmillan Press, London, pp. 143–157

Round, A. and Wallis, D. I. (1987). Further studies on the blockade of 5-HT depolarizations of rabbit vagal afferent and sympathetic ganglion cells by MDL 72222 and other antagonists. *Neuropharmacology*, **26**, 39–48

Sanger, G. J. and King, F. D. (1988). From metoclopramide to selective gut motility stimulants and 5-HT$_3$ receptor antagonists. *Drug Des. Deliv.*, **3**, 273–295

Sharp, T., Bramwell, S. R. and Grahame-Smith, D. G. (1989). 5-HT$_1$ agonists reduce 5-hydroxytryptamine release in rat hippocampus *in vivo* as determined by brain microdialysis. *Br. J. Pharmacol.*, **96**, 283–290

Shirakawa, J., Takeda, K., Taniyama, K. and Tanaka, C. (1989). Dual effects of 5-hydroxytryptamine on the release of gamma-aminobutyric acid from myenteric neurones of the guinea-pig ileum. *Br. J. Pharmacol.*, **98**, 339–341

Smith, W. L., Callaham, E. M. and Alphin, R. S. (1988). The emetic activity of centrally administered cisplatin in cats and its antagonism by zacopride. *J. Pharm. Pharmacol.*, **40**, 142–143

Sokoloff, L., Reivich, M., Kennedy, C., Des Rosiers, M. H., Patlack, C. S., Pettigrew, K. D., Sakurada, O. and Shinohara, M. (1977). The [^{14}C]deoxyglucose method for the measurement of local cerebral glucose utilization: theory, procedure, and normal values in the conscious and anesthetized albino rat. *J. Neurochem.*, **28**, 897–916

Talley, N. J., Phillips, S. F., Haddad, A., Miller, L. J., Twomey, C., Zinsmeister, A. R. and Ciociola, A. (1989). Effect of selective 5-HT$_3$ anatagonists (GR 38032F) on small intestinal transit and release of gastrointestinal peptides. *Dig. Dis. Sci.*, **34**, 1511–1515

Treisman, M. (1977). Motion sickness: an evolutionary hypothesis. *Science, N.Y.*, **197**, 493–495

Verbeuren, T. J. (1989). Synthesis, storage, release and metabolism, of 5-hydroxytryptamine in peripheral tissues. In *The Peripheral Actions of 5-Hydroxytryptamine* (ed. J. R. Fozard). Oxford University Press, Oxford, pp. 1–25

Waeber, C., Dixon, K., Hoyer, D. and Palacios, J. M. (1988). Localization by autoradiography of neuronal 5-HT$_3$ receptors in the mouse CNS. *Eur. J. Pharmacol.*, **151**, 351–352

Waeber, C., Hoyer, D. and Palacios, J. M. (1989). 5-Hydroxytryptamine$_3$ receptors in the human brain: autoradiographic visualization using [^{3}H]ICS205 930. *Neuroscience*, **31**, 393–400

Wang, S. C. and Borison, H. L. (1952). A new concept of organization of the central emetic mechanism: recent studies on the sites of action of apomorphine, copper sulphate and cardiac glycosides. *Gastroenterology*, **22**, 1–12

Wang, S. C., Renzi, A. A. and Chinn, H. I. (1958). Mechanism of emesis following X-irradiation. *Am. J. Physiol.*, **193**, 335–359

Watling, K. T., Aspley, S., Swain, C. J. and Saunders, J. (1988). [^{3}H]quaternised ICS 205-930 labels 5-HT$_3$ receptor binding sites in rat brain. *Eur. J. Pharmacol.*, **149**, 397–398

Young, R. W. (1986). Mechanisms and treatment of radiation-induced nausea and vomiting. In *Nausea and Vomiting: Mechanisms and Treatment* (ed. C. J. Davis, G. V. Lake-Bakaar and D. G. Grahame-Smith). Springer-Verlag, Berlin, pp. 94–109

4

Excitatory Amino Acid Receptors and Phosphoinositide Breakdown: Facts and Perspectives

MAX RÉCASENS, EBRAHIM MAYAT and JANIQUE GUIRAMAND

Laboratoire de Neurobiologie de l'Audition (Université Montpellier II), INSERM Unité 254, Hôpital St Charles, 3104 rue A. Broussonnet, 34059 Montpellier Cedex 1, France

Contents

Current Aspects of the Neurosciences, Vol. 3. Edited by N. N. Osborne. © The Macmillan Press Ltd 1991

1. *Historical Introduction*

Membrane Phosphoinositides as Precursors of Second Messengers

Although phosphoinositides were isolated from brain membranes by Folch in
1949, stimulated phosphoinositide metabolism by neuroactive substances was
discovered in 1953 by Hokin and Hokin, who showed that the incorporation
of ^{32}P into phospholipids of the pancreas was augmented by acetylcholine. In
1961, Dittmer and Dawson (Dawson and Dittmer, 1961; Dittmer and
Dawson, 1961) identified these polyphosphoinositides as phosphatidylinosi-
tol-4-phosphate (PIP) and phosphatidylinositol-4,5-bisphosphate (PIP$_2$).
However, the notion that phosphoinositide metabolism is associated with
receptor function was only proposed in 1969 by Durell and co-workers, while
a few years later (1975) Michell assumed a close relation between phosphoinositide metabolism and intracellular calcium. Finally, the missing link
(inositol trisphosphate) between membrane receptor-coupled phosphoinositide metabolism and the changes in intracellular calcium originating from
internal stores was discovered by Berridge and Irvine in 1984.

Excitatory Amino Acids (EAAs) and Phosphoinositide Metabolism

The first evidence that EAA receptor activation leads to the breakdown of
phosphoinositides to generate second messengers was reported by Sladeczek
and his colleagues in 1985. It was the result of a fruitful collaboration between
F. Sladeczek, who had learned the technique of inositol phosphate measurements from C. Kirk during his stay in Montpellier, S. Weiss and M. Sebben,
who developed the primary culture of striatal neurons, and M. Récasens, who
worked on EAA receptors for several years with a young student, J.-P. Pin,
in the laboratory of J. Bockaert. During the same period, the group of
Nicoletti, Costa and their colleagues reported the stimulating effects of EAA

agonists on the formation of inositol phosphates (IPs) in rat hippocampal slices (1986b) and in cerebellar granule cells (1986d). Since then, several reports have confirmed and extended these studies to other models. However, the characterization and the physiological role of these EAA receptors linked to phosphoinositide metabolism remained somewhat confusing.

Few reviews have dealt with this topic (Sladeczek *et al.*, 1988; Smart, 1989). In this chapter a complete analysis of the data reported so far is presented. It may help to clarify the various apparent discrepancies in this field. Subsequent chapters will then be devoted to the interpretation of the data in order to emphasize the emerging ideas concerning the physiological and pathophysiological role of this second messenger system linked to EAA receptors.

2. *Phosphoinositide Metabolism: Background*

The aim of this section is to remind the reader of the fundamentals of phosphoinositide metabolism. More details on this topic can be found in various excellent reviews (Berridge, 1984; Berridge and Irvine, 1984, 1989; Nishizuka, 1984a, b and 1988; Hokin, 1985; Fischer and Agranoff, 1987). The main precursor of membrane polyphosphoinositides is phosphatidylinositol (PI). It is composed of two molecules of fatty acids (usually stearic and arachidonic acids), one molecule of sn-glycero-3-phosphoric acid and one molecule of inositol (Figure 1). The inositol molecule is bound by the hydroxyl group in position 1 to the sn-glycero-3-phosphoric acid. This chemical structure clearly indicates that a large variety of PI may exist, depending both on the type of fatty acids bound to the sn-glycero-3-phosphoric acid and on the position of the hydroxyl group of inositol attached to the phosphoric part of the sn-glycero-3-phosphoric acid. These PI are successively phosphorylated in positions 4 and 5 of the inositol molecule to yield PIP and PIP_2. Thus, several types of PIP_2 exist in the membranes. The phosphorylation reactions described above are catalysed by specific kinases, while the reverse reactions are catalysed by phosphomonoesterases.

Stimulation of cell-surface receptors increases the breakdown of PIP_2, which produces at least two types of second messengers: diacylglycerol (DAG) and inositol-1,4,5-trisphosphate (IP_3). DAG represents a family of compounds. These messengers are, in fact, the result of a complex transduction mechanism, which involves a receptor, a precursor (PIP_2), a coupling G protein and an enzyme called phospholipase C (PLC), phosphoinositidase C (PIC) or phosphodiesterase. It must be emphasized that several G proteins (Lochrie and Simon, 1988) and PLC (Katan *et al.*, 1988; Suh *et al.*, 1988; Meldrum *et al.*, 1989) exist. The mechanisms by which IP_3 and DAG trigger their effects are schematically summarized in Figure 2. IP_3 probably acts on an endoplasmic reticulum receptor to release calcium, which, in turn, activates several proteins (calmodulin, IP_3 kinase, calpain, etc.). DAG

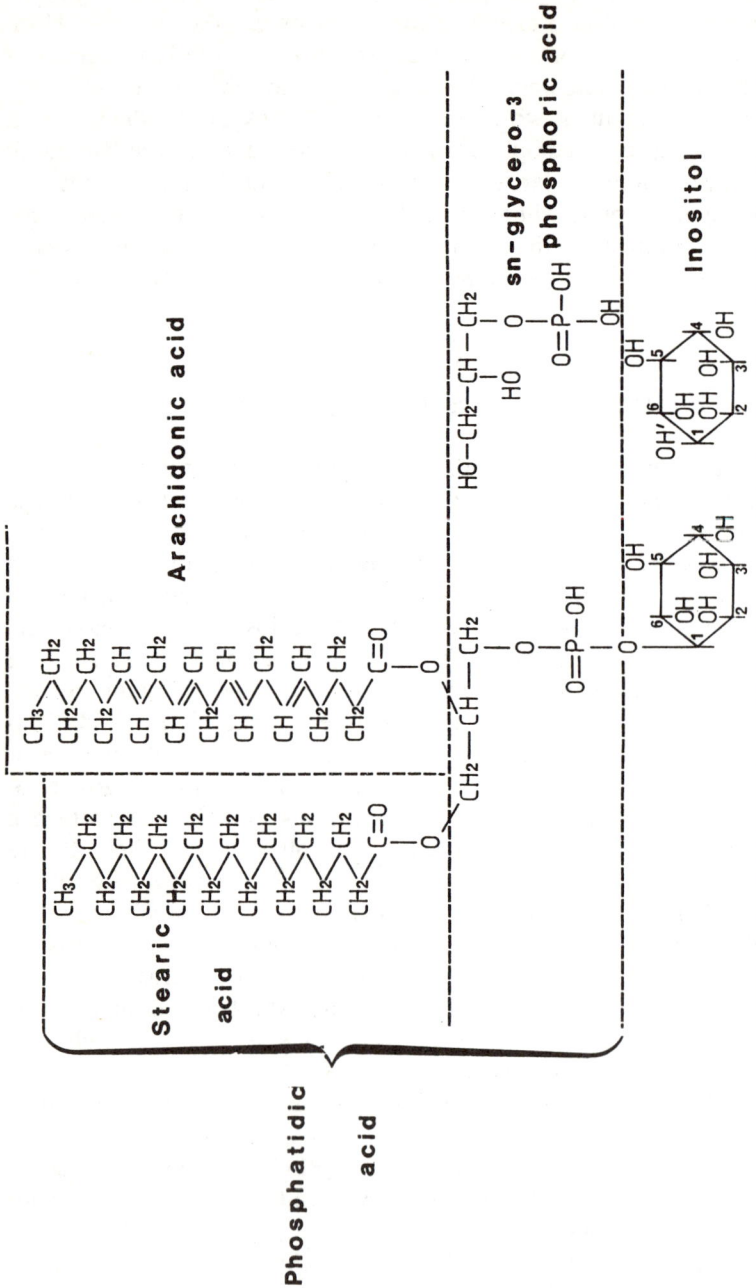

Figure 1 Phosphatidylinositol (PI) is composed of two molecules of fatty acids (usually stearic and arachidonic acids), one molecule of sn-glycero-3 phosphoric acid and one molecule of D-myoinositol. The new IUPAC convention for inositol phosphate nomenclature is described in the review article of Berridge and Irvine (1989)

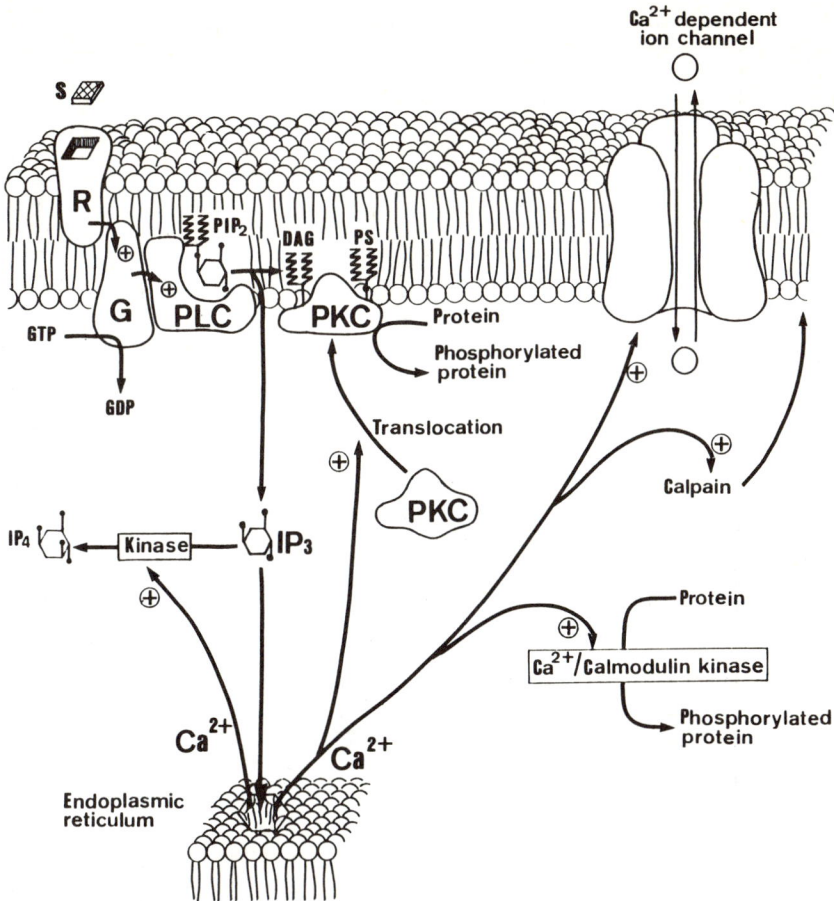

Figure 2 Schematic diagram of the mechanism of action of neuroactive substances on the polyphosphoinositide transduction system. A neuroactive substance (S) binds to its receptor (R). This binding stimulates phospholipase C (PLC) activity via a coupling G protein (G) on GTP binding. PLC then catalyses the breakdown of phosphatidylinositol-4,5-bisphosphate (PIP_2) to yield D-myoinositol-1,4,5-trisphosphate (IP_3) and diacylglycerol (DAG). IP_3 induces calcium release from the endoplasmic reticulum. The rise in intracellular calcium activates a large number of proteins, some of which are shown here—namely IP_3 kinase, calmodulin, calpain, calcium-dependent ion channels and protein kinase C (PKC). The latter enzyme is translocated to the cell membrane, where it is activated by the concerted action of DAG and phosphatidylserine (PS)

activates the membrane C kinases, which favour the phosphorylation of some proteins. The second-messenger role of IP_3 and DAG has recently been reviewed by Berridge and Irvine (1989) and Nishizuka (1988), respectively. IP_3 is catabolized either into inositol-1,3,4,5-tetrakisphosphate (IP_4) or into inositol-1,4-bisphosphate (IP_2), which is successively dephosphorylated into

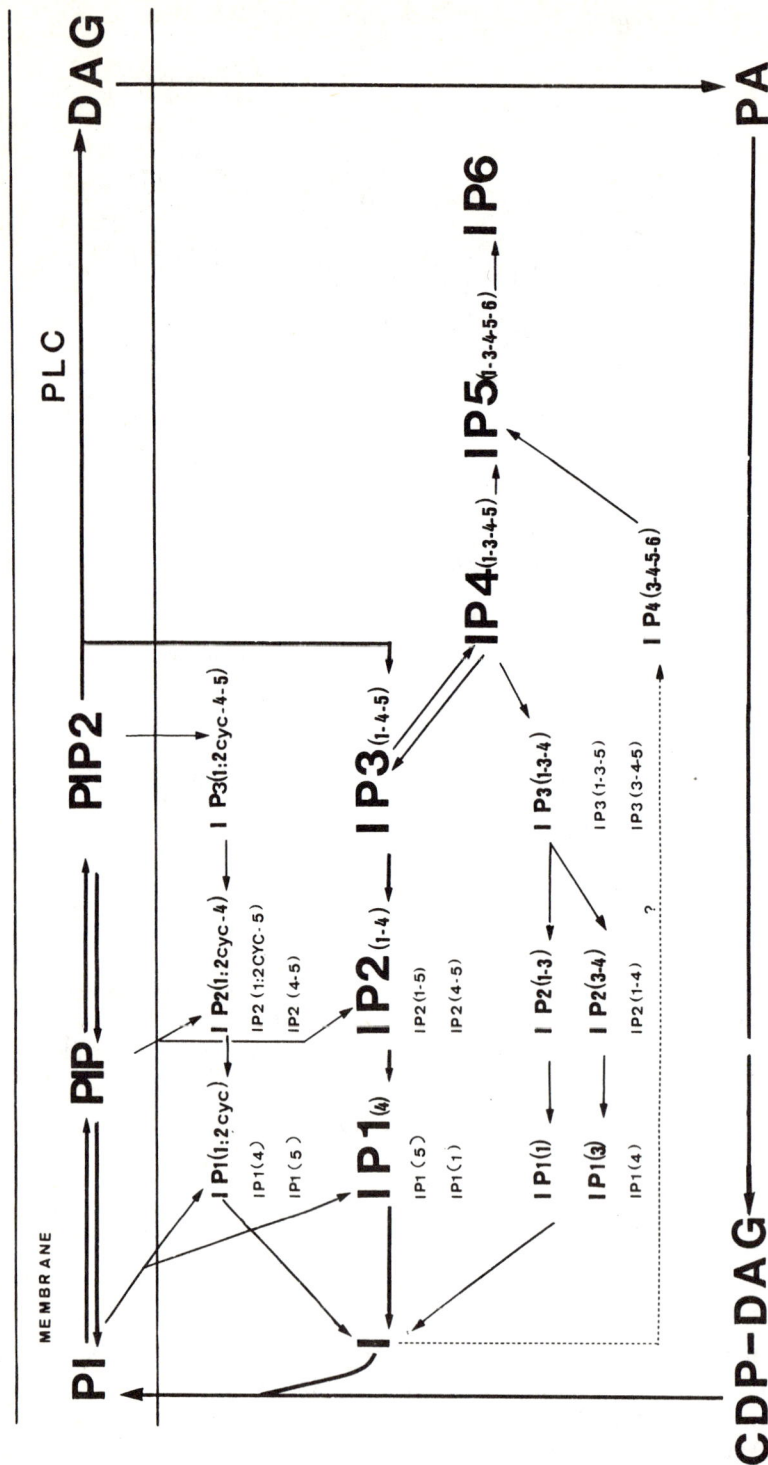

Figure 3 Summary of the known (solid arrows) and putative (dashed arrows) metabolic pathways of inositol phospholipids. The compounds in large type correspond to identified metabolites, whereas those in small type could, theoretically, exist. PI, PIP, PIP₂ are phosphatidylinositol, phosphatidyl-4-phosphate and phosphatidylinositol-4,5-bisphosphate, respectively. IP refers to inositol phosphate. The numbers in parentheses correspond to the position of the phosphate substituents on the inositol molecule. 1:2cyc denotes the phosphate cyclization between carbons 1 and 2 of the inositol molecule. PLC, phospholipase C; DAG, diacylglycerol; PA, phosphatidic acid; CDP-DAG, cytidine-diphosphate diacylglycerol

inositol-4-monophosphate (IP_1) and inositol (Figure 3). The kinase-catalysed phosphorylation (from inositol to inositol pentakisphosphate, IP_5) as well as the phosphatase-catalysed dephosphorylation (from inositol hexakisphosphate, IP_6, to IP_1) could occur at any step of IP metabolism. Several isomers (depending on the position of the phosphate(s) moiety) of each inositol phosphate, as well as related cyclic compounds, can be found. IPs may also be directly formed from PI and/or PIP breakdown. This results in the existence of a large number of IPs, most of which, together with their respective pathways, have now been identified in eukaryotic cells (Majerus *et al.*, 1988; Shears, 1989; for review, see Berridge and Irvine, 1989).

In all, phosphoinositide metabolism is not a single transduction system, but represents a pleiad of transduction systems generating a tremendous number of messengers for which many postulated functions have now been ascribed. Here we concentrate on the IPs produced by EAA.

3. Pharmacology of EAA Receptor Subtypes Linked to Phosphoinositide Metabolism

Introduction

The classification of the EAA receptors involved in IP formation is apparently controversial. For example, ibotenate (IBO), a rigid structural analogue of glutamate (Glu), is the most potent agent in stimulating IP accumulation in the presence of lithium chloride in adult rat hippocampal slices (Nicoletti *et al.*, 1986b). This response is blocked by 2-amino-4-phosphonobutyrate (APB). However, other authors found that EAA agonists are inactive in this same area (Baudry *et al.*, 1986). In other models, namely striatal neurons (Sladeczek *et al.*, 1985), cerebellar granule cells (Nicoletti *et al.*, 1986d), *Xenopus* oocytes injected with rat brain mRNA (Sugiyama *et al.*, 1987) and rat brain synaptoneurosomes (Récasens *et al.*, 1987b), quisqualate (QA), another Glu agonist, proved to be the most efficient agent for stimulating inositol phospholipid hydrolysis. This response is not blocked by APB. These discrepancies probably originate from various factors, which could be identified as: (1) the experimental model used; (2) the anatomical origin of the model (hippocampus, cortex, striatum, cerebellum, etc.) or the nature of the cells in primary culture (glials or neurons); (3) the age of the animals or that of the cells; (4) to a lesser extent, the species; and, finally, (5) the technique used to measure IP formation. One could arbitrarily consider that the main variability factor is the experimental model. In fact, in slices or even in cells in culture, IP synthesis may result from several events: the direct effects of the neuroactive substances tested, but also indirect effects due to intracellular or extracellular regulations. An example of such a regulation is the induced release by EAA of other substances, themselves stimulating or inhibiting IP formation. Consequently, we shall present the current situation concerning the EAA receptors linked to IP turnover, model by model.

Besides their stimulating effects on IP formation, it was reported that EAA inhibit IP synthesis elicited by other neuroactive substances (Baudry *et al.*, 1986; Nicoletti *et al.*, 1986a; Schmidt *et al.*, 1987). Here there is also some controversy, probably originating from the same variability factors as those described above. For instance, Baudry *et al.* (1986) reported that the carbachol-stimulated IP formation, but not the noradrenaline-induced response, is inhibited by EAA in adult hippocampal slices. Nicoletti *et al.* (1986a) found the contrary. Thus, the same framework as that proposed for the stimulatory effect of EAA will be followed in presenting the inhibitory EAA action.

Current Knowledge on the Pharmacology of EAA-stimulated IP Formation

Rat Brain Slices

Hippocampal Slices
Most of the work on EAA-stimulated IP formation has been performed on adult rat hippocampal slices (Baudry *et al.*, 1986; Iadarola *et al.*, 1986; Nicoletti *et al.*, 1986b, c; Jope and Li, 1989; Schoepp and Johnson, 1988a, b, 1989a; Table 1) or neonatal rat hippocampal slices (Nicoletti *et al.*, 1986a; Chen *et al.*, 1988; Palmer *et al.*, 1988, 1989; Schoepp, 1989; Schoepp and Johnson, 1989b; Table 2).

The main findings in adult rat hippocampal slices is that IBO is the most potent EAA agonist in magnitude, inducing an IP response 3–5 times higher than QA (Nicoletti *et al.*, 1986b; Schoepp and Johnson, 1988a). Conversely, on the basis of their EC_{50} values, QA possesses the highest apparent affinity, being about 20 times more potent than IBO (Table 1). Both the IBO- and the QA-elicited IP responses are inhibited by APB and some other drugs (2-amino-3-phosphonopropionate (APP), L-serine-*O*-phosphate (SOP)). The only discrepancy which appears in Table 1 is that Glu and homocysteate (HCA) stimulate IP formation in the experiments performed by Nicoletti *et al.* (1986b), weakly in those done by Schoepp and Johnson (1988a and 1989a) and not at all in those conducted by Baudry *et al.* (1986) and Jope and Li (1989). The different results obtained by Nicoletti and co-workers compared with those found by the others could be easily explained by the method used to measure the accumulation of the IPs, as elegantly demonstrated by Jope and Li (1989). Nicoletti and his colleagues incorporated the [^{3}H]inositol into the hippocampal slices for 1 h, incubated them with lithium chloride for 20 min and stimulated with the agonists for a further 40 min. The other authors extensively washed the slices between [^{3}H]inositol incorporation and stimulation. Moreover, the difference between the slight IP stimulation by HCA and Glu observed by Schoepp and Johnson as compared with the lack of stimulation reported by Baudry *et al.* and Jope and Li for these same

Table 1 Pharmacology of EAA-stimulated IP formation in adult hippocampal slices

Ref.	Agonists (1 mM)		Antagonists (1 mM)		Inactive agonists	Inactive antagonists	Method[c]
	Magnitude of stimulation (%)[a]	Potency, EC_{50} (µM)	Magnitude of inhibition (%)[b]	Potency, IC_{50} (µM)			
Nicoletti et al. (1986b)	IBO (870) QA (200) HCA (200) L-Glu (140) L-Asp (155)	110 n.d. n.d. n.d. n.d.	DL-APB (99)	300	KA NMDA Quinolinate	DL-APV GDEE γ-DGG	A
Baudry et al. (1986)	IBO, QA: not tested				KA NMDA L-Glu HCA		B
Schoepp and Johnson (1988a, b; 1989a)	IBO (450) QA (220) L-Glu (123) HCA (143)	148 7.7 n.d. n.d.	DL-APB (82) L-APB (77) DL-APP (79) L-α-AA (69) L-SOP (78)	489 160–250 120 530 390	KA NMDA AMPA NAAG	D-APB L-APV D-APV D-SOP	B
Jope and Li (1989)	IBO, QA: not tested				L-Glu		A and B

[a]The magnitude of stimulation is expressed as the percentage of stimulation of the control value, and the agonists were all tested at 1 mM.
[b]The magnitude of inhibition is expressed as the percentage of the 10^{-3} IBO stimulated IP formation with an antagonist concentration of 10^{-3} M.
[c]The main difference between method A and method B is that in method A [^{3}H]inositol is maintained throughout the experiment (incorporation and stimulation), while in method B free [^{3}H]inositol is washed (twice or three times) after 1 h of incorporation.
n.d. = not determined.

Table 2   Pharmacology of EAA-stimulated IP formation in neonatal rat hippocampal slices

Ref.	Agonists (1 mM)		Antagonists (1 mM)		Inactive agonists	Inactive antagonists	Method Age (days)
	Magnitude of stimulation (%)[a]	Potency, EC_{50} (μM)	Magnitude of inhibition (%)[b]	Potency, IC_{50} (μM)			
Nicoletti et al. (1986a)	IBO (1450) QA (1200) L-Asp (1040) L-Glu (800) APB[c] (126) SOP[c] (128)	15 300			KA NMDA Quinolinate		A, 6–8
Palmer et al. (1988, 1989)	QA[d] (1500–2000) IBO (1500–2000) AMPA (400) KA (300) trans-ACPD (2000)	2 25	NMDA (75)	30	NMDA	CNQX	B, 10–13
Chen et al. (1988)	QA[d] (1000)	0.5					A, 8
Schoepp (1989)	IBO (1200) QA[d] (1150) Glu (750)		PDB[e] (80)				B, 7

Schoepp and Johnson (1989b)	IBO (1125)	27			L-APB (25)	1915	NMDA	DL-APB	B, 7
	QA^d (1100)	1.9			L-APP (80)	369		CNQX	
	Glu (625)	458							
	Asp (600)								
	AMPA^f (350)								
	HCA^f (300)								
	KA^f (200)								

[a] The magnitude of stimulation is expressed as the percentage of stimulation of the control values.

[b] The inhibition by 1 mM antagonists is expressed as a percentage of the maximal IP response induced by IBO (10^{-3}, 10^{-4} M), QA (10^{-4} M) or Glu (10^{-4} M).

[c] APB and SOP are weak stimulating agents of IP turnover in 6-day-old hippocampal slices and became antagonists of IBO-, QA- and Glu-evoked IP accumulation in 15-day-old hippocampal slices (Nicoletti et al., 1986a).

[d] [QA] = 10^{-4} M; at 10^{-3} M the QA-induced IP response is inhibited, irrespective of author(s) (about 700% of the control value in Palmer et al., 1988).

[e] PDB: phorbol, 12,13-dibutyrate.

[f] It must be noted that AMPA-, HCA- and KA-elicited IP formation are inhibited by neither L-APB nor DL-APP.

substances undoubtedly originates from the duration of the stimulation and the temperature at which the experiment was conducted.

Finally, in adult rat brain hippocampal slices an IBO–QA-sensitive receptor, blockable by APB and APP, is linked to IP formation.

In neonatal rat hippocampal slices, the pharmacology of the main EAA receptor coupled to the phosphoinositide turnover is similar to that found in adult hippocampal slices, with three differences: (1) QA is as potent as IBO in magnitude for stimulating IP accumulation; (2) APB is not an inhibitor of IP synthesis produced by IBO or QA (Table 2); (3) KA, HCA and AMPA significantly augment IP synthesis in young animals. This augmentation is not blocked by APB or APP.

To sum up, an IBO–QA-sensitive receptor, only blocked by APP (not by APB), is present in neonatal rat hippocampal slices. In addition, KA, HCA and AMPA induce an IP accumulation which is not inhibited by APB and APP.

Cortical Slices

Several reports have dealt with EAA-induced IP formation in neonatal and adult rat cortex slices (Nicoletti *et al.*, 1986a, b; Akiyama *et al.*, 1987; Godfrey *et al.*, 1988; Gonzales and Moerschbaecher, 1989; Noble *et al.*, 1989). Their findings are shown in Table 3. In adult rat cortex slices, IBO and QA are generally found to be the most potent agonists in magnitude. However, Jope and Li (1989) reported that QA is unable to enhance IP synthesis. None of the EAA antagonists, including APB and APP, was tested (Table 3). The reason is that the main aim of these papers was to investigate the inhibitory effect of EAA on neurotransmitter-evoked IP formation.

In 6-day-old animals the stimulatory action of EAA is greatly increased (Nicoletti *et al.*, 1986a) when compared with that found in adult rats. This finding is similar to that observed in the hippocampal slices.

In summary, a QA–IBO-sensitive receptor is linked to IP production, although its pharmacology remains to be fully established.

Striatal Slices

Few experiments on EAA-induced IP turnover have been conducted in adult striatal slices. There is no report which concentrates mainly on this model, but only scattered results in the subsections of Nicoletti *et al.* (1986b, 1987a) and Jope and Li (1989) (Table 4).

One paper (Doble and Perrier, 1989) is entirely devoted to EAA-elicited IP formation in neonatal striatal slices, while two others are partially dedicated to this model (Nicoletti *et al.*, 1986a; Chen *et al.*, 1988; Table 4). The two main EAA agonists, in adult and neonatal striatal slices, are IBO and QA. As in other brain slices, the IP accumulation is higher in young animals than in the adult. EAA antagonists have not yet been tested in adult slices. In neonatal slices, Doble and Perrier (1989) report that a barbiturate (quinalbarbitone) inhibits both QA- and IBO-elicited IP accumulation. This

Table 3 Pharmacology of EAA-stimulated IP formation in rat cortex slices

Ref.	Agonists (1 mM)		Antagonists (1 mM)		Inactive agonists	Inactive antagonists	Method, Age
	Magnitude of stimulation (%)[e]	Potency, EC_{50} (µM)	Magnitude of inhibition (%)	Potency, IC_{50} (µM)			
Nicoletti et al. (1986b)	IBO (131)				QA		A, adult
Akiyama et al. (1987)	IBO (191)						A, adult
Godfrey et al. (1988)	IBO[a] (179), QA[b] (227), Glu (140), NMDA (121)	30, 20			KA, Asp		B, adult
Noble et al. (1989)	IBO[c] (121), QA (127), KA (115), Glu (120)						B, adult
Jope and Li (1989)					Glu, QA, NMDA		A, adult
Gonzales and Moerschbaecher (1989)					NMDA		B, adult
Nicoletti et al. (1986a)	Glu (458), IBO[a] (383)						A, 6 days
Schoepp and Hillman (1990)[d]	QA[c] (620), IBO[c] (480), trans-ACPD (1000)		APP (87)[d], APP (93)[d]; APB (30)[d], APP (91)[d]; APB (36)[d]		APB[d]		B, 7 days

[a] [IBO] = 0.5 mM.
[b] [QA] = 0.3 mM.
[c] [IBO] or [QA] = 0.1 mM.
The first three groups of workers used frontal cortex, pyriform cortex/amygdala and cortex slices, while the last three authors performed their experiments in cerebral cortex slices.
[d] The antagonists APP and APB were tested at 1 mM against the stimulatory effects of 0.1 mM QA, IBO and trans-ACPD.
[e] The magnitude of stimulation is expressed as the percentage of stimulation of the control values.

Table 4   Pharmacology of EAA-stimulated IP formation in rat striatal slices

Ref.	Agonists (1 mM)		Antagonists (1 mM)		Inactive agonists	Inactive antagonists	Method, Age
	Magnitude of stimulation (%)	Potency, EC_{50} (μM)	Magnitude of inhibition (%)	Potency, IC_{50} (μM)			
Nicoletti et al. (1986b, 1987a)	IBO (219) QA (138)				Glu		A, adult
Jope and Li (1989)					Glu		A, adult
Nicoletti et al. (1986a)	IBO[a] (432) Glu (384)						A, 6 days
Chen et al. (1988)	QA (177) QA[b] (442)						A, 7 days
Doble and Perrier (1989)	IBO (1283)	6.8	Quinalbarbitone L-SOP[c]	660 250	KA	APB	A, 8–10 days
			Quinalbarbitone	100	NMDA	APV	
	QA[b] (1166)	0.26				DαAA	
	L-Glu (903)	120				Kyn	
	L-Asp (1103)	130				PCA	
	D-Glu (233)	1000				CPP	
	D-Asp (730)	1000				GDEE	
	AMPA (250)					CNQX	
						γ-DGG	
						GAMS	
						PCP	
						MK 801	

[a] [IBO] = 0.5 mM.
[b] [QA] = 0.1 mM.
[c] It should be noted that quinalbarbitone inhibits both QA- and IBO-induced IP formation, while L-SOP inhibits only the IBO-elicited IP response. Quinalbarbitone also blocks Carb-induced IP formation.
The inactive antagonists were tested at 10^{-2} M (except for PCP and MK 801: 10^{-4} M) against the IP response elicited by 10^{-6} M QA or 10^{-5} M IBO.

Table 5 Pharmacology of EAA-stimulated IP formation in rabbit retinal slices

Ref.	Agonists (0.5 mM)		Antagonists (1 mM)		Inactive agonists (1 mM)	Inactive antagonists (1 mM)	Method, Age
	Magnitude of stimulation (%)	Potency, EC_{50} (µM)	Magnitude of inhibition (%)	Potency, IC_{50} (µM)			
Osborne (1990)	QA (317) IBO (210) KA (201) Glu (193) NMDA (188) Asp (172)	0.1				APV APB GDEE PDA	B, adult

Results are expressed as the percentages of the control value.

barbiturate is slightly more efficient with the IP formation induced by QA. Quinalbarbitone also blocks carbachol-stimulated IP formation. L-SOP inhibits only QA-evoked IP response, without affecting that of IBO. APB is inactive in this respect, which is in agreement with the previous findings in other neonatal brain slices.

In all, in adult striatal slices an IBO–QA-sensitive receptor appears to be coupled to phosphoinositide turnover, but the precise pharmacology, particularly concerning the antagonists, remains to be established. In neonatal rat striatal slices, an IBO–QA receptor, which seems less selective than that described in the adult, is linked to IP formation. It could be blocked by a non-selective antagonist, quinalbarbitone, and to a lesser extent by L-SOP.

Rabbit Retinal Slices
Recently the stimulatory actions of EAA on IP metabolism in rabbit retinal slices were reported (Osborne, 1990). QA is the most potent agonist in magnitude, followed in decreasing order by IBO, KA, Glu, NMDA and Asp. None of the classical antagonists tested (APV, APB, GDEE) have an effect (Table 5) on this stimulated IP metabolism.

Thus, a QA-sensitive receptor, not blocked by any EAA antagonists tested, is coupled to PLC in rabbit retinal slices.

Brain Cells

Neuronal Cells
Sladeczek and colleagues (1985) were the first to show that QA and Glu increase the IP accumulation in the presence of lithium chloride. Their experiments were performed in mouse striatal neurons in primary culture. Since then, EAA-induced IP synthesis has been measured in striatal neurons (Schmidt *et al.*, 1987; Ambrosini and Meldolesi, 1989; Weiss, 1989; Weiss *et al.*, 1989), in hippocampal neurons (Ambrosini and Meldolesi, 1989), in cerebellar granule cells (Nicoletti *et al.*, 1986d, 1987b; Wroblewski *et al.*, 1987; Nicoletti and Canonico, 1989) and in rabbit retinal neurons (Osborne, 1990). In striatal, hippocampal, retinal and cerebellar neurons, QA and Glu are the most potent EAA agonists in magnitude, while IBO tested at the same concentration as Glu or QA is a powerless agonist (Table 6). The apparent affinity of QA is 25 times higher than that of Glu in striatal neurons (Sladeczek *et al.*, 1985). However, the apparent affinity is similar for both compounds in cerebellar granule cells (Nicoletti *et al.*, 1986d). NMDA and KA enhance, albeit weakly, IP synthesis. Among the numerous antagonists used, none were able to inhibit the IP accumulation generated by QA. 2-Amino-5-phosphonovalerate (APV) inhibits the NMDA- and (a low concentration of) Glu-stimulated IP formation, as well as that of KA. The IP response caused by these three agonists is also blocked by phencyclidine (PCP).

In neuronal cells a QA-sensitive receptor is responsible for the major IP production, which cannot be blocked by any of the known antagonists. A NMDA–KA receptor, which is activated by low Glu concentrations and blocked by APV or PCP, is also present.

Glial Cells

EAAs also induce an increase in the breakdown of polyphosphoinositides in astrocyte-enriched cultures prepared from the cerebral cortex of newborn rats (Pearce *et al.*, 1986; Milani *et al.*, 1989). QA is the most efficient EAA agonist in stimulating IP formation (with respect to the maximal response and the apparent affinity), followed by Glu and IBO (Table 7). Gamma-D-glutamylglycine at 20 mM completely inhibits the IP response elicited by these three compounds, as does a pretreatment of the astrocytes by phorbol-12-myristate-13-acetate (PMA). The antagonists PCP, DNQX and APB are inefficient in blocking the effect of these three EAAs. NMDA, Asp and HCA are inactive agonists, while KA significantly increases IP accumulation.

Thus, a QA–Glu-activated receptor increases IP turnover in astrocytes from the cerebral cortex. This increase is inhibited by 20 mM γ-DGG and not by APB. NMDA does not induce an IP response, while KA does. The antagonistic profile has not yet been determined.

Brain Synaptoneurosomes

The increase in the IP turnover triggered by EAAs has also been examined in rat brain synaptoneurosomes (Récasens *et al.*, 1987b, 1988b; Dudek *et al.*, 1989; Guiramand *et al.*, 1989a, b). In this brain membrane preparation obtained from 6–9-day-old rats (synaptoneurosomes: synaptosomes attached with resealed postsynaptic membranes), QA induces maximal IP accumulation, as do Glu and IBO. Its apparent affinity is 20 and 40 times higher than that of Glu and IBO, respectively (Table 8). AMPA is ineffective up to concentrations of 0.1 mM. At 1 mM none of the numerous antagonists tested, APB and CNQX included, inhibit the QA- or Glu-induced IP formation. At 10 mM GAMS decreases by 34% the IP accumulation produced by QA. NMDA and KA also slightly increase the phosphoinositide turnover. The NMDA effect is blocked by APV. Similar results were obtained in synaptoneurosomes prepared from adult rat brains, except that all the EAA-induced IP responses are reduced—in particular, the QA one (160% as opposed to 250% of the control value).

Finally, in synaptoneurosomes a QA receptor is linked to IP synthesis. No antagonist has yet been found for this receptor. NMDA also stimulates the IP accumulation via a receptor blocked by APV.

Xenopus **Oocytes**

The leading work in this field was performed by Sugiyama and colleagues (1987), who induced the expression of the EAA receptors by injecting *Xenopus* oocytes with rat-brain mRNA. They then recorded the variations in membrane currents caused by bath-applied EAAs and compared them with

Table 6 Pharmacology of EAA-stimulated IP formation in neuronal cells in primary cultures

Ref.	Agonists (1 mM)		Antagonists (1 mM)				Method, age (days in vitro)
	Magnitude of stimulation (%)	Potency, EC_{50} (μM)	Magnitude of inhibition (%)	Potency, IC_{50} (μM)	Inactive agonists (1 mM)	Inactive antagonists (1 mM)	
Striatal neurons							
Sladeczek et al. (1985)	Glu* (400) Asp* (265) CA (254) CSA (248) HCA (227) QA*** (400) NMDA* (146) KA (130)	4 0.16 15 10				APV	B, 11–14
Weiss et al. (1989)	QA*** (375) Glu (350)	0.16 50			AMPA	Kyn γ-DGG GDEE APB	B, 15
Ambrosini and Meldolesi (1989)	Glu** (205) QA** (194) NMDA* (111)					APV (10 μM) MK-801 (100 μM) γ-DGG (10 μM)	B, 7–9
Hippocampal neurons							
Ambrosini and Meldolesi (1989)	Glu* (177) QA** (185)					APV (10 μM) MK-801 (100 μM)	B, 7–9

	Agonists		Antagonists		
Cerebellar granule cells					
Nicoletti et al. (1986b, 1987b)	Glu* (457)	10–20	DL-APV, PDA, γ-DGG	GDEE, DL-APB APV, PDA, γ-DGG	B, 7–9
	QA* (304)	50		GDEE, DL-APB	
	KA* (239)	10–20	DL-APV, PDA, γ-DGG	GDEE, DL-APB	
	Asp* (200)	10–20	DL-APV, PDA	DL-APB	
	IBO* (165)				
	NMDA* (126)	200			
	Quinolinate* (128)				
Wroblewski et al. (1987)	Glu** (627)			PCP	B, 7–9
	QA* (581)			PCP	
	KA* (527)		PCP (45)		
	Asp* (382)		PCP (64)		
	NMDA* (364)		PCP (73)		
Rabbit retinal culture					
Osborne (1990)	QA (305)				B, 3–5
	IBO (192)				
	KA (190)				

The concentrations of the agonists were 1 mM, except: *100 μM, **10 μM, ***1 μM.
The experiments by Wroblewski et al. were performed in Mg^{2+}-free medium.
PCP was assayed at a concentration of 500 nM.
If nothing is indicated, the antagonists were tested against the concentration of the EAA agonists indicated in the 'Agonists' column.
Results are expressed as the percentages of the control value.

Table 7 Pharmacology of EAA-stimulated IP formation in astroglial cells in cultures

Ref.	Agonists (1 mM)		Antagonists (1 mM)		Inactive agonists	Inactive antagonists	Method, Age (days)
	Magnitude of stimulation (%)[a]	Potency, EC_{50} (μM)	Magnitude of inhibition (%)	Potency, IC_{50} (μM)			
Pearce *et al.* (1986)	Glu (275) QA (350) KA (172)	40–50	GAMS (60)		NMDA Asp HCA		B, 14–21
Milani *et al.* (1989)	Glu (500) QA (400) IBO (250) KA (170) APB (120)	40 5 40	γ-DGG[b] PMA[c]			PCP (1 μM) DNQX (100 μM) APB (1000 μM) α-PDD[d]	B, 14

[a] The magnitudes of stimulation are expressed as percentages of the control value.
[b] γ-DGG assayed at 20 mM totally blocked Glu-, QA- and IBO (0.5 mM)-induced IP formation, as well as pretreatment of the astrocytes with 100 nM of PMA.
[c] PMA: phorbol-12-myristate-13-acetate.
[d] α-PDD: α-phorbol-12,13-didecanoate.

Table 8 Pharmacology of EAA-stimulated IP formation in rat brain synaptoneurosomes

Ref.	Agonists (1 mM)		Antagonists		Inactive agonists (1 mM)	Inactive antagonists (0.5 mM)	Method, Age
	Magnitude of stimulation (%)[a]	Potency, EC_{50} (µM)	Magnitude of inhibition (%)	Potency, IC_{50} (µM)			
Récasens et al. (1987b, 1988b)[b]	Glu (254) QA (250) NMDA (180) KA (150) AMPA (155) CSA (214)	23 0.12 1000 1000 1000 7	DL-APV[d]		GDEE GAMS[c] FG9065 γ-DGG DL-APB DL-APV[d]		B, 6–9 days
Récasens et al. (unpublished results)	HCSA (234) CA (208) HCA (208)	13 17 9					
Guiramand et al. (1989a, b, and unpublished results)[b]	Glu (144) QA (140) IBO (152) NMDA (132) KA (120)				DL-APB		B, adult (6 months)
Dudek et al. (1989)[b]	Glu (230) AMPA						B, 7 days
	Glu (128) AMPA (135) NMDA (105) KA (112)					APV Kyn	B, 21 days and adult

[a] Magnitudes of stimulation are expressed as the percentages of the control value.
[b] The studies of Récasens et al. and Guiramand et al. were performed on synaptoneurosomes from rat forebrain, while that of Dudek was conducted on rat neocortex synaptoneurosomes.
[c] GAMS tested at 10 mM slightly inhibits the QA-elicited IP response (34%).
[d] DL-APV at 10 mM and 50 mM significantly inhibits only NMDA (10^{-3} M)-induced IP formation by 38% and 80%, respectively.

those produced by the direct injection of IP_3 into the oocytes. In this model, IP_3 activates a chloride current, as do QA and Glu. Several papers have confirmed and extended their findings (Fong *et al.*, 1988; Ito *et al.*, 1988a; Kawai *et al.*, 1988; Oosawa and Yamagishi, 1989; Sugiyama *et al.*, 1989). QA is most potent in stimulating IP formation, followed by IBO, Glu and HCSA (homocysteinesulphinate), respectively. Joro spider toxin (JSTX) does not inhibit QA-induced IP response, even though it blocks QA-induced depolarization. None of the classical EAA antagonists listed in Table 9 block the IPs accumulation. In addition, NMDA and KA have no effect on the chloride current.

In summary, in *Xenopus* oocytes injected with rat brain mRNA a QA receptor, not blocked by any of the classical EAA antagonists, is coupled to IP metabolism.

Advantages and Drawbacks of the Various Models

Before discussing the characterization of the EAA receptors linked to IP metabolism, it is relevant to mention the advantages and disadvantages of each model and of the techniques used (Table 10).

In slices and in cells in culture, the IP formation induced by neuroactive substances results from both direct and indirect effects. The direct effect is the action of the neurotransmitter on its receptor, which is coupled to phosphoinositide metabolism. The indirect effects could be numerous. For instance, the neurotransmitter tested may induce the release of other neuroactive substances, which in turn may stimulate or inhibit IP formation. This released neurotransmitter may also induce ion fluxes, which directly activate the enzymes involved in IP metabolism. Calcium and sodium do so in relation to the PLC enzymes (Renard *et al.*, 1987; Gusovsky and Daly, 1988a, b; Nakanishi *et al.*, 1988). This illustrates intercellular or extracellular regulations which occur in such models.

Intracellular modulations may also interfere with the IP response. The rise in intracellular calcium, triggered by IP_3, could induce the translocation of PKC, which is activated at the membrane level of diacylglycerol. The stimulation of PKC is known to inhibit IP formation (Labarca *et al.*, 1984; Leeb-Lundberg *et al.*, 1985; Schoepp and Johnson, 1988b). Thus, slices and cultured cells are essential to study regulations, but rather inconvenient for measuring the direct effect of a substance on IP metabolism.

The similarity between these two models is limited to the above description. In fact, there are also specific properties for each of these two models. Slices contain both neuronal and glial cells which have made their differentiation and connections *in vivo*. Cells in culture differentiate and establish connections *in vitro*. They are prepared from embryonic rat brain (neurons, except cerebellar granule cells) and newborn rat brain (glial cells). Thus, slices are advantageous to study regulations and to extrapolate the results to a

Table 9 Pharmacology of EAA-receptors expressed in *Xenopus* oocytes by injection of rat-brain messenger RNA

Ref.	Agonists (1 mM)		Antagonists (1 mM)		Inactive EAA agonists (1 mM)	Inactive EAA antagonists (1 mM)
	Magnitude of stimulation (%)	Potency, EC_{50} (μM)	Magnitude of inhibition (%)	Potency, IC_{50} (μM)		
Sugiyama *et al.* (1987, 1989); Ito *et al.* (1988a)	Glu	81			NMDA	JSTX
	QA	2.2			KA	KA
	GDEE	n.d.			AMPA	APP
	IBO	43			Willardiine	APB
	HCSA	81			L-SOP	APV
						L-SOP
					L-Asp	GDEE
					L-CSA	HA966
					L-CA	D-α-AA
					L-HCA	DAP
					Quinolinate	DAS
					Domoic acid	MK801
						CNQX
						GAMS
						Kyn
						PDA
Fong *et al.* (1988)	Glu					APV
	QA					D-α-amino hexanedioic acid

JSTX, Joro spider toxin; HA966, 3-amino-1-hydroxypynolidone; DAP, D-α-aminopimelic acid; DAS, DL-α-aminosuberic acid; PDA, *cis*-2,3-piperidine dicarboxylic acid.

Table 10   Advantages and disadvantages of the various models used to study IP accumulation

Model	Presence of cell–cell interactions	Presence of intracellular regulation	Homogeneous incorporation of [³H]inositol	Complete incorporation of [³H]inositol	Conceivability of developmental study
Slices	Yes	Yes	No (not necessary)	No	Yes
Cells in cultures	Yes	Yes	Yes	Yes	No (or *in vitro*)
Synapto-neurosomes	No	Yes (limited)	Yes	No	Yes
Xenopus oocytes injected with rat brain mRNA	No	Yes	—	—	No or limited

mature physiological system, as compared with cells in culture. Moreover, slices allow the investigation of the developmental changes that take place *in vivo*, whereas cells in culture only allow investigation of changes occurring *in vitro*. On the other hand, it is possible to obtain cultures enriched either in neurons or in glial cells. This favours the study of the contribution of each cell type to a physiological response.

The cells-in-culture model is the only one with which [³H]inositol incorporation into inositol phospholipids could be performed at a steady state level. In fact, the radioactive inositol could be added to the medium several days before the experiments. In contrast, slices maintain their responsiveness for only a few hours, which is not sufficient to accomplish the saturated labelling of membrane phosphoinositides by [³H]inositol. In addition, the labelling is not homogeneous throughout the slice, owing to the difficulty of achieving the diffusion of the radioactive inositol into the thickness of the slice.

Slices, even prepared from the same brain area, are slightly different from one another with respect to their cellular organizations, while cells in culture constitute a more homogeneous preparation.

The usual choice of a given brain structure (hippocampus, striatum, cortex, etc.) enables the study of the specific receptors linked to the IP turnover in this particular brain area, but precludes the characterization of other receptors, poorly or not at all expressed in that brain region.

To overcome most of the difficulties indicated above (indirect effects, lack of homogeneity in the labelling, etc.), we have chosen to study the IP metabolism elicited by EAAs on a membrane preparation known as synaptoneurosomes. This preparation was described for the first time by Hollingsworth and colleagues in 1985. It consists of synaptosomes with attached resealed postsynaptic entities (neurosomes), and exhibits usefulness for

Knowledge of nature of cell	Simplicity of preparation	Cost	Time-scale	Study on whole brain and/or specific areas	Ease of interpretation
No	Yes	Inexpensive	From several seconds to 1 h	Possible; slices not necessarily identical	Not easy
Yes	No	Expensive	From several seconds to 1 h	Possible	Easier
No	Yes	Inexpensive	From several seconds to 1 h	Possible	Easy
No	No	Inexpensive	ms range	'Possible'*	Easy

*It is possible to prepare whole rat brain mRNAs, but nobody knows if their expression in oocytes exactly reflects the receptors found in the whole brain.

studying transduction systems (Hollingsworth *et al.*, 1985, 1986; Gusovsky *et al.*, 1986; Heuschneider and Schwartz, 1989). Cell–cell interactions as well as most of the intracellular regulations are eliminated. Although this preparation contains membranes and inside-out resealed entities, the [^{3}H]inositol incorporation does not take place in such membrane contaminants, since the soluble enzymes involved in the IP cycle are no longer present. The incorporation corresponds, in fact, to a purification step where only membrane vesicles containing the complete multienzymic machinery involved in IP turnover could be labelled. The choice could be made to prepare synaptoneurosomes from a specific brain region or from whole brain. In the latter case, one may expect that most of the EAA receptors linked to the IP cycle are present. This model is also convenient for studying developmental changes (Guiramand *et al.*, 1989b). Synaptoneurosomes are homogeneous, and easy and inexpensive to prepare. Despite their numerous advantages, this model has some disadvantages, like the two other models. As opposed to cells in culture, but like slices, synaptoneurosomes could be maintained in good condition for only a few hours. This hinders the complete labelling of the membrane phosphoinositides, which in turn decreases the sensitivity of the IP measurement. Responsive glial membrane vesicles could also be present, making it difficult to determine the origin (neuronal versus glial) of the IP response.

The last model which has been used to investigate the phosphoinositide turnover is the *Xenopus* oocyte injected with rat brain mRNA. This experimental model completely differs from the other models described above. First, no direct measurement of IP accumulation was performed. Membrane currents induced by EAA agonists are recorded and compared with the chloride current elicited by IP$_3$, injected into the oocytes. The expression of rat brain mRNA in *Xenopus* oocytes may lead to the formation of heterologous complexes (for instance, expressed rat brain EAA receptors coupled to G protein and PLC from the oocytes) which could differ in their responsiveness to EAAs from the original complex present in the rat brain. Moreover, the chloride current measured in the oocytes may be modulated by intracellular components, specific to the oocytes. The expression of a given EAA receptor subtype in the *Xenopus* oocytes could lead to the unmasking of receptor function (Kawai *et al.*, 1988). These authors demonstrate that the sensitivity to EAAs of oocyte membranes injected with mRNA of lobster muscle is entirely different from that in the original muscle. NMDA, inactive at the lobster muscle membrane, induced current responses in the oocyte membranes. The opposite may also occur. NMDA causes no current responses in *Xenopus* oocytes injected with rat brain mRNA (Sugiyama *et al.*, 1987), while it induces sodium and calcium currents in rat brain.

Despite these drawbacks, this model is very useful in studying a specific receptor, since various types of EAA agonists induce different types of ionic currents (Sugiyama *et al.*, 1987). The instantaneous changes in chloride currents may be measured, thanks to the sensitivity of electrophysiological recordings, while only long-lasting modifications could be observed with biochemical radioassays.

In short, each experimental model could be useful, depending on the purpose of the study.

Evaluation of the Techniques Used to Measure IP Formation

The techniques used to measure IP formation may also be responsible for some discrepancies concerning the pharmacology of the EAA receptors coupled to the PLC. The main difference between the radioassays developed by the various authors is the presence of a washing step between [^{3}H]inositol incorporation and agonist stimulation (method B) or its absence (method A) (see the legend to Table 1). Method A is more sensitive than method B, because of the permanent presence of [^{3}H]inositol. However, this could lead to an erroneous quantification of the IPs formed. The constant presence of radioactive inositol facilitates its continuous incorporation into membrane phospholipids. This results in a continuous non-linear increase in IP formation. This process of amplification will be more significant as the agonist potency increases. With the first method (A) one would expect a permanent increase in IP accumulation, while with the second method the accumulation will saturate as soon as the radioactive precursor pool of phosphoinositides is exhausted.

Some relatively unimportant parameters may also explain the different magnitudes of stimulation of EAA agonists, such as the incubation time and the temperature. In some reports, lithium chloride has been added at the same time as the radioactive inositol, which will undoubtedly lead to a weaker incorporation of [^{3}H]inositol into the membrane phospholipids than that obtained in the absence of lithium.

All these experimental parameters must be taken into account before analysing and comparing the various data.

What is the Nature of the EAA Receptors Coupled to Phosphoinositide Metabolism

Ionotropic EAA Receptors

Receptor subtypes for EAAs in brain have been classified as NMDA, QA and KA on the basis of the selective excitation of neurons by these compounds (Watkins and Evans, 1981; Fagg *et al.*, 1986). Another EAA receptor subtype has been proposed to explain the antagonistic effects of APB at a number of excitatory synapses (Fagg *et al.*, 1982; McLennan, 1983; Monaghan *et al.*, 1983a, b). Remarkable reviews are devoted to the classification of EAA receptors linked to ion channels (Watkins and Evans, 1981; Fagg *et al.*, 1986; Watkins and Olvermann, 1987; Stone and Burton, 1988). Here a summary of the main pharmacological characteristics of the EAA receptor subtypes mediating channel opening (ionotropic EAA receptors) is presented (Table 11). The NMDA receptor is the best-characterized EAA receptor for which selective competitive (APV and CPP: 3-[+]-2-(carboxypiperazin-4-yl)-propyl-1-phosphonic acid) and non-competitive antagonists (magnesium, PCP, ketamine and MK 801) are known. Magnesium blocks the Glu-activated ion channel at resting potential (Mayer *et al.*, 1984; Nowak *et al.*, 1984). The NMDA receptor complex possesses a modulatory site, activated by glycine, as recently discovered by Johnson and Ascher (1987). The glycine receptor site is blocked by 7-chlorokynurenic acid (Kemp *et al.*, 1988) or by D-cycloserine (Hood *et al.*, 1989a). A polyamine recognition site might be present on the NMDA receptor complex (Carter *et al.*, 1989; Williams, K. *et al.*, 1989). The ion channel associated with the NMDA receptor is permeable to calcium, potassium and sodium (Mayer and Westbrook, 1985; MacDermott *et al.*, 1986; Ascher and Nowak, 1988a; Ascher *et al.*, 1988). The pharmacology of QA and KA is less developed. Glutamate diethylester (GDEE), γ-D-glutamylglycine (γ-DGG) and α-D-glutamyl-aminomethylsulphonate (GAMS) are weak antagonists with relatively different specificities towards the non-NMDA receptor subtypes. Recently, more selective antagonists (CNQX—6-nitro-7-cyanoquinoxaline-2,3-dion—and DNQX—6,7-dinitro-quinoxaline-2,3-dion) have been synthesized by Honoré and colleagues (1988) and Drejer and Honoré (1988). The only known non-competitive antagonists of the ionotropic QA receptor have been extracted from spider venoms (Kawai *et al.*, 1982; Abe *et al.*, 1983; Aramaki *et al.*, 1986). The channels associated with QA and KA receptors appear to be selective for sodium and potassium ions (Ascher and Nowak, 1988b). A fourth class of EAA receptors has been postulated on the basis of the inhibitory effect of

Table 11 Characteristics of the ionotropic EAA receptor subtypes

Ionotropic receptor subtype	Selective agonists	Endogenous agonists	Competitive antagonists	Non-competitive antagonists	Modulatory effectors	Antagonists of modulatory effectors	Ion permeability
NMDA	NMDA (IBO)	Glu Asp HCA CSA	APV APH CPP CGS 19755[f]	Ketamine PCP, TCP MK 801 SKF 10047 Mg^{2+}	Glycine ACC^c	7-chloro-kynurenate Kynurenate Cycloleucine[a] HA 966[b] $ACBC^d$ $I2CA^e$ (CNQX) (DNQX)	Ca^{2+} K^+ Na^+
QA, preferably AMPA	AMPA QA	Glu	GDEE GAMS γ-DGG CNQX DNQX	JSTX			Na^+ K^+
KA	KA Domoate	Glu?	GDEE GAMS γ-DGG CNQX DNQX	(JSTX)			Na^+ K^+
APB		Glu?	APB				K^+? Cl^-?

[a] Snell and Johnson (1988).
[b] HA 966: 1-hydroxy-3-aminopyrrolidone-2 (Drejer et al., 1989).
[c] ACC: 1-aminocyclopropane-1-carboxylic acid (Nadler et al., 1988; Marvizon et al., 1989).
[d] ACBC: 1-aminocyclobutane-1-carboxylate (Hood et al., 1989b).
[e] I2CA: Indole-2-carboxylic acid (Huettner, 1989).
[f] CGS 19755: cis-4-phosphonomethyl-2-piperidine carboxylic acid (Murphy et al., 1988).

APB on the neurotransmission in the hippocampus (Yamamoto *et al.*, 1983; Lanthorn *et al.*, 1984). This compound also mimics the endogenous photoreceptor transmitter action onto ON bipolar cells, blocking ON activity while leaving OFF activity relatively unaffected (Slaughter and Miller, 1981; Nawy and Copenhagen, 1987) or enhanced (Arkin and Miller, 1987). The binding sites of APB have been characterized (Monaghan *et al.*, 1983a, b), although some of these sites may correspond to sodium-independent, chloride-dependent uptake (Pin *et al.*, 1984; Récasens *et al.*, 1987a) or diffusion (Kessler *et al.*, 1987).

The main endogenous substance thought to activate these receptors is Glu (Fonnum, 1984). Asp and acidic, sulphur-containing amino acids (CSA, HCA, etc.) may also be involved (Baba *et al.*, 1982; Récasens *et al.*, 1982; Do *et al.*, 1986; Lehman *et al.*, 1988).

Metabotropic EAA Receptors
Two main facts emerge from the observation of the various tables presenting the pharmacology of the metabotropic EAA receptors. First, there is an apparent difference between the pharmacology of the EAA-induced IP formation in adult animals and that in young animals, whatever the experimental model used (see Tables 1 and 2 for a striking example). Second, a disparity appears between the hippocampus and the other brain areas. Coming back to the first point, one can say that in young rats, all the active EAAs produce a much larger IP synthesis than they do in the adult. Some weak or inactive EAA agonists in the adult become significantly active in the young animals in most experimental models (Glu, Asp, KA, etc.). Moreover, APB, which is a good antagonist of the IBO-induced IP formation in adult hippocampal slices, is a weak agonist in neonatal hippocampal slices (Nicoletti *et al.*, 1986a; Schoepp and Johnson, 1989b). This brings us to the second point: hippocampus versus other brain areas. APB was not found to be an antagonist in rat forebrain synaptoneurosomes (Récasens *et al.*, 1988b), in striatal neurons in primary culture (Sladeczek, personal communication), in glial cells (Milani *et al.*, 1989) and in *Xenopus* oocytes injected with rat brain mRNA (Sugiyama *et al.*, 1989). In adult cortical and striatal slices, the effect of APB has not yet been tested. In the hippocampus from adult rats, IBO is far more potent than QA in inducing IP accumulation (Table 1). However, in adult rat brain cortex slices, Godfrey *et al.* (1988) report a similar potency of QA and IBO in activating IP metabolism. These results could be explained by the existence of either several EAA metabotropic receptors or a single one. Even though the pharmacological profiles are not identical in the hippocampus, as opposed to the other models, it cannot be excluded that a single EAA receptor subtype is coupled to the PLC. The pharmacological differences may stem from cell–cell or intracellular regulations, specific to the hippocampus.

On the sole basis of the pharmacology summarized in the tables, at first

Table 12   Characteristics of the EAA metabotropic receptor subtypes

Type of receptor	Agonists	Main antagonists	Activator	Main inactive agonists	Main inactive antagonists	Location
QA_m	$QA>Glu^b = IBO$ $(10^{-4}-10^{-2} \text{M})$	None (APP)?		AMPA NMDA KA	APB APV CNQX L-SOP	Brain synaptoneurosomes Striatal neurons Astroglial cells *Xenopus* oocytes injected with rat brain mRNA Retinal slices and culture
'IBO-QA'[b]	$IBO>QA^b$	(APP) APB L-SOP 'Quinalbarbitone'[c]		NMDA KA	APV CNQX	Hippocampal slices Striatal slices (from adults and newborns)
NMDA	NMDA Glu^a $(10^{-6}-10^{-5} \text{M})$	APV PCP	lycine		APB L-SOP	Striatal neurons Brain synaptoneurosomes Cortex slices

[a] High concentrations of Glu appear to activate the QA receptor, while low Glu concentrations activate probably the NMDA receptor.
[b] It must be emphasized that the different pharmacological profiles between the QA_m and the 'IBO–QA' receptor subtypes may originate from indirect regulations. The 'IBO–QA' receptor has only been characterized in slices, where cell–cell interactions occur.
[c] Quinalbarbitone is not a specific EAA antagonist, but it blocks the IP's metabolism whatever the receptor type activated (adrenergic, cholinergic, etc.).

glance, it could be proposed that the activation of four distinct EAA receptors could lead to an increase in IPs synthesis (but see Table 12).

1. A QA-sensitive receptor which could be fully activated by high concentrations of Glu or IBO or weakly stimulated by AMPA and is not blocked by any of the EAA antagonists so far tested. This QA receptor appears to be present in adult and neonatal rat forebrain synaptoneurosomes, in *Xenopus laevis* oocytes injected with rat brain mRNA, in striatal and retinal neurons in primary culture, in rabbit retinal slices and probably in astroglial cells in culture.
2. An IBO receptor, which can be partially activated by QA and inhibited by APB, APP, L-SOP. It appears to be exclusively located in the adult hippocampus. This receptor may be identical with the QA receptor described above.
3. An IBO–QA-sensitive receptor, significantly stimulated by Glu and Asp, and blocked essentially by APP and quinalbarbitone but not by APB. This receptor is present in neonatal hippocampal and striatal slices. It may correspond to the immature state of the IBO receptor described above.
4. A NMDA receptor, activated by low concentrations of Glu and blocked by APV and PCP. It is present in striatal neurons, cerebellar granule cells and rat brain synaptoneurosomes.

A question that arises from these considerations is: if such a multitude of metabotropic EAA receptors exist, why have they not been detected in EAA binding experiments? This question is examined below.

Are There Relationships between EAA Binding and EAA Receptors Linked to IP Formation?

Interpretations of Glu binding experiments were for a long time partially erroneous. This was due to the fact that a large part of the Glu binding, measured in the presence of chloride ions, corresponds to a Na^+-independent, Ca^{2+}/Cl^--dependent uptake mechanism, as we demonstrated (Pin *et al.*, 1984a; Récasens *et al.*, 1987a). Simultaneously, a better correspondence between EAA electrophysiological data and Glu binding experiments using purified synaptic membranes was found (Fagg and Matus, 1984). However, using crude membrane preparations and specific precautions to avoid artefacts of uptake, we characterized a Glu binding site (Pin *et al.*, 1984b), the pharmacology of which did not correspond at all to that found in electrophysiology. This Glu binding was not displaced by NMDA, KA or the classical EAA antagonists, but partially by QA and an anion blocker, DIDS (Récasens *et al.*, 1987a). A subpopulation of these Glu binding sites may correspond to the QA receptor, linked to IP metabolism, that we defined in rat forebrain synaptoneurosomes (Récasens *et al.*, 1988a). Similar pharmacological profiles of the Glu binding have been reported in rat brain slices (Cha *et al.*, 1988) and for partially purified Glu binding protein (Brose *et al.*, 1989).

What is the Correspondence between EAA Ionotropic and Metabotropic Receptors?

Apart from the NMDA receptor, there is no evident pharmacological correspondence between EAA receptors associated with ion channels and those coupled to PLC. However, a different pharmacology does not necessarily mean that different receptors exist. Electrophysiological studies with patch-clamp techniques allow the measurement of instantaneous changes in membrane currents or voltage, due to the frequency and the duration of channel opening elicited by EAA agonists. IP accumulation results both from the affinity of the agonist for the receptor and the efficacy *vis-à-vis* the transduction mechanism. IP production is usually measured after several minutes of stimulation. Under these conditions, a series of events, including not only the stimulation step but also all the regulatory processes, occurs. These regulations are all the more important since the complexity of the experimental model increases (from synaptoneurosomes to slices). Together with the transduction mechanism(s), they must be better known before electrophysiological and biochemical data can be compared. This will be the aim of the following sub-sections.

Molecular Mechanisms Involved in the Phosphoinositide Transduction System and Its Regulation

Introduction

This sub-section is devoted to the understanding of the data concerning the sequential steps which lead from the EAA receptor activation to the synthesis of the various phosphoinositide metabolites. Since EAAs are known to depolarize neurons, one of the first steps of this phosphoinositide transduction mechanism could be the release by EAAs of substances, which themselves stimulate or inhibit IP turnover. Another possibility is EAA-triggered ion fluxes. The possible implication of G proteins and the regulatory actions of ions and PKC on this EAA-elicited IP response are also examined.

Is EAA-induced Release of Neurotransmitters Responsible for the EAA-elicited IP Formation?

EAAs are able to stimulate the release of Glu (Campochiaro *et al.*, 1985; Gallo *et al.*, 1987; Laroche *et al.*, 1987; Lopez-Colomé and Roberts, 1987; Young *et al.*, 1988) and a number of other neuroactive substances, including acetylcholine (Lehman and Scatton, 1982), dopamine (Roberts and Anderson, 1979; Cheramy *et al.*, 1986), noradrenaline (Jones *et al.*, 1987; Ransom and Deschenes, 1988; Schmidt and Taylor, 1988), GABA (Drejer *et al.*, 1987; Pin *et al.*, 1988; Weiss, 1988; Harris and Miller, 1989), taurine (Butcher *et al.*, 1987; Menéndez *et al.*, 1989), somatostatin (Tapia-Arancibia and Astier, 1989), cholecystokinin (Yaksh *et al.*, 1987) and gonadotrophin-releasing hormone (Gay and Plant, 1987). To address the question as to whether the

EAA effects on IP metabolism are direct or not, the following means of action have been used: (1) the effect of TTX; (2) the influence of the absence of external calcium; (3) the inhibition by appropriate antagonists of substance(s) possibly liberated by EAAs; (4) the additivity of the EAA-induced IP response with that of the possibly released substances.

In cortex slices (Godfrey *et al.*, 1988), in neonatal rat striatal slices (Doble and Perrier, 1989), in striatal neurons (Sladeczek *et al.*, 1985), in cerebellar granule cells (Nicoletti *et al.*, 1987b) and in synaptoneurosomes (Récasens *et al.*, 1987b), TTX (0.3–3 μM) fails to inhibit the IP formation elicited by QA and IBO. However, Ambrosini and Meldolesi (1989) reported that TTX (0.5 μM) 'greatly reduced the size of the phosphoinositide hydrolysis responses induced by the activation of individual receptors in neuronal cells and that, under the latter conditions, a few agonists (such as NMDA) became almost ineffective'.

Thus, one could assert that TTX-sensitive, voltage-dependent Na^+ channels are not responsible for the IBO- or QA-enhanced phosphoinositide hydrolysis observed by the different authors cited above, except in the experiments of Ambrosini and Meldolesi. This represents the first evidence suggesting that the EAA-produced IP responses did not result from the EAA-elicited release of other neurotransmitters.

In the absence of calcium, most authors observed a decrease in both the basal and the QA-, IBO- or Glu-induced IP accumulation in synaptoneurosomes (Récasens *et al.*, 1987b), in neonatal rat striatal slices (Doble and Perrier, 1989), in cerebellar granule cells (Nicoletti *et al.*, 1986d) and in astrocytes (Pearce *et al.*, 1986). The further addition of EGTA (0.5–1 mM) dramatically reduces or even abolishes the IP responses. Ambrosini and Meldolesi (1989) found that the absence of calcium and the presence of 1 mM EGTA reduce the (10 μM) QA-induced IP formation, but not the basal IP formation in TTX-treated hippocampal and striatal neurons. Simultaneous decreases in the basal and EAA-stimulated IP formations in the absence of calcium further support the idea that the QA- or IBO-elicited IP turnover is not due to the calcium-dependent release of other substances. This parallel decrease probably reflects the need of PLC for calcium in order to be maximally activated (Bennett and Crooke, 1987; Berridge, 1987; Katan and Parker, 1987; Renard *et al.*, 1987; Eberhard and Holz, 1988).

In various studies antagonists of neuroactive substances capable of being released by EAA have been tested. Atropine, which inhibits the IP formation elicited by muscarinic agonists, does not antagonize EAA-induced IP formation in adult and neonatal rat hippocampal slices (Nicoletti *et al.*, 1986a, b), in striatal slices (Doble and Perrier, 1989), in neurons (Sladeczek *et al.*, 1985) and in rat forebrain synaptoneurosomes (Guiramand *et al.*, 1989a). In addition, mepyramine, phentolamine, ketanserin and bicuculline, which block histaminergic (H_1), alpha-1-adrenergic, serotonergic (5-HT_2) and $GABA_A$ receptors, respectively, do not affect the IP formation elicited by IBO in adult rat hippocampal slices (Nicoletti *et al.*, 1986b). Similarly,

Osborne (1990) found that prazosin, ketanserin and atropine do not affect the QA-induced IP formation in rabbit retinal slices. Although it appears to be difficult to inhibit all the putative neuroactive substances which can be liberated by EAAs, the above findings further strengthen the possibility that the IBO and QA actions on IP metabolism do not occur via released compounds.

Finally, IBO- or QA-elicited IP formation is additive with that produced by carbachol in hippocampal slices (Schoepp and Johnson, 1988a) or in synaptoneurosomes (Guiramand *et al.*, 1989a) or with that induced by noradrenaline (Schoepp and Johnson, 1988a).

Taken together, these data strongly suggest that QA- or IBO-induced IP accumulation is not due to the release of an endogenous compound.

However, this conclusion cannot be extended to NMDA-stimulated IP turnover, for the following reasons: (1) NMDA is the most potent EAA agonist to trigger the release of acetylcholine (Lehman and Scatton, 1982; Snell and Johnson, 1986), noradrenaline (Jones *et al.*, 1987; Ransom and Deschenes, 1988; Schmidt and Taylor, 1988; Fink *et al.*, 1989) and dopamine (Cheramy *et al.*, 1986; Clow and Jhamandas, 1988); (2) the spontaneous release of endogenous Glu could occur in slices or cells in culture and be blocked by APV (Gallo *et al.*, 1982; Nicoletti *et al.*, 1987b); (3) TTX blocked NMDA-induced IP accumulation in striatal and hippocampal neurons (Ambrosini and Meldolesi, 1989); (4) NMDA weakly stimulates IP formation in the various models, although the presence of magnesium and an insufficient concentration of glycine may have inhibited the stimulatory effect of NMDA.

In summary, the direct stimulation of IP metabolism by NMDA is less evident than that by QA or IBO. Further studies are necessary to ascertain the mechanism of NMDA action.

Is EAA-induced Depolarization Responsible for EAA-elicited IP Formation?

Depolarizing agents (potassium) or agents that enhance sodium influx increase IP formation in rat and guinea-pig forebrain synaptoneurosomes (Gusovsky *et al.*, 1986; Récasens *et al.*, 1987b; Gusovsky and Daly, 1988a; Guiramand *et al.*, 1989a) as well as in cerebellar granule cells (Nicoletti *et al.*, 1987b). These agents can be divided into five categories: (1) agents activating voltage-dependent sodium channels (batrachotoxin, aconitin or veratridine); (2) compounds that inhibit the Na^+/K^+ ATPase, such as ouabain; (3) scorpion venoms that increase the activation or slow the inactivation of sodium channels (toxins from *Leiurus quinquestriatus*, and *Centruroides* and *Tityus* species); (4) substances that cause the repetitive firing of sodium channel-dependent action potentials (pumiliotoxin B and pyrethroids); (5) sodium ionophores (monensin). When testing the combination of two sodium channel agents, each belonging to a different category (scorpion venom + batrachotoxin; scorpion venom + pumiliotoxin B; scorpion venom + monensin; batrachotoxin + pumiliotoxin B), the IP responses were not additive

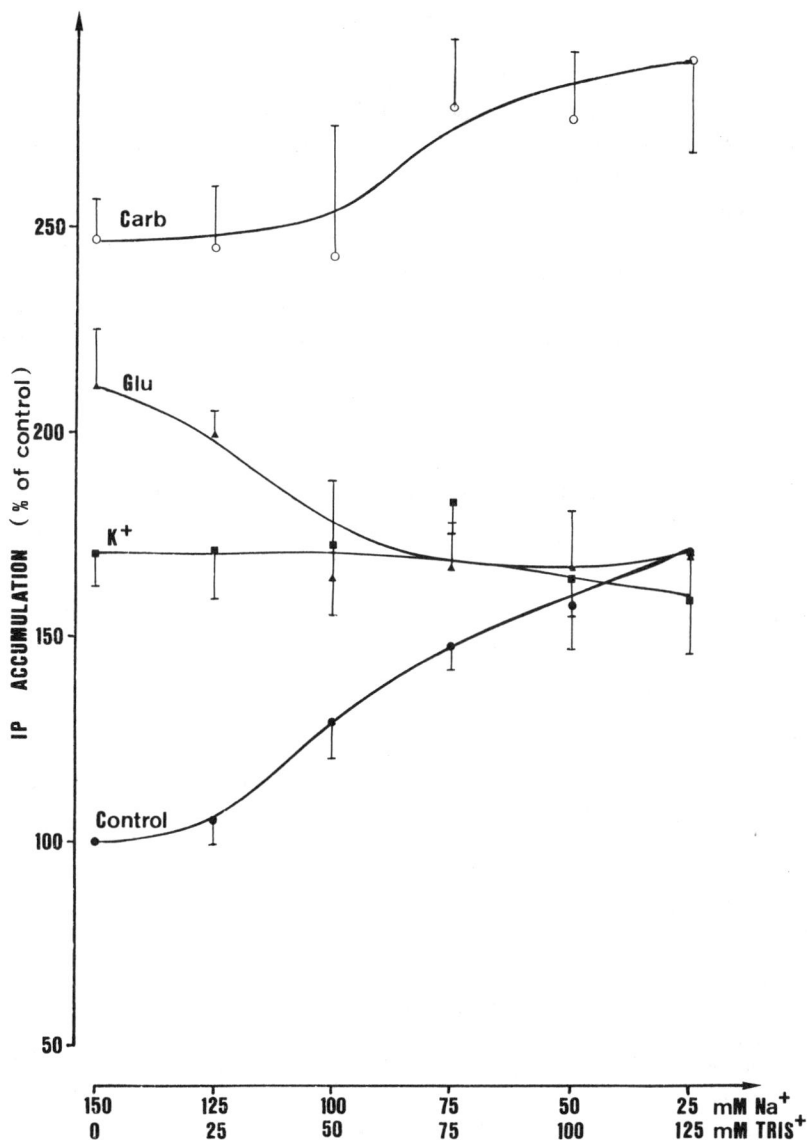

Figure 4 Effect of the replacement of buffer sodium ions by Tris$^+$ ions on IP formation induced by Glu, potassium and Carb in 8-day-old rat forebrain synaptoneurosomes. Synaptoneurosomes were incubated at 37 °C for 1 h in the presence of [^{3}H]myoinositol. After washing the excess of radioactive inositol with modified Krebs–Ringer buffers, synaptoneurosomes were resuspended in these modified Krebs–Ringer buffers and incubated for 10 min in the presence of 10 mM lithium chloride, followed by a further 20 min stimulation period with or without the neuroactive substance indicated above. Water-soluble radiolabelled IPs were extracted, purified and radioassayed according to the method of Récasens *et al.* (1987b). Results are the means ± SEM of six separate experiments, each performed in triplicate. Results are expressed as the percentages of the basal IP formation obtained with normal Krebs–Ringer buffer

(Gusovsky *et al.*, 1987). These data seem to indicate that depolarization and/or sodium influx could be responsible for IP formation.

Since EAA agonists are known to depolarize cells, their action on phosphoinositide metabolism could result from these depolarizing properties. In fact, we found that QA-induced IP synthesis is not additive with potassium-evoked IP response in rat brain synaptoneurosomes (Guiramand *et al.*, 1989a). On the contrary, the combination of potassium and carbachol produces a more than additive response in synaptoneurosomes, as was found in cortex slices (Baird and Nahorski, 1986; Court *et al.*, 1986). This result clearly indicates the interdependence of QA- and potassium-induced IP formation. This probably means that both compounds share at least one common step in the multistep mechanism which leads from QA receptor activation to the increased synthesis of IPs. The most likely common step is depolarization and/or sodium influx. The replacement of external Na^+ ions by $Tris^+$ (tris(hydroxymethyl)aminomethane) or by N-methyl-D-glucamine$^+$ leads to a marked elevation of the basal IP formation, in addition to which no further IP stimulation could be evoked by Glu or QA (Rècasens *et al.*, 1988a; Figure 4). Conversely, the carbachol-induced IP formation parallels the basal IP formation (Figure 4). Similar data are obtained in neonatal rat striatal slices, where sodium chloride was replaced by choline chloride (Doble and Perrier, 1989). External sodium ions are a prerequisite for the enhanced IP accumulation elicited by QA. EAAs induce sodium fluxes in striatal (Luini *et al.*, 1981) and hippocampal slices (Baudry *et al.*, 1983). The order of potency of sodium flux is NMDA ($50 \mu M$) > KA ($100 \mu M$) > QA $\gg$ Glu ($1 mM$) (Baudry *et al.*, 1983). There is apparently no correlation between the extent of sodium flux and the magnitude and potency of the IP response elicited by these EAA agonists. A similar lack of correlation between sodium fluxes and IP formation, triggered by agents increasing the sodium intracellular concentration, was reported in synaptoneurosomes (Gusovsky *et al.*, 1987). However, one could propose that a small fraction of sodium channels or transporters is responsible for the EAA- or sodium-agents-enhanced phosphoinositide breakdown, while the whole population of sodium channels or transporters are involved in the net sodium fluxes. A second possibility is that only a small fraction of the maximal sodium ion influx in distinct localizations is necessary to induce maximal IP responses (Gusovsky *et al.*, 1987). Since high concentrations of ethylisopropylamiloride or amiloride are required to inhibit the Glu- or QA-induced IP formation (data not shown), the Na^+/Ca^{2+} and Na^+/H^+ exchangers might be involved in the IP response elicited by EAA. TTX potently inhibits the sodium influx elicited by scorpion venom, batrachotoxin and veratridine into guinea-pig cortical synaptoneurosomes (Gusovsky *et al.*, 1987), while being 100 times less potent in blocking the IP formation produced by these compounds. In rat forebrain synaptoneurosomes, TTX ($2 \mu M$) blocks about 90% of the IP formation elicited by $1 \mu M$ veratridine, but does not affect the EAA- or carbachol-induced IP responses (Récasens *et al.*, 1987b). These findings may indicate that the sodium

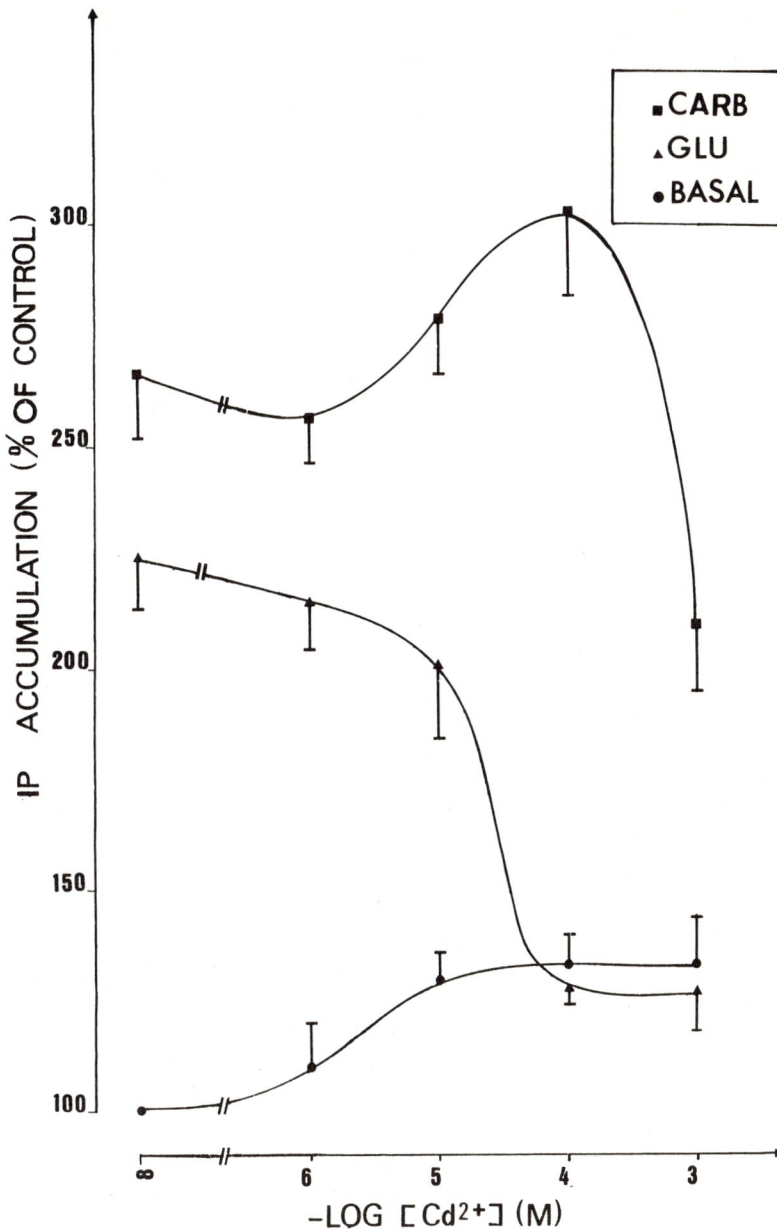

Figure 5 The influence of cadmium ions on IP accumulation in synaptoneurosomes prepared from 8-day-old rat forebrain synaptoneurosomes. Experimental conditions were similar to those described in Figure 4, except that normal Krebs–Ringer buffer was used in all cases. Results are the means ± SEM of six separate experiments, each performed in triplicate. Results are expressed as the percentages of the basal IP formation

channels probably involved in the IP formation produced by EAA or agents enhancing sodium fluxes are relatively TTX-resistant. Such a type of sodium channel has already been described (Renaud *et al.*, 1983; Bowers, 1985) and is known to be blocked by Cd^{2+} (Bowers, 1985; Frelin *et al.*, 1986). Cd^{2+} ions inhibit the phosphoinositide breakdown evoked by scorpion venom in guinea-pig synaptoneurosomes, with an IC_{50} value of 80 μM (Gusovsky *et al.*, 1987). Here we report that this ion blocks the Glu-elicited IP formation in rat forebrain synaptoneurosomes with an IC_{50} value of 25 μM, but does not modify the carbachol-elicited IPs response at concentrations up to 200 μM (Figure 5).

In conclusion, Glu induced IP synthesis via a QA-sensitive receptor. Limited depolarization and/or sodium fluxes induced by this receptor activation is a necessary step for the triggering of the enhanced phosphoinositide breakdown. This step is TTX-resistant and cadmium-sensitive. Nothing is known concerning the sodium requirements for the 'other' EAA metabotropic receptors.

What Are the Influences of Calcium Ions?

Since 'membrane depolarization' seems to play a role in the EAA-induced IP formation, it is conceivable that voltage-dependent calcium channels are involved. Three subtypes of these calcium channels (L, N and T) have been defined in nervous tissue (Nowycky *et al.*, 1985). The L type is blocked by 1,4-dihydropyridines (such as nifedipine), phenylalkylamines (such as verapamil) and benzothiazepine (diltiazem), high concentrations of Cd^{2+} and ω-conotoxine. The N channel is inhibited only by ω-conotoxin and Cd^{2+}. No effective antagonist is known for the T type. In rat forebrain synaptoneurosomes, nifedipine or verapamil as well as ω-conotoxin did not affect the Glu-dependent IP formation (unpublished results). This excludes the possibility that Glu activates PLC by increasing intracellular calcium via the L and N channels. Moreover, this indicates that the inhibition by Cd^{2+} of Glu-induced IP synthesis (Figure 5) did not result from an effect of this ion on the calcium influx via L and N channels. However, this does not preclude the possibility of calcium influx via voltage-dependent T-type channels or other, yet unknown calcium channels. Nevertheless, the simultaneous decrease in the basal and EAA-stimulated IP response observed on lowering the external concentration of calcium rather suggests the non-involvement of calcium channels. The low external concentration of calcium may induce a general decrease in intracellular calcium, possibly via an effect on the electrogenic and voltage-dependent Na^+/Ca^{2+} exchanger (Barcenas-Ruiz *et al.*, 1987), thus inhibiting PLC.

The role of calcium in NMDA-stimulated IP synthesis may be of another nature, because of the specific properties of the NMDA channel. NMDA channels are permeable to calcium ions (Ascher and Nowak, 1986, 1988a; MacDermott *et al.*, 1986; Mayer *et al.*, 1987; for a review, see Ascher, 1988), which could activate PLC. Actually, NMDA-stimulated IP formation appears to possess all the pharmacological properties of the ionotropic NMDA receptor. Mg^{2+} dependency and blockade by APV have been found in synaptoneurosomes (Récasens *et al.*, 1987b, 1988a), striatal neurons (Sladeczek *et al.*, 1985) and cerebellar granule cells (Nicoletti *et al.*, 1987b; Wroblewski *et al.*, 1987). Recently Nicoletti and Canonico (1989) have shown that glycine potentiates the IP formation induced by EAAs. However, several authors report that NMDA fails to stimulate inositol phospholipid hydrolysis in neonatal rat striatal slices (Doble and Perrier, 1989), in adult and neonatal hippocampal slices (Nicoletti *et al.*, 1986a, b; Schoepp and Johnson, 1989b), in astroglial cells (Milani *et al.*, 1989) and in oocytes injected with rat brain mRNA (Sugiyama *et al.*, 1987). These apparent discrepancies probably result from the experimental model used. NMDA may indirectly stimulate to varying degrees the IP formation by releasing endogenous substances. These discrepancies could also be explained by the fact that predepolarization of the membrane is necessary for the full action of NMDA on its receptor in a magnesium-containing medium, particularly if the IP stimulation occurs via a calcium influx. The extent of predepolarization required for fully activating the NMDA receptor may be different according to the various experimental models, and NMDA alone would not be sufficient to trigger it. Another interesting possibility is that NMDA is efficiently linked to PLC only in a short transient period of time. Guiramand *et al.* (1989b) have shown that a peak of IP stimulation by NMDA occurs in 12-day-old rat forebrain synaptoneurosomes. In slices, however, NMDA has been tested without effect either in adult or in 6–9-day-old rats. In this period of time the maximal NMDA effect is masked. This also argues against the fact that the NMDA-induced release of neuroactive compounds is responsible for NMDA-elicited IP formation, since this release increases with age.

Does EAA-elicited Phosphoinositide Breakdown Involve a G Protein?

That G proteins are involved in the receptor-stimulated breakdown of phosphoinositides was first suggested by Gomperts (1983). Despite extensive work in this field, it is yet unknown whether G proteins interact directly with the PLC enzymes or via yet unappreciated intermediates. Moreover, the identity of the G protein(s) implicated in the regulation of the PLC enzymes remains a matter of speculation (Chuang, 1989). The best indirect evidence so far reported concerning the involvement of a G protein in the EAA-evoked phosphoinositide breakdown is the inhibitory effect of pertussis toxin. Pertussis toxin catalyses ADP ribosylation of the $alpha_i$ subunit of the G_i protein (Brass *et al.*, 1988) or the $alpha_o$ subunit of the G_o protein (for review, see Gilman, 1987). This toxin, injected 20 h before the experiments, blocks the oscillating chloride currents, triggered by EAA, in *Xenopus* oocytes injected with rat brain mRNA (Sugiyama *et al.*, 1987). In this model, Glu receptors are not directly coupled to the endogenous chloride channels but indirectly activate these via the IP_3–Ca^{2+} messenger system (Oosawa and Yamagishi, 1989). Ambrosini and Meldolesi (1989) reported that a 3 h pretreatment with pertussis toxin results in a 55% or 75% inhibition of QA-induced IP responses in hippocampal and striatal neurons, respectively. Rat cultured hippocampal cells treated for 24 h with pertussis toxin (10 μg per ml) show a Glu- or QA-elicited intracellular calcium mobilization half that of the control as measured by means of fura-2 fluorescence (Furuya *et al.*, 1989). Surprisingly, the pertussis toxin effect was not tested by all the other authors. The inhibitory effects observed with the long-lasting treatment of pertussis toxin may be due, for instance, to the variation in cAMP levels resulting from prolonged alpha$_i$ inactivation or from ADP ribosylation of other G proteins involved in other cellular signalling systems (Brass *et al.*, 1988).

Thus, it is far from being demonstrated that G proteins are directly linked to the IP formation produced by EAAs.

Does Kinase C (PKC) Activation Regulate EAA-stimulated IP Accumulation?
The second class of intracellular messengers generated by PIP$_2$ hydrolysis—namely the diacylglycerides—are endogenous activators of PKC. The synergistic interaction between the PKC and the IP$_3$–Ca^{2+} pathways underlies a variety of cellular responses to external stimuli (Nishizuka, 1984b; Kikkawa and Nishizuka, 1986). In addition to this positive forward action, PKC may provide negative feedback control (Kikkawa and Nishizuka, 1986; Nishizuka, 1988). Numerous receptors coupled to the phosphoinositide transduction mechanisms are subject to feedback desensitization as a result of PKC activation (for a review, see Kikkawa and Nishizuka, 1986). Phorbol esters, which directly activate PKC, inhibit the EAA-stimulated phosphoinositide hydrolysis in neonatal and adult rat hippocampal slices (Schoepp and Johnson, 1988b; Schoepp, 1989), in cortical slices (Godfrey *et al.*, 1988), in neuronal cultures (Canonico *et al.*, 1988; Ambrosini and Meldolesi, 1989) in striatal neurons (Manzoni *et al.*, 1990) and in astroglial cells (Milani *et al.*, 1989). The EAA agonists used are IBO in the hippocampus and QA or Glu in the other models. EAA-induced IP response is preferentially inhibited as compared with the carbachol-evoked response. However, NMDA-induced IP accumulation is not affected by phorbol esters in cerebellar neurons (Canonico *et al.*, 1988).

In *Xenopus* oocytes injected with rat brain mRNA, phorbol esters suppress receptor-mediated responses (Ito *et al.*, 1988a). The extent of inhibition by PKC activators does not depend on the type of receptors stimulated (serotonergic, muscarinic or glutamatergic). Injection of IP$_3$ in the oocytes elicits chloride currents. Phorbol esters enhance this IP$_3$-produced response. Taken together, these results suggest that the inhibition by PKC activators of the chloride current elicited by receptor agonists in the oocytes occurs at a step situated after the receptor activation and before the synthesis of IP$_3$.

In summary, PKC activation produces a feedback inhibition of EAA-stimulated IP accumulation.

Conclusion

The preliminary analyses of the pharmacology of the EAA-elicited IP responses suggest the existence of four EAA metabotropic receptor subtypes. Closer examination of these IP responses suggests that these different pharmacological profiles arise from the various experimental models and techniques used. Thus, most, if not all, of the findings could be explained by the existence of two major receptor subtypes coupled to phosphoinoisitide metabolism—namely a QA and a NMDA receptor (Table 12). The former, tentatively called QA_m, appears to be distinct from the ionotropic QA receptor (QA_i). No antagonist has yet been found for this QA_m receptor. The NMDA receptor involved in stimulating phosphoinositide metabolism seems to be identical with the ionotropic NMDA receptor. A third metabotropic EAA receptor, activated by IBO, could also exist in the hippocampus, although direct evidence for the clear-cut difference between this receptor and the QA_m one remains to be established (Table 12).

4. *What Are the Receptor Types Coupled to Phosphoinositide Breakdown and Inhibited by EAAs? What Types of EAA Receptors Are Responsible for This Inhibition?*

Introduction

Besides their action as stimulating agents of phosphoinositide breakdown, EAAs were reported to inhibit the IPs produced by other neuroactive substances. Some other receptors (dopamine D2 and adenosine A1, in particular) inhibited receptor-mediated IP synthesis (for a review, see Linden and Delahunty, 1989). Here we present the current findings concerning the inhibition of the agonists-receptor-mediated IP synthesis by EAAs and the characterization of the EAA receptors involved.

Properties of the Receptors Stimulating IP Accumulation and Inhibited by EAAs and the Characterization of These EAA Receptors

Muscarinic Receptors
The stimulation of muscarinic receptors leads to an enhanced formation of IPs (Michell, 1980; Fischer, 1986; Nathanson, 1987). This IP accumulation is inhibited by EAAs in hippocampal slices (Baudry *et al.*, 1986), in cortex slices (Godfrey *et al.*, 1988; Gonzales and Moerschbaecher, 1989; Noble *et al.*, 1989), in neonatal rat brain striatal slices (Doble and Perrier, 1989), in rabbit retinal slices (Osborne, 1990) and in striatal neurons in primary culture (Schmidt *et al.*, 1987). NMDA and KA are the most potent inhibitors in

Table 13 Inhibitory action of EAAs on muscarinic-receptor-mediated phosphoinositide hydrolysis

Ref.	EAA inhibition		Reversal of inhibition		Substances which failed to reverse	External ion effects			Model	Method
	Magnitude (%)[a]	Potency IC_{50} (µM)	Magnitude (%)	Potency IC_{50} (µM)		Ions	Effect			
Baudry et al. (1986) (carbachol, 0.5 mM)	NMDA (85) HCA (78) Glu (90) KA (Veratridine)	20 40 1500 50	APV (80) DαAA (50) Ketamine	400 2000		Ca^{2+} Na^+	No Yes		Hippocampal slices	B
Godfrey et al. (1988) (carbachol, 1 mM)	NMDA KA IBO Glu QA		APV, MK 801		APB APV, MK 801 APB				Cortex slices	B
Noble et al. (1989)	NMDA (93)	14	APV (74)						Cortex slices	B
Osborne (1990) (carbachol, 0.5 mM)	NMDA (23) KA (35)		APV 'GDEE, APV'		APB, GDEE APB				Rabbit retinal slices	B

[a]The magnitude of inhibition is expressed as the percentage of the muscarinic agonist stimulation over the basal values.

magnitude, with an IC_{50} of about 50 μM whatever the experimental model tested (Table 13). QA, which is inactive in striatal neurons (Schmidt *et al.*, 1987) in inhibiting the carbachol-induced IPs response, was not tested in the other models. The NMDA inhibition of the carbachol-elicited IPs formation could be reversed by classical competitive NMDA antagonists (APV, D-αAA, CPP) as well as by uncompetitive antagonists (ketamine, PCP, MK 801). Drugs interacting with the NMDA receptor through the sigma opiate receptor subtype (cyclazocine, etoxadrol, etc.) also reverse the NMDA inhibition. The KA inhibition is not removed by any of the classical NMDA antagonists, or by GDEE, APB, CNQX, GAMS, etc.

Taken together, these data indicate that the increased IP formation produced by carbachol is inhibited by EAAs via their interaction with two receptor subtypes—the NMDA and the KA subtypes.

Adrenergic Receptors
The stimulation of phosphoinositide breakdown by noradrenaline has been shown to be inhibited by EAAs in cortical, hippocampal and striatal slices (Nicoletti *et al.*, 1986a; Godfrey *et al.*, 1988; Jope and Li, 1989; Li and Jope, 1989). Glu, Asp and QA are the most potent agonists in producing this inhibition, the reversal of which has not yet been studied. APB and SOP, antagonists of IBO-induced IP formation in hippocampal slices, also inhibit the noradrenaline-evoked IP response in these slices (Nicoletti *et al.*, 1986a). Thus, APB and SOP behave as EAA agonists such as Glu, Asp and QA (Table 14). Sulphur-containing amino acids (HCA, SOS, CSA, cysteine, cystine) also inhibit the noradrenaline-evoked IP accumulation in rat prefrontal cortex slices (Li and Jope, 1989). In contrast to what was observed for carbachol-induced IP formation, the noradrenaline IP response was not blocked by NMDA, IBO or KA in hippocampal slices (Nicoletti *et al.*, 1986a; Table 14), although there was an inhibitory effect of KA in cortex slices (Godfrey *et al.*, 1988).

The apparently contradictory reports of Baudry *et al.* (1986), who observed an inhibition by EAAs of the IP formation induced by carbachol, but not by noradrenaline, and of Nicoletti and colleagues (1986a), who found exactly the opposite in the same model, could be explained in part by the methods used in each of these studies. This situation was particularly well described in the paper of Jope and Li (1989). These authors demonstrate that EAAs inhibit the incorporation of [³H]inositol into membrane phospholipids. Glu and QA specifically inhibit this incorporation into a pool of membrane phosphoinositides, the breakdown of which is triggered by the activation of adrenergic receptors. NMDA and KA also inhibit the incorporation of tritiated inositol into membrane lipids, but probably in a pool, which is not affected by adrenergic agonists. Nicoletti and co-workers stimulate the slices by noradrenaline, while [³H]inositol is still present in the incubation medium. In this case, so long as the noradrenaline-mediated phosphoinositide breakdown increases, the replenishment of the tritiated phosphoinositide pool

Table 14 Inhibitory action of EAAs on adrenergic-receptor-mediated phosphoinositide hydrolysis

Ref.	EAA inhibition		Reversal of EAA inhibition		Lack of EAA inhibition	Model	Method
	Magnitude (%)[c]	Potency IC$_{50}$ (µM)	Magnitude (%)	Potency IC$_{50}$ (µM)			
Godfrey et al. (1988); [NA] = 0.3 mM	KA (50)		NT			Cortex slices	B
Nicoletti et al. (1986a)[a]; [NA] = 0.1 mM	Glu (79) Asp (86) QA (86) APB (82) SOP (85)		NT		KA NMDA IBO	Hippocampal slices	A
Jope and Li (1989); [NA] = 0.2 mM	Glu (68) Cysteine HCA		NT			Striatal cortical and hippocampal slices	A
Li and Jope, 1989	CSA				Glu		B
Baudry et al.[a] (1986)			NT		Glu	Hippocampal slices	B
Osborne (1990)					KA NMDA QA	Rabbit retinal slices	B

Reference	Agonist		Inhibitors			Tissue	
Gonzales and Moerschbaecher (1989)	NMDA (70) (0.1 mM)	10	APV	120	GDEE	Cortex slices	B
			DαAA (82)	260	Nalorphine		
			Ketamine	23	Haloperidol		
			PCP	4	Dexoxadrol		
			MK 801	0.8			
			Kyn (98)				
			Cyclazocine	26			
			Etoxadrol	24			
			N(+)-ANM[b]	41			
Doble and Perrier (1989)	NMDA (61) (1 mM)		APV	123	GDEE	Neonatal striatal slices	A
			DαAA	141	CNQX		
			Kyn	107	DGG		
			CPP	7	γ-GT		
			PCP	1	GAMS		
			Ketamine	28	PCA		
			N-ANM[b]	10	APB		
			MK 801	0.2	SOP		
Schmidt et al. (1987)[a]	NMDA (46)	56	APV			Striatal neurons	B
	Glu (45)	24	APV				
	KA						

[a] Baudry found that K$^+$ ions did not inhibit carbachol-induced IP formation, while Schmidt reported that QA is ineffective. Nicoletti and co-workers (1986a) did not detect any inhibition by Glu, Asp, APB, SOP of carbachol-elicited IP response in adult hippocampal slices. Unless otherwise stated, slices were prepared from rat brains.

Animals used in these experiments were rats, except as indicated.

[b] N-ANM: N-allylnormetazocine.

[c] The magnitude of inhibition is expressed as the percentage of adrenergic agonist stimulation over the basal value.

NT: not tested.

sensitive to adrenergic agonists occurs in the absence of EAAs. The presence of EAAs impedes the incorporation of [³H]inositol into this phospholipid pool, which explains the EAA-produced inhibition. Baudry and his colleagues, who washed the slices after the incorporation of [³H]inositol and before the stimulation with noradrenaline, did not observe the inhibition by EAAs.

The findings of Jope and Li satisfactorily explained the lack of inhibition by EAAs, observed by Baudry *et al.*, of the noradrenaline-induced IP accumulation and the blocking effect of EAAs reported by Nicoletti *et al.* for this same IP response. However, these findings did not account for the inhibition by EAAs of carbachol-elicited IP formation reported by Baudry and co-workers and the absence of effect of these EAA agonists described by Nicoletti and his colleagues.

Other Receptors

NMDA inhibits K^+- and histamine-induced IP formation in hippocampal slices (Baudry *et al.*, 1986; Table 15). KA blocks K^+- and serotonin-elicited IP accumulation in cortex slices (Godfrey *et al.*, 1988; Noble *et al.*, 1989; Table 15). NMDA has also been shown to inhibit the QA stimulation of phosphoinositide breakdown (Palmer *et al.*, 1988; Table 15). The potency of various EAA agonists as well as the reversibility of their inhibitions have not been thoroughly examined. Further studies are required to analyse the EAA effects on IP formation induced by these neuroactive substances.

Mechanisms of EAA Inhibition of IP Formation Induced by Various Neuroactive Substances

Although there is no clear evidence of the mode(s) of EAA action to inhibit IP formation triggered by some neurotransmitters or other neuroactive substances, speculative proposals are presented in this subsection.

Baudry *et al.* (1986) reported that the EAA inhibition of IP accumulation by carbachol is not affected by the absence of extracellular calcium, but is eliminated by the absence of extracellular sodium ions. This could lead to the proposal that depolarization induced by EAAs causes a substantial sodium influx, which in turn produces the inhibition observed. However, K^+ depolarization promotes ion fluxes, including sodium ion fluxes. K^+ does not inhibit carbachol-induced IP responses (Baudry *et al.*, 1986; Guiramand *et al.*, 1989a). Thus, one could suspect that a different location of the sodium influx for K^+- and EAA-induced depolarization is responsible for the distinct effect of these compounds. It is conceivable that a local sodium influx alters the intracellular calcium level. This rise in intracellular calcium may favour the translocation of PKC from the cytosol to the membrane, where the enzyme could be activated by diacylglycerides (Nishizuka, 1988; Weiss *et al.*, 1989). The activation of PKC may in turn inhibit the IP cycle stimulated by

Table 15 Inhibitory action of EAA and K$^+$ on the phosphoinositide metabolism stimulated by miscellaneous neuroactive substances

Ref.	Neuroactive substances	Type of receptor or of action	EAA-inhibitory		Model	Method
			Magnitude	Potency IC_{50} (μM)		
Baudry et al. (1986)	K$^+$ (50 mM) Histamine (100 μM)	Depolarization H$_1$?	NMDA NMDA		Hippocampal slices	B
Godfrey et al. (1988)	K$^+$ (20 mM) Serotonin (0.1 mM)	Depolarization 5-HT$_2$	KA (100) KA		Cortex slices	B
Schmidt et al. (1987)[a]	Neurotensin				Striatal neurons	B
Palmer et al. (1988)[b]	QA	QA	NMDA (75) KA (25)		Hippocampal slices	B
Noble et al. (1989)	Serotonin (1 mM)		NMDA (78)		Cortex slices	B

[a] Glu did not inhibit neurotensin-evoked IP synthesis.
[b] Palmer and co-workers have shown that CPP reverses the NMDA inhibition of QA-induced IP accumulation.

carbachol (Gonzales *et al.*, 1987; Lenox *et al.*, 1988).

By analogy with the adenylate cyclase transduction systems, receptor–receptor interactions offer a second means whereby EAA may block carbachol-elicited IP turnover. PLC may be dually regulated via distinct G proteins ($G_{p(s)}$ stimulating PLC and $G_{p(i)}$ inhibiting PLC), which are activated via one type of receptor and inhibited via another type.

A third possibility is that EAAs, which are known to be potent neurotoxic compounds (Rothman, 1985; Choi, 1987; Garthwaite and Garthwaite, 1989a) kill specific cells containing either muscarinic or adrenergic receptors. For instance, Schmidt *et al.* (1987) indicate that NMDA significantly increases the activity of lactate dehydrogenase in the incubation medium of striatal neurons. This increased activity probably results from the release of the cytosolic lactate dehydrogenase from dead striatal neurons. QA exposure of hippocampal slices leads to the degeneration of pyramidal neurons (Garthwaite and Garthwaite, 1989b). However, this explanation does not hold for cortical slices. In fact, Jope and Li (1989) indicated that preincubation of rat brain slices with Glu for 1 h under conditions identical with those that were used to measure the synthesis of IPs, does not alter the inhibitory effect of Glu on noradrenaline-induced IP accumulation. Glu uptake by glial cells may account for the protection of neuronal cells from the neurotoxic effects of this agent in slices. Glial cells are almost absent in neurons in primary culture. Another eventuality must be taken into account, which is that Glu may preferentially kill cells containing muscarinic receptors rather than those possessing adrenergic receptors, because of a higher density of Glu receptors in the former than in the latter.

A last hypothesis would be the inhibitory action of substances released by EAAs on carbachol- or noradrenaline-induced IP accumulation. In all these studies, drugs were applied for at least 10 min, which is too long a time for these slow, indirect actions to be ruled out. Along this line, adenosine and dopamine have been shown to trigger receptor-mediated inhibition of IP production by neuroactive substances in a large variety of tissues (for a review, see Linden and Delahunty, 1989). In fact, EAAs are able to cause the release of both dopamine (Roberts and Anderson, 1979; Cheramy *et al.*, 1986) and adenosine (Hoehn and White, 1990).

Conclusion

EAAs are able to inhibit receptor-mediated IP accumulation. NMDA and KA inhibit the carbachol-induced IP response, while QA inhibits noradrenaline-elicited IP formation. With the exception of perhaps the classical NMDA receptor, the EAA receptor subtypes involved in these inhibitory effects are not yet well characterized. Inhibition by NMDA is reversed by competitive (APV, CPP, etc.) and non-competitive (PCP, MK-801, etc.) antagonists. NMDA and KA also inhibit histamine- and serotonin-evoked IP responses.

Although several mechanisms of action have been proposed for these inhibitory effects of EAAs, further studies are required to establish the piece of biochemical machinery involved. The physiological meanings of such a mechanism have not even been approached.

5. *Physiological and Pathophysiological Roles of EAA Receptors Coupled to Phosphoinositide Metabolism*

When approaching integrated functions or dysfunctions of cells or organs, it is illusory to believe that a single mechanism is responsible for the large-scale modifications observed. Nevertheless, we shall examine in this section the possible specific involvement of the EAA receptors linked to the phosphoinositide metabolism in cell physiology and in integrated functions.

EAA Metabotropic Receptors and Development

The evolution of EAA-stimulated IP turnover during postnatal development was investigated in rat forebrain synaptoneurosomes (Dudek *et al.*, 1989; Guiramand *et al.*, 1989b), and in rat hippocampal (Nicoletti *et al.*, 1986a) and cortical slices (Schoepp and Hillman, 1990). We found that EAAs, in contrast to some other neuroactive substances, stimulate the accumulation of IPs in synaptoneurosomes during a narrowly defined period of postnatal development. QA-induced IP formation peaks in synaptoneurosomes prepared from 8-day-old rat forebrains, while that of NMDA reaches its maximal value in 12-day-old animals. Carbachol-, noradrenaline- and K^+-induced IP formations plateau in synaptoneurosomes prepared from adult rats. The specific developmental profile of EAA-induced IP accumulation appears to result from a modification in the number of receptors coupled to this transduction system, since no change in the apparent affinity of EAAs for stimulating IP turnover was observed (Guiramand *et al.*, 1989b). However, variations in the efficiency of the coupling between EAA receptors and phosphoinositide turnover could not be excluded. These data confirm the existence of two distinct EAA receptors, which are linked to IP metabolism in rat brain synaptoneurosomes—namely, a QA_m and an NMDA receptor. In addition, an IBO-sensitive receptor, possibly distinct from QA_m, is linked to IP turnover in hippocampal slices (Nicoletti *et al.*, 1986a). The existence of distinct EAA metabotropic receptor subtypes is supported by the fact that QA, IBO and *trans*-ACPD exhibit different efficacies towards cortical phosphoinositide-coupled EAA receptors during development (Schoepp and Hillman, 1990). However, all these EAA-elicited IP formations are inhibited by the same antagonist APP.

The physiological role associated with these transient increases in IP formation by EAA agonists is still unknown. Nevertheless, some hypotheses

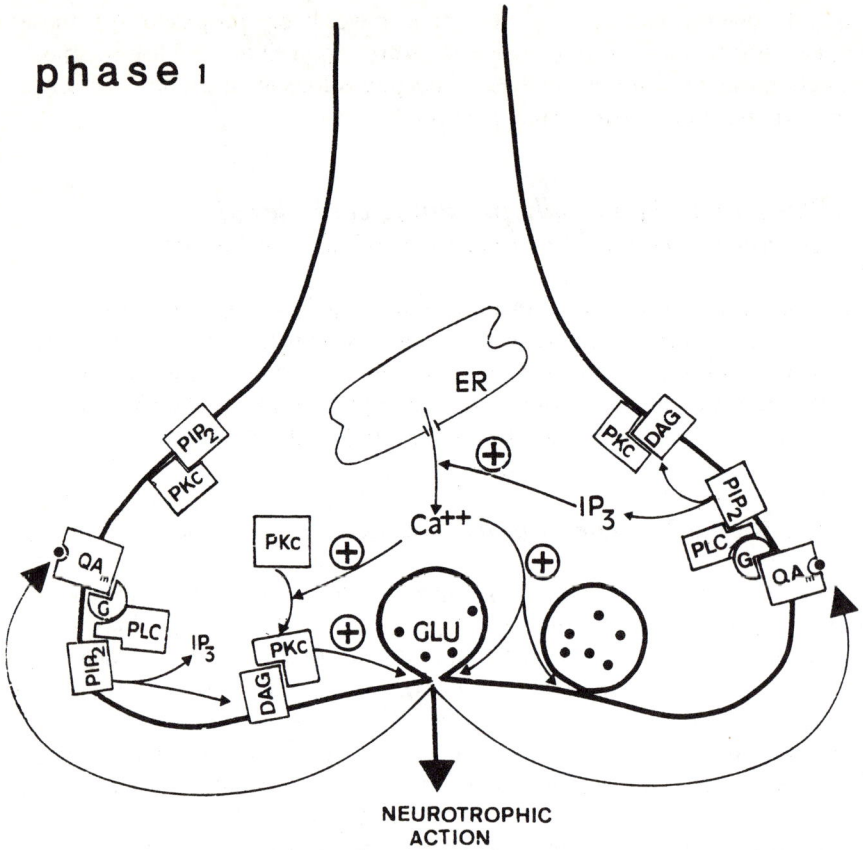

Figure 6   The possible EAA mechanisms which are involved in the establishment and the maintenance of the synapse. Phase 1: The increase in the number of metabotropic QA (QA_m) receptor subtypes, which peaks in 8-day-old rat brain (Guiramand *et al.*, 1989b) may allow the presynaptic maintenance of a constantly elevated Glu release. This released Glu may activate the presynaptic QA_m receptor, which in turn activates PKC (activation of PKC is known to augment presynaptic release: Malenka *et al.*, 1986; Shapira *et al.*, 1987; Daschmann *et al.*, 1988) and produces a rise in intracellular calcium (calcium is needed for vesicular release). This self-maintained Glu release serves as a target signal, a guide and a trophic factor for developing nerve fibres. Phase 2: The setting-up of several synaptic contacts with the nerve terminals which emit the guiding signal (sustained Glu release) leads to an increase in the postsynaptic density of Glu ionotropic and metabotropic receptors and the subsequent modifications of the neuroarchitecture of the postsynaptic areas. This may also cause a decrease in the Glu content in the synaptic cleft and a resultant diminution in the intensity of the emitted signal. The excessive stimulation of the postsynaptic NMDA receptor subtype, the density of which is maximal at 12 days (Guiramand *et al.*, 1989b), may in turn trigger toxic effects via the augmentation of calcium influx through the NMDA-associated ion channel. Consequently, some newly formed synaptic contacts may be eliminated. Phase 3: Concomitantly or following a certain time-lapse, the proliferation of glial cells and/or the growth of their extensions around the newly established synapses may

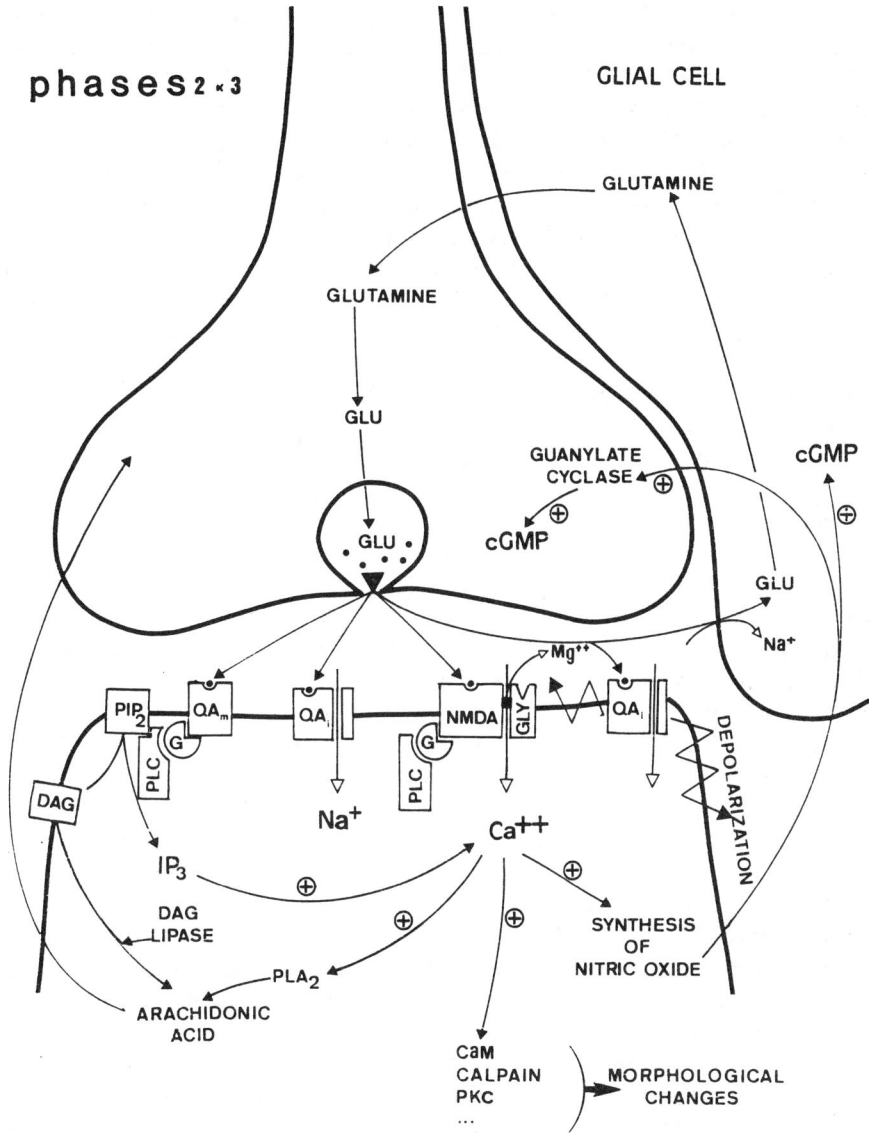

drastically reduce the intrasynaptic Glu concentration. Indeed, glial cells possess efficient, high-affinity Glu uptake mechanisms. These successive events ultimately culminate in the installation of the functional, mature synapse.

CaM, calmodulin; cGMP, cyclic GMP; DAG, diacyglycerol; ER, endoplasmic reticulum; G, GTP-binding protein; Glu, glutamate; IP_3, inositol-1,4,5-trisphosphate; PIP_2, phosphatidylinositol-4,5-bisphosphate; PKC, protein kinase C; PLA_2, phospholipase A_2; PLC, phospholipase C; NMDA, *N*-methyl-D-aspartate; NO, nitric oxide; QA_i, ionotropic quisqualate receptor; QA_m, metabotropic quisqualate receptor

may be proposed. The development of many parts of the vertebrate nervous system is characterized by an initial abundance of synaptic connections, followed or accompanied by a period of synapse elimination (Purves and Lichtman, 1980; Jackson and Parks, 1982; Mariani, 1983). Decreasing or blocking neuronal activity delays synapse elimination (Jackson, 1983; Thompson, 1983). The specific developmental pattern of EAA-induced IP response corresponds to a transitory intense biosynthesis of second messengers such as IPs and diacylglycerol, triggered first by QA or Glu and a few days later by NMDA receptor activation (Dudek *et al.*, 1989; Guiramand *et al.*, 1989b). Glu-induced IP formation increases the intracellular level of calcium (Murphy and Miller, 1988), which in turn may activate the release of neurotransmitters, including Glu from the presynaptic terminals (possibly via translocation and/or activation of PKC). Activation of PKC is known to augment both spontaneous and evoked neurotransmitter release (Wakade *et al.*, 1985; Eusebi *et al.*, 1986; Malenka *et al.*, 1986; Zurgil *et al.*, 1986; Shapira *et al.*, 1987; Daschmann *et al.*, 1988; Shuntoh *et al.*, 1989). This self-maintained neurotransmitter release of Glu could represent a target signal, a guide and a trophic factor for fibres arriving to make synapses. For instance, NMDA promotes the survival of cerebellar granule cells in culture (Balazs *et al.*, 1988a, b, 1989). After the arrival of the fibres, the postsynaptic membrane could be activated via QA and NMDA receptors. A high density of NMDA receptors is present at that time (Dupont *et al.*, 1987; Hamon and Heinemann, 1988; Tremblay *et al.*, 1988; Guiramand *et al.*, 1989b). The activation of NMDA receptors and the subsequent increase in intracellular Ca^{2+} may serve to modify the cytoarchitecture of the postsynaptic area (Lassing and Lindberg, 1985, 1988; Mattson *et al.*, 1988b). The cessation of these plastic events may occur as a result of the growth of extensions of some glial cells around the newly formed Glu synapses and/or glial cell proliferation during that period of development. The glial cells would serve to remove Glu from the extracellular space via an efficient Glu uptake mechanism (Henn *et al.*, 1974; Balcar *et al.*, 1977; Hertz *et al.*, 1978). The resulting diminution of extracellular Glu may in turn decrease the self-stimulation of the presynaptic Glu release, and the 'mature' synapse will be established (Figure 6). The local absence of surrounding glial cells may probably result in an excessive Glu stimulation of the postsynaptic fibres. This Glu overstimulation will undoubtedly trigger toxicity in the postsynapse and its subsequent elimination (Rothman, 1985; Choi, 1987). NMDA postsynaptic receptors are thus indispensable both for the modulation of the cytoarchitecture of the postsynapse and for the eventual triggering of toxicity in this scheme of synapse establishment (Figure 6). Another possible effect of the postsynaptic feedback on the presynaptic Glu release is the diffusion from the Glu-stimulated postsynaptic area of substances which are able to inhibit this presynaptic release. NMDA, for instance, is known to trigger the synthesis of arachidonic acid (Dumuis *et al.*, 1988) and of nitric oxide (NO), also known as endothelium-derived relaxing factor (Garthwaite *et al.*, 1988).

EAA Receptors and Long-term Potentiation (LTP)

Definition and Current Hypotheses

Brief trains of high-frequency electrical stimulation, delivered to monosynaptic pathways, result in a long-lasting increase in synaptic efficacy or strength. This phenomenon, termed long-term potentiation (LTP), was first observed in the dentate gyrus of the hippocampus (Lomo, 1966, 1971; Bliss and Lomo, 1973). The cellular mechanisms underlying LTP have recently been reviewed for the CA1 region of the hippocampus (Linden and Routtenberg, 1989; Malenka *et al.*, 1989a). The sequential steps leading to the establishment and the maintenance of LTP are: an increased release of Glu, following high-frequency electrical stimulation; an activation of the ionotropic QA receptor, which depolarizes the postsynaptic membrane (Muller *et al.*, 1988); a stimulation of the postsynaptic NMDA receptor complex (Collingridge *et al.*, 1983), whose blockade by physiological concentrations of Mg^{2+} ions is relieved by depolarization (Nowak *et al.*, 1984); an influx of Ca^{2+} through the voltage-gated associated NMDA channels; an activation by Ca^{2+} of calmodulin and subsequently of calcium–calmodulin kinase (Malenka *et al.*, 1989b); a modification via multistep mechanisms of the postsynaptic QA receptor (Davies *et al.*, 1989); and/or a sustained increase of Glu release (Bliss *et al.*, 1986; Errington *et al.*, 1987; Williams, J. H. *et al.*, 1989). The latter multistep mechanisms include a rapid increase in the level of immediate early gene messenger RNA *zif*/268 (Cole *et al.*, 1989) and/or c-*fos* (Szekely *et al.*, 1989).

Alternative effects of Ca^{2+} have also been proposed such as the stimulation of PKC (Lovinger *et al.*, 1986, 1987; Malinow *et al.*, 1988; Borst *et al.*, 1989; for a review, see Linden and Routtenberg, 1989) or proteases such as calpain (Lynch and Baudry, 1987).

The Possible Role of EAA Metabotropic Receptors

However, it now appears that different mechanisms may underlie LTP at different synapses. For instance, LTP at the mossy-fibre synapses in the CA3 region of the hippocampus does not seem to require the activation of NMDA receptors (Harris and Cotman, 1986). The rise in intracellular calcium, which is a key step in the triggering of LTP (Lynch *et al.*, 1983), is not necessarily produced by the influx of this ion through NMDA channels. The new Glu metabotropic receptor that we have characterized in rat forebrain synaptoneurosomes (Récasens *et al.*, 1988b) could also increase intracellular calcium, by releasing it from internal stores (Murphy and Miller, 1988). This receptor seems to be identical with that described by Sugiyama and colleagues (1987). The possible involvement of this receptor subtype in LTP is not yet substantially documented, but pertussis toxin suppresses LTP at hippocampal mossy-fibre synapses in the CA3 region (Ito *et al.*, 1988b; Goh and Pennefather, 1989). 'Another possibility' is the involvement of the metabotropic hippocampal IBO receptor, defined by Nicoletti and co-workers (1986b).

Recently it was reported that spatial learning potentiates EAA-induced IP formation (Nicoletti *et al.*, 1988). LTP is a phenomenon correlated with certain forms of learning (Swanson *et al.*, 1982).

The synaptic events underlying LTP may also be of another nature. Rather than resulting solely from changes at existing synapses, as described above, LTP may also originate from modifications in the number of functional synaptic connections. These synaptic connections may be latent and become functional as a result of stimuli (Miles and Wong, 1987). They may also stem from dendritic spine sprouting, which creates new synaptic contacts. The scheme that we have proposed above could be relevant. The EAA-induced phosphoinositide transduction system could allow, presynaptically, the maintenance of increased Glu release and, postsynaptically, the morphological changes mediated by intracellular calcium mobilization and PKC activation.

Kindling and EAA-induced Phosphoinositide Hydrolysis

Kindling is a process induced by brief, repeated subconvulsive electrical stimulations during a period of several days in the limbic brain regions. It results in the progressive and permanent intensification of electrical discharges, which culminate in generalized seizures (Goddard *et al.*, 1969). The neurochemical changes responsible for the appearance and the persistence of kindling are not well understood. Since inhibitory postsynaptic potentials are not reduced (Jibiki *et al.*, 1981; Tuff *et al.*, 1983), an enhanced excitatory transmission must be essential. The evidence supporting this hypothesis is as follows: veratrine-induced endogenous Glu release is augmented (Leach *et al.*, 1985); L-[^{3}H]Glu binding to QA-sensitive sites is increased in hippocampal synaptic membranes (Savage *et al.*, 1982); [^{3}H]D-Asp uptake is undetectable in kindled tissue (Leach *et al.*, 1987); NMDA (APV, APH, CPP, MK 801) and non-NMDA (APB, GAMS) antagonists inhibit the development of electrical kindling (Peterson *et al.*, 1983; Croucher *et al.*, 1988; Gilbert, 1988). Recently the involvement of the EAA metabotropic receptor has been proposed to be responsible for the long-lasting seizure susceptibility of amygdala/piriform cortex-kindled rats (Iadarola *et al.*, 1986; Akiyama *et al.*, 1987, 1989; Yamada *et al.*, 1989). Indeed, amygdala kindling (stage 3–4) enhances the IBO stimulation of IP synthesis in rat hippocampal slices (Iadarola *et al.*, 1986; Akiyama *et al.*, 1987), but also in the amygdala (Akiyama *et al.*, 1987). This stimulation is blocked by APB in the hippocampus (Iadarola *et al.*, 1986). The maximal increase in IBO-induced IP formation is observed in the hippocampus and amygdala, 1 day after the last electrical stimulation. In the hippocampus of amygdala-kindled animals the increment of IBO-elicited IPs returns to normal within 1 week (Akiyama *et al.*, 1989). In the amygdala the IBO-induced IP response is still present, although weaker, 1 month after the last seizure. When kindling is induced by electrical stimulation of the hippocampus (hippocampus-kindled rats), the IBO-induced IP response is also maximal 1 day after the last seizure, both in the hippocampus and in the amygdala. Even in this case, the increased IP response elicited by IBO lasts longer in the amygdala (still present after 1 month) than in the hippocampus. These results indicate that IP turnover evoked by EAA agonists increases in a long-lasting manner in the amygdala, regardless of the primary kindled area (amygdala or hippocampus). These findings suggest that the long-lasting seizure susceptibility originates primarily from the changes in the neuronal activity in the amygdala.

It could be hypothesized that electrical stimulation produces an excessive Glu release, which is partially maintained as a result of the activation of presynaptic IBO receptors coupled to phosphoinositide metabolism. Glu receptor activation may lead to the modification of presynaptic calcium channels, as was also shown for the postsynaptic calcium channels (Krishtal *et al.*, 1989). Postsynaptic metabotropic receptors could also be activated, inducing a change in the biochemical properties of the ionotropic QA receptor via intracellular calcium mobilization. Another alternative is the overstimulation of the postsynaptic NMDA receptor, which can result in a massive influx of calcium.

Nerve Sprouting or Regeneration

Lesions of nerve fibres lead to the degeneration of certain cells from which the fibres originate and of some others which are the target cells of these fibres. Lesion sequelae are then partially compensated by plastic phenomena, including glial cell proliferation and extension, nerve sprouting and new synaptic connections. Adaptive changes, which do not necessarily involve important morphological changes, also occur in the intact surrounding cells. An example is the 'receptor plasticity' which corresponds to hypo- or hypersensitivity of the receptors following the lesion.

The involvement of EAA metabotropic receptors coupled to PLC in these plastic events has been suggested by Nicoletti and colleagues (1987a). They found that chemical or surgical lesions of three glutamatergic pathways potentiate the increase of IPs elicited by EAA (IBO, Glu, QA, but not NMDA). Interestingly enough, the increased IP response in the hippocampus and the striatum of lesioned animals has a pharmacological profile similar to that observed in 6-day-old rats. One could postulate that the absence of Glu stimulation, due to the degeneration of the presynaptic fibres, results in the hypersensitivity of the postsynaptic neurons. This hypersensitivity probably arises from an increase in the number of postsynaptic receptors responsive to the usual stimuli (Glu). It could also be explained by the reversal of the feedback inhibition by PKC activation. Indeed, PKC activation by phorbol esters inhibit EAA-induced IP formation (Godfrey *et al.*, 1988; Schoepp and Johnson, 1988b; Milani *et al.*, 1989; Schoepp, 1989; Manzoni *et al.*, 1990).

Cell Growth, Differentiation, Survival and Death

The link between cell life and EAA-induced phosphoinositide breakdown has not yet been experimentally taken up. However, several reports indicate that this transduction system, in general, could be involved in the essential physiological functions of the cell—namely mitosis, growth, differentiation, survival and death (Pardee, 1989).

Subtoxic concentrations of Glu, QA and KA reduce the growth rates and lengths of dendrites without altering axonal growth in cultured hippocampal pyramidal cells (Mattson *et al.*, 1988a). NMDA receptor activation stimulates neurite outgrowth from cerebellar granule cells (Pearce *et al.*, 1987; Balazs *et al.*, 1988a) and promotes cell survival (Balazs *et al.*, 1988b). Exposure of young rat hippocampal slices to QA leads to severe 'dark cell degeneration' of pyramidal neurons (Garthwaite and Garthwaite, 1989b). This toxicity is not blocked by CNQX, which suggests that the QA metabotropic receptor is involved in the triggering of pyramidal cell death. These findings indicate that EAAs actively participate in the physiological changes that occur in the cell during its life, but the extent of the contribution made by the EAA metabotropic receptors in these events remains to be determined.

EAA Metabotropic Receptors and Pathologies

Three facts may explain the involvement of EAA in numerous pathological disorders, such as Alzheimer's disease (Greenamyre *et al.*, 1988), epilepsy (Meldrum *et al.*, 1983; Aram and Lodge, 1987), Huntington's chorea (Beal *et al.*, 1986), hypoglycaemia-induced neuronal damage (Wieloch, 1985), hepatic encephalopathy (Moroni *et al.*, 1983) and ischaemic brain damage (Simon *et al.*, 1984). First, EAA receptors are present on most, if not all, neuronal cells. Second, the intracellular Glu concentration is about 10 mM. Third, extracellular concentrations of Glu, exceeding 0.01 mM, induce neuronal damage to cells possessing a high density of EAA receptors. Taken together, these facts indicate that an excessive Glu release leads inexorably to the death of surrounding cells enriched in EAA receptors. Massive Glu release is caused by overstimulation of some pathways (epilepsy), by persistent depolarization (as is the case in ischaemia, where there is a lack of energy for the maintenance of ionic gradients on the two sides of the cell membrane) or by cell degeneration, as occurs in trauma or ageing. In the last two cases Glu release comes from both its neurotransmitter and metabolic pools. In kindled animals (Iadarola *et al.*, 1986; Akiyama *et al.*, 1987, 1989; Yamada *et al.*, 1989), after transient ischaemia (Chen *et al.*, 1988; Seren *et al.*, 1989) or lesions of putative glutamatergic pathways (Nicoletti *et al.*, 1987a), an increase in EAA-induced IP response has been observed. At least three hypotheses may be proposed to explain why IP formation is augmented:

1. The excessive Glu release produced in these pathological states may induce a considerable stimulation of the presynaptic EAA metabotropic receptor. This may serve to maintain a continuously enhanced Glu release, as we proposed in the developmental scheme shown in Figure 6. This will lead to the expression of toxicity in the postsynapse, mainly via NMDA receptor activation. In fact, NMDA antagonists protect against ischaemic damage (Simon *et al.*, 1984). However, the involvement of other EAA receptors is also possible.

2. Postsynaptic EAA metabotopic receptors may be involved in the expression of EAA neurotoxicity. Indeed, we have hypothesized that these receptors are involved in the establishment of the shape of the postsynaptic element during development. The functioning of these receptors is probably inhibited later on by the setting up of the synaptic activity. This includes the activation of NMDA receptors which trigger an influx of Ca^{2+}, subsequently causing PKC translocation to the cell membrane. PKC may in turn inhibit EAA-induced IP formation. In the established synapse, Glu may preferentially act on the ionotropic NMDA receptor rather than on the EAA metabotropic receptors, owing to their respective affinities. The excessive, external Glu concentration may remove this feedback inhibition and trigger postsynaptic morphological changes and toxicity, via an overmobilization of intracellular calcium.

3. Enhanced IP accumulation observed after an ischaemic episode may also result from the proliferation of glial cells in the damaged area. Glial cells possess EAA metabotropic receptors (Pearce *et al.*, 1986; Milani *et al.*, 1989). However, APB blocks EAA-elicited IP formation after lesions of putative glutamatergic pathways (Nicoletti *et al.*, 1987a), and not that evoked by EAA in astrocytes (Milani *et al.*, 1989). Nevertheless, this evidence cannot be relied upon, since dose-dependent inhibitions by APB have not yet been performed in glial cells.

In conclusion, it seems that the permanent 'repression' of the EAA metabotropic receptors, in adult animals, may be one of the guarantors for the efficient functioning of the glutamatergic synapse.

6. Conclusion

It is now clear that the previous classification into three receptor subtypes must be reviewed. At least four receptors are responsible for the EAA actions: three ionotropic EAA receptor subtypes, which could be named NMDA, AMPA (ionotropic QA receptor: QA_i) and KA and one metabotropic receptor, where QA is the most potent agonist. This receptor is tentatively named QA or QA_m. It must be noted that a nomenclature based on the name of the most selective ligand is not the best choice, since the discovery of each

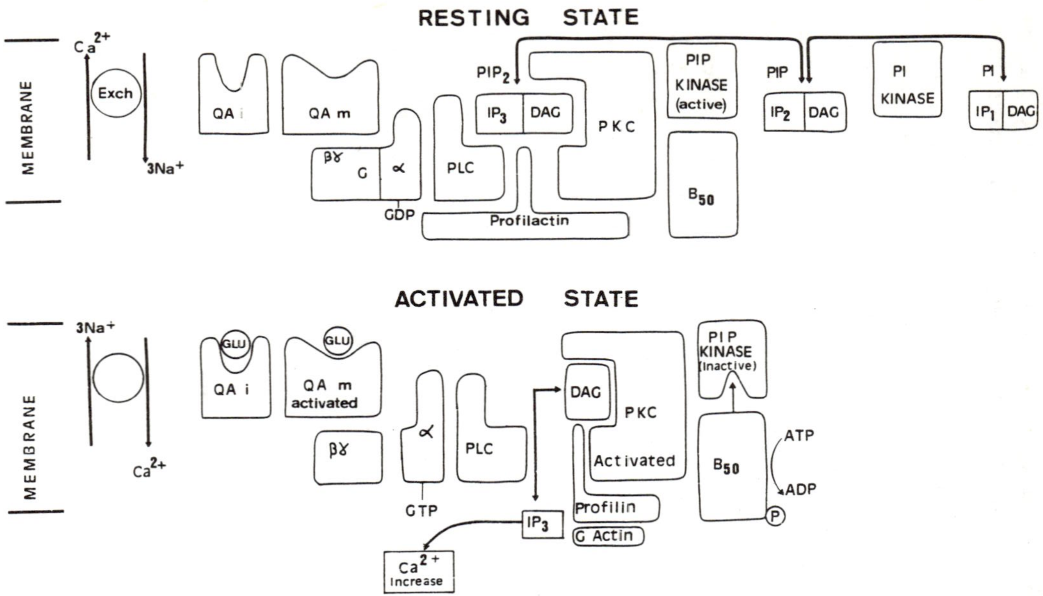

Figure 7 Effects of EAA metabotropic receptor activation on the membrane molecular events. Glu binding to the QA_m receptor activates PLC via a G protein. The G protein is a heterotrimer composed of α, β and γ subunits. The replacement of GDP by GTP on the α subunit leads to the dissociation of the α subunit from the $\beta-\gamma$ complex and the resultant α subunit binds to the PLC enzyme. The PLC enzyme, thus activated, catalyses the breakdown of PIP_2 into IP_3 and DAG and causes the dissociation of the profilactin complex to release G-actin into the cytosol. DAG activates PKC, which phosphorylates the B_{50} protein, which in turn inhibits the PIP kinase (note that DAG, PIP_2 and phorbol ester all compete for the same activator-receiving region of PKC: Chauhan et al., 1989). The functioning of the Na^+/Ca^{2+} exchanger is locally reversed by depolarization.

B_{50}, 50 kD substrate protein of PKC; DAG, diacylglycerol; Exch, Na^+/Ca^{2+} exchanger; G, GTP binding protein; IP_1, inositol-1-phosphate; IP_2, inositol-1,4-phosphate; IP_3, inositol-1,4,5-trisphosphate; PI, phosphatidylinositol; PIP, phosphatidylinositol-4-phosphate; PIP_2, phosphatidylinositol-4,5-bisphosphate; PLC, phospholipase C; PKC, protein kinase C; QA_i, ionotropic quisqualate receptor; QA_m, metabotropic quisqualate receptor

new ligand with improved potency will oblige nomenclature modification. On the other hand, one must follow the traditional terminology in this field. The existence of other receptors have been proposed on the basis of the antagonistic properties of APB in some hippocampal pathways and on the stimulating action of IBO on IP metabolism in adult rat hippocampal slices. This stimulating effect on the phosphoinositide turnover is blocked by APB (Nicoletti *et al.*, 1986b). However, we did not find an inhibitory effect of APB in neonatal and adult rat forebrain synaptoneurosomes. Sugiyama and his colleagues (1989), using *Xenopus* oocytes injected with rat brain mRNA, reported findings similar to ours. Consequently, it must be first demonstrated that the blocking action of APB does not result from an indirect effect of this compound in slices before it can be concluded that a new IBO metabotropic receptor exists.

The putative molecular mechanisms by which the activation of the EAA metabotropic receptor (QA_m) generates the two second messengers, trigger cellular responses and then return to its resting state, are summarized in Figures 7 and 8. None of the various steps proposed have yet been demonstrated. There is merely an indication of some of the future directions that could be explored.

Finally, our data and those presented in this chapter suggest that the main physiological function of the EAA-metabotropic receptor is fully expressed during a narrow period of the development. At this stage, the activation of such a receptor may play a key role for the establishment, the regression and the stabilization of some synapses, as presented in Figure 6. After this period, the role of EAA-metabotropic receptors may be essential for limited plastic events (though of fundamental importance), such as LTP. They may also play a key role in the compensatory phenomena that occur after neuronal damage, whatever the origin.

Further research in this fascinating field will surely yield promising insights into the plasticity phenomena that accompany many essential higher brain functions.

Acknowledgements

We should like to thank Professor P. Ascher, who kindly agreed to provide general comments on this review. Helpful discussion with Professor R. Pujol is deeply appreciated. We are also indebted to F. Lebrun, I. Sassetti, M. Gallego, S. Bartolami and M. Vignes, who recently joined our group and generously provided their assistance in the preparation of this review. We also thank A. Bara for the layout of the tables and the abbreviations section.

Some of the work presented in this review was supported by grants from CNAMTS-INSERM, MRES, Air Liquide, IPSEN and Institut H. Beaufour.

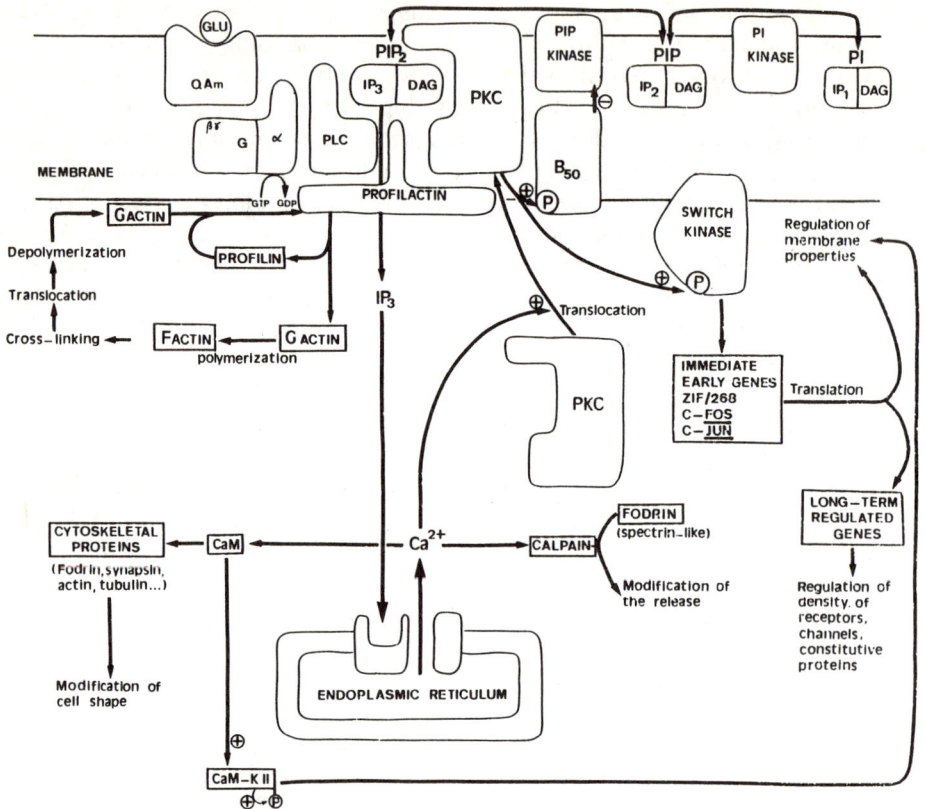

Figure 8 Perspectives on the putative membrane and intracellular changes that occur following the activation of the metabotropic quisqualate receptor. The ultimate activation of PLC after glutamate binding to QA_m may cause the dissociation of the profilactin complex to liberate G-actin. The latter, in the presence of high intracellular concentrations of calcium, triggered by IP_3, can polymerize to form F-actin, which in turn can undergo cross-linkage, thus leading to microfilament assembly. The calcium increase activates a number of cellular proteins, including calpain I, calmodulin, protein kinase C, adducin, etc. Calpain, a calcium-dependent neutral protease, is known to degrade spectrin, fodrin (a spectrin-like protein) and MAP2. The calcium augmentation also favours the translocation and the activation of PKC, which phosphorylates, among other proteins, the B_{50}, which in turn inactivates the PIP-kinase. This effect corresponds to a negative feedback mechanism on the stimulation of phosphoinositide metabolism. Calmodulin activated by calcium causes the de-polymerization of microtubules and affects other cytoskeletal proteins. All in all, one may conclude that the rise in intracellular calcium, following QA_m activation, may induce the partial degradation of the existing cytoskeleton (via, for instance, calpain and calmodulin) and immediate reorganization via profilactin. Long-term changes may occur following QA_m stimulation by at least two pathways, which are linked to switch kinase and calcium–calmodulin kinase. The phosphorylation of switch kinases, catalysed by PKC, enables them to act on immediate early genes, whose ultimate translation may change the properties of certain membrane proteins. The translation products of the immediate early genes may also affect the expression of long-term regulated genes, which eventually could modify the density of membrane proteins.

Abbreviations

α-AA	α-amino adipate
ACBC	1-amino cyclobutane-1-carboxylate
ACC	1-aminocyclopropane-1-carboxylic acid
AMPA	α-amino-3-hydroxy-5-methyl-4-isoxazole propionic acid
APB	2-amino-4-phosphonobutyrate
APH	amino-phosphono-heptanoate
APP	2-amino-3-propionate
APV	2-amino-5-phosphonovalerate
Asp	aspartate
CA	cysteate
CGS 19755	*cis*-4-phosphonomethyl-2-piperidine-carboxylic acid
CNQX (FG 9065)	6-nitro-7-cyanoquinoxaline-2,3-dion
CPP	3-[+]-2-(carboxypiperazin-4-yl)-propyl-1-phosphonic acid
CSA	cysteine sulphinate
DAG	diacylglycerol
DAP	D-α-aminopimelic acid
DAS	D-α-aminosuberic acid
γ-DGG, gamma-DGG	gamma-D-glutamylglycine
DIDS	4,4′-diisothiocyanatostilbene-2,2′-disulphonic acid
DNQX	6,7-dinitro-quinoxaline-2,3-dion
EAA	excitatory amino acid
FG 9065	*see* CNQX
GAMS	alpha-D-glutamylaminomethylsulphonate
GDEE	glutamate diethylester
Glu	glutamate
γ-GT	γ-glutamyltaurine
HA 966	1-hydroxy-3-aminopyrrolidone-2
HCA	homocysteate
HCSA	homocystein sulphinate
IBO	ibotenate
I2CA	indole-2-carboxylic acid
IP	inositol phosphate
IP_1	inositol-4-monophosphate
IP_2	inositol-1,4-bisphosphate
IP_3	inositol-1,4,5-trisphosphate
IP_4	inositol-1,3,4,5-tetrakisphosphate
IP_6	inositol hexakisphosphate or phytate
JSTX	Joro spider toxin
KA	kainate
Kyn	kynurenate
MK 801	[+]-5-methyl-10,11-dihydro-5*H*-dibenzo [a,c] cyclohepten-5,10-imine maleate
mRNA	messenger ribonucleic acid
NAAG	*N*-acetyl-aspartyl-glutamate
NANM	*see* SKF 10047
NMDA	*N*-methyl-D-aspartate
PCA (PDA)	2,3-*cis*-piperidine carboxylic acid
PCP	phencyclidine

Figure 8 (*continued*)   Calcium–calmodulin kinase II (CaM-K II) may undergo activation by autophosphorylation, which is a manifestation of a permanent change after stimuli (a possible explanation for LTP). This sustained enzymic activation may lead to the persistent changes in the properties of certain membrane proteins.

The abbreviations used in this figure have been defined in the captions to Figures 6 and 7

PDA (PCA)	2,3-*cis*-piperidine dicarboxylate
PDB	phorbol 12,13-dibutyrate
α-PDD	α-phorbol-12,13-didecanoate
PI	phosphatidylinositol
PIC	phosphoinositidase C
PIP	phosphatidylinositol-4-phosphate
PIP$_2$	phosphatidylinositol-4,5-bisphosphate
PKC	protein kinase C
PLC	phospholipase C
PMA	phorbol 12-myristate 13-acetate
QA	quisqualate
SKF 10047	*N*-allyl-normetazocine (NANM)
SOP	L-serine-*O*-phosphate
SOS	serine-*O*-sulphate
TCP	1-(1-(2-thienyl)-cyclohexyl) piperidine
Trans-ACPD	*trans*-1-amino-cyclopentyl-1,3-dicarboxylic acid
Tris	Tris(hydroxymethyl)aminomethane
TTX	Tetrodotoxin

References

Abe, T., Kawai, N. and Miwa, A. (1983). Effects of a spider toxin on the glutaminergic synapse of lobster muscle. *J. Physiol.*, **339**, 243–252

Akiyama, K., Yamada, N. and Sato, M. (1987). Increase in ibotenate-stimulated phosphatidylinositol hydrolysis in slices of the amygdala/pyriform cortex and hippocampus of rat by amygdala kindling. *Exp. Neurol.*, **98**, 499–508

Akiyama, K., Yamada, N. and Otsuki, S. (1989). Lasting increase in excitatory amino acid receptor-mediated polyphosphoinositide hydrolysis in the amygdala/pyriform cortex of amygdala-kindled rats. *Brain Res.*, **485**, 95–101

Ambrosini, A. and Meldolesi, J. (1989). Muscarinic and quisqualate receptor-induced phosphoinositide hydrolysis in primary cultures of striatal and hippocampal neurons. Evidence for differential mechanisms of activation. *J. Neurochem.*, **53**, 825–833

Aramaki, Y., Yasuhara, T., Higashijima, T., Yoshioka, M., Miwa, A., Kawai, N. and Nakajima, T. (1986). Chemical characterization of spider toxin, JSTX and NSTX. *Proc. Jap. Acad. Sci.*, **62**, 359–362

Aram, J. A. and Lodge, D. (1987). NMA receptors and different types of epileptiform activity in rat cortical slices. *J. Physiol. (Lond.)*, **382**, 89P

Arkin, M. S. and Miller, R. F. (1987). Subtle actions of 2-amino-4-phosphonobutyrate (APB) on the OFF pathway in the mudpuppy retina. *Brain Res.*, **426**, 142–148

Ascher, P. (1988). Divalent cations and the NMDA channel. *Biomed. Res.*, **9**, Suppl. 2, 31–37

Ascher, P. and Nowak, L. (1986). Calcium permeability of the channels activated by *N*-methyl-D-aspartate (NMDA) in mouse central neurones. *J. Physiol. (Lond.)*, **377**, 43P

Ascher, P. and Nowak, L. (1988a). The role of divalent cations in the *N*-methyl-D-aspartate responses of mouse central neurones in culture. *J. Physiol. (Lond.)*, **399**, 247–266

Ascher, P. and Nowak, L. (1988b). Quisqualate- and kainate-activated channels in mouse central neurones in culture. *J. Physiol. (Lond.)*, **399**, 227–245

Ascher, P., Bregestovski, P. and Nowak, L. (1988). *N*-Methyl-D-aspartate-activated ion channels of mouse central neurones in magnesium-free solutions. *J. Physiol. (Lond.)*, **399**, 207–226

Baba, A., Lee, E., Tatsuno, T. and Iwata, H. (1982). Cysteine sulfinic acid in the central nervous system: Antagonistic effect of taurine on cysteine sulfinic acid-stimulated formation of cyclic AMP in guinea pig hippocampal slices. *J. Neurochem.*, **38**, 1280–1285

Baird, J. G. and Nahorski, S. R. (1986). Potassium depolarization markedly changes muscarinic receptor stimulated inositol tetrakisphosphate accumulation in rat cerebral cortical slices *Biochem. Biophys. Res. Commun.*, **141**, 1130–1137

Balcar, V. J., Borg, J. and Mandel, P. (1977). High affinity uptake of L-glutamate and L-aspartate by glial cells. *J. Neurochem.*, **28**, 87–93

Balazs, R., Hack, N. and Jorgensen, O. S. (1988a). Stimulation of the *N*-methyl-D-aspartate receptor has a trophic effect on differentiating cerebellar granule cells. *Neurosci. Lett.*, **87**, 80–86

Balazs, R., Hack, N., Jorgensen, O. S. and Cotman, C. W. (1989). *N*-Methyl-D-aspartate promotes the survival of cerebellar granule cells: pharmacological characterization. *Neurosci. Lett.*, **101**, 241–246

Balazs, R., Jorgensen, O. S. and Hack, N. (1988b). *N*-Methyl-D-aspartate promotes the survival of cerebellar granule cells in culture. *Neuroscience*, **27**, 437–451

Barcenas-Ruiz, L., Beuckelmann, D. J. and Wier, W. G. (1987). Sodium-calcium exchange in heart: Membrane currents and changes in $[Ca^{2+}]_i$. *Science, N.Y.*, **238**, 1720–1722

Baudry, M., Evans, J. and Lynch, G. (1986). Excitatory amino acids inhibit stimulation of phosphatidylinositol metabolism by aminergic agonists in hippocampus. *Nature*, **319**, 329–331

Baudry, M., Kramer, K., Fagni, L., Récasens, M. and Lynch, G. (1983). Classification and properties of acidic amino acid receptors in hippocampus. II. Biochemical studies using a sodium efflux assay. *Mol. Pharmacol.*, **24**, 222–228

Beal, M. F., Kowall, N. W., Ellison, D. W., Mazurek, M. F., Swartz, K. J. and Martin, J. B. (1986). Replication of the neurochemical characteristics of Huntington's disease by quinolinic acid. *Nature*, **321**, 168–171

Bennett, C. F. and Crooke, S. T. (1987). Purification and characterization of a phosphoinositide-specific phospholipase C from guinea pig uterus. *J. Biol. Chem.*, **262**, 13789–13797

Berridge, M. J. (1984). Inositol trisphosphate and diacylglycerol as second messengers. *Biochem. J.*, **220**, 345–360

Berridge, M. J. (1987). Inositol trisphosphate and diacylglycerol: two interacting second messengers. *Ann. Rev. Biochem.*, **56**, 159–193

Berridge, M. J. and Irvine, R. F. (1984). Inositol trisphosphate, a novel second messenger in cellular signal transduction. *Nature*, **312**, 315–321

Berridge, M. J. and Irvine, R. F. (1989). Inositol phosphates and cell signalling. *Nature*, **341**, 197–205

Bliss, T. V. P. and Lomo, T. (1973). Long lasting potentiation of synaptic transmission in the dentate area of the anaesthetized rabbit following stimulation of the perforant path. *J. Physiol. (Lond.)*, **232**, 331–356

Bliss, T. V. P., Douglas, R. M., Errington, M. L. and Lynch, M. A. (1986). Correlation between long-term potentiation and release of endogenous amino acids from dentate gyrus of anaesthetized rats. *J. Physiol. (Lond.)*, **377**, 391–408

Borst, J. G. G., Melchers, B. P. C. and Lopes da Silva, F. H. (1989). Effect of different concentrations of phorbol ester on tetanus-induced long-term potentiation in the rat hippocampus. *Neurosci. Res. Commun.*, **4**, 11–16

Bowers, C. W. A. (1985). A cadmium-sensitive, tetrodotoxin-resistant sodium channel in bullfrog autonomic axons. *Brain Res.*, **340**, 143–147

Brass, L. F., Woolkalis, M. J. and Manning, D. R. (1988). Interactions in platelets betwen G proteins and the agonists that stimulate phospholipase C and inhibit adenylyl cyclase. *J. Biol. Chem.*, **263**, 5348–5355

Brose, N., Halpain, S., Suchanek, C. and Jahn, R. (1989). Characterization and partial purification of a chloride- and calcium-dependent glutamate-binding protein from rat brain. *J. Biol. Chem.*, **264**, 9619–9625

Butcher, S. P., Lazarewicz, J. W. and Hamberger, A. (1987). *In vivo* microdialysis studies on the effects of decortication and excitotoxic lesions on kainic acid-induced calcium fluxes, and endogenous amino acid release, in the rat striatum. *J. Neurochem.*, **49**, 1355–1360

Campochiaro, P., Ferkany, J. W. and Coyle J. T. (1985). Excitatory amino acid analogs evoke release of endogenous amino acids and acetylcholine from chick retina *in vitro*. *Vision Res.*, **25**, 1375–1386

Canonico, P. L., Favit, A., Catania, M. V. and Nicoletti, F. (1988). Phorbol esters attenuate glutamate-stimulated inositol phospholipid hydrolysis in neuronal cultures. *J. Neurochem.*, **51**, 1049–1053

Carter, C., Rivy, J.-P. and Scatton, B. (1989). Ifenprodil and SL 82.0715 are antagonists at the polyamine site of the *N*-methyl-D-aspartate (NMDA) receptor. *Eur. J. Pharmacol.*, **164**, 611–612

Cha, J.-H. J., Greenamyre, T., Nielsen, E. O., Penney, J. B. and Young, A. B. (1988). Properties of quisqualate-sensitive L-[³H]glutamate binding sites in rat brain as determined by quantitative autoradiography. *J. Neurochem.*, **51**, 469–478

Chauhan, A., Chauhan, V. P. S., Deshmukh, D. S. and Brockerhoff, H. (1989). Phosphatidylinositol 4,5-bisphosphate competitively inhibits phorbol ester binding to protein kinase C. *Biochemistry*, **28**, 4952–4956

Chen, C.-K., Silverstein, F. S., Fisher, S. K., Statman, D. and Johnston, M. V. (1988). Perinatal hypoxic-ischemic brain injury enhances quisqualic acid-stimulated phosphoinositide turnover. *J. Neurochem.*, **51**, 353–359

Cheramy, A., Romo, R., Godeheu, G., Baruch, P. and Glowinski, J. (1986). *In vivo* presynaptic control of dopamine release in the cat caudate nucleus. II. Facilitatory or inhibitory influence of L-glutamate. *Neuroscience*, **19**, 1081–1090

Choi, D. W. (1987). Ionic dependence of glutamate neurotoxicity. *J. Neuroscience*, **7**, 369–379

Chuang, D.-M. (1989). Neurotransmitter receptors and phosphoinositide turnover. *Ann. Rev. Pharmacol. Toxicol.*, **29**, 71–110

Clow, D. W. and Jhamandas, K. (1988). Characterization of L-glutamate action on the release of endogenous dopamine from the rat caudate putamen. *J. Pharmacol. Exp. Ther.*, **248**, 722–728

Cole, A. J., Saffen, D. W., Baraban, J. M. and Worley, P. F. (1989). Rapid increase of an immediate early gene messenger RNA in hippocampal neurons by synaptic NMDA receptor activation. *Nature*, **340**, 474–476

Collingridge, G. L., Kehl, S. J. and McLennan (1983). Excitatory amino acids in synaptic transmission in the Schaffer collateral-commissural pathway of the rat hippocampus. *J. Physiol. (Lond.)*, **334**, 33–46

Court, J. A., Fowler, C. J., Candy, J. M., Hoban, P. R. and Smith, C. J. (1986). Raising the ambient potassium ion concentration enhances carbachol stimulated phosphoinositide hydrolysis in rat brain hippocampal and cerebral cortical miniprisms. *Naunyn-Schmiedebergs Arch. Pathol. Exp. Pharmacol.*, **334**, 10–16

Croucher, M. J., Bradford, H. F., Sunter, D. C. and Watkins, J. C. (1988). Inhibition of the development of electrical kindling of the prepyriform cortex by daily focal injections of excitatory amino acid antagonists. *Eur. J. Pharmacol.*, **152**, 29–38

Daschmann, B., Allgaier, C., Nakov, R. and Hertting, G. (1988). Staurosporine counteracts the phorbol ester-induced enhancement of neurotransmitter release in hippocampus. *Arch. Int. Pharmacodyn. Ther.*, **296**, 232–245

Davies, S. N., Lester, R. A. J., Reyman, K. G. and Collingridge, G. L. (1989). Temporally distinct pre- and post-synaptic mechanisms maintain long-term potentiation. *Nature*, **338**, 500–503

Dawson, R. M. C. and Dittmer, J. C. (1961). Evidence for the structure of brain triphosphoinositide from hydrolytic degradation studies. *Biochem. J.*, **81**, 540–545

Dittmer, J. C. and Dawson, R. M. C. (1961). The isolation of a new lipid, triphosphoinositide and monophosphoinositide from ox brain. *Biochem. J.*, **81**, 535–540

Do, K. Q., Mattenberger, M., Streit, P. and Cuenod, M. (1986). *In vitro* release of endogenous excitatory sulfur-containing amino acids from various rat brain regions. *J. Neurochem.*, **46**, 779–786

Doble, A. and Perrier, M. L. (1989). Pharmacology of excitatory amino acid receptors coupled to inositol phosphate metabolism in neonatal rat striatum. *Neurochem. Int.*, **15**, 1–8

Drejer, J. and Honoré, T. (1988). New quinoxalinediones show potent antagonism of quisqualate responses in cultured mouse cortical neurons. *Neurosci. Lett.*, **87**, 104–108

Drejer, J., Honoré, T. and Schousboe, A. (1987). Excitatory amino acid-induced release of ^{3}H-GABA from cultured mouse cerebral cortex interneurons. *J. Neurosci.*, **7**, 2910–2916

Drejer, J., Sheardown, M., Nielsen, E. and Honoré, T. (1989). Glycine reverses the effect of HA-966 on NMDA responses in cultured rat cortical neurons and in chick retina. *Neurosci. Lett.*, **98**, 333–338

Dudek, S. M., Bowen, W. D. and Bear, M. F. (1989). Postnatal changes in glutamate stimulated phosphoinositide turnover in rat neocortical synaptoneurosomes. *Dev. Brain Res.*, **47**, 123–128

Dumuis, A., Sebben, M., Haynes, L., Pin, J.-P. and Bockaert, J. (1988). NMDA receptors activate the arachidonic cascade system in striatal neurons. *Nature*, **336**, 68–70

Durell, J. Garland, J. T. and Friedel, R. O. (1969). Acetylcholine action: biochemical aspects. Two major approaches to understanding the mechanism of action of acetylcholine are examined. *Science, N.Y.*, **165**, 862–866

Dupont, J.-L., Gardette, R. and Crepel, F. (1987). Postnatal development of the chemosensitivity of rat cerebellar Purkinje cells to excitatory amino acids. An *in vitro* study. *Dev. Brain Res.*, **34**, 59–68

Eberhard, D. A. and Holz, R. W. (1988). Intracellular Ca^{2+} activates phopholipase C. *Trends Neurosci.*, **11**, 517–520

Errington, M. L., Lynch, M. A. and Bliss, T. V. P. (1987). Long-term potentiation in the dentate gyrus: induction and increased glutamate release are blocked by D(-)aminophosphonovalerate. *Neuroscience*, **20**, 279–284

Eusebi, F., Molinaro, M. and Caratsch, C. G. (1986). Effects of phorbol ester on spontaneous transmitter release at frog neuromuscular junction. *Pflügers Arch.*, **406**, 181–183

Fagg, G. E., Foster, A. C., Mena, E. E. and Cotman, C. W. (1982). Chloride and calcium ions reveal a pharmacologically distinct population of L-glutamate binding sites in synaptic membranes: correspondence between biochemical and electrophysiological data. *J. Neurosci.*, **2**, 958–965

Fagg, G. E., Foster, A. C. and Ganong, A. H. (1986). Excitatory amino acid mechanisms and neurological function. *Trends Pharmacol. Sci.*, **7**, 357–363

Fagg, G. E. and Matus, A. (1984). Selective association of N-methyl-D-aspartate and quisqualate types of L-glutamate receptor with postsynaptic densities. *Proc. Natl Acad. Sci. USA*, **81**, 6876–6880

Fink, K., Göthert, M., Molderings, G. and Sclicker, E. (1989). N-Methyl-D-aspartate (NMDA) receptor mediated stimulation of noradrenaline release, but not release of other neurotransmitters in the rat brain cortex: receptor location, characterization and desensitization. *Naunyn-Schmiedebergs Arch. Pathol. Exp. Pharmacol.*, **339**, 514–521

Fischer, S. K. (1986). Inositol lipids and signal transduction at CNS muscarinic receptors. *Trends Pharmacol. Sci.* (Suppl.), 61–65

Fischer, S. K. and Agranoff, B. W. (1987). Receptor activation and inositol lipid hydrolysis in neural tissues. *J. Neurochem.*, **48**, 999–1016

Fong, T. M., Davidson, N. and Lester, H. A. (1988). Properties of two classes of rat brain acidic amino acid receptors induced by distinct mRNA populations in *Xenopus* oocytes. *Synapse*, **2**, 657–665

Folch, J. (1949). Brain diphosphoinositide, a new phosphatide having inositol metadiphosphate as a constituent. *J. Biol. Chem.*, **177**, 505–519

Fonnum, F. (1984). Glutamate: a neurotransmitter in mammalian brain. *J. Neurochem.*, **42**, 1–11

Frelin, C., Cognard, C., Vigne, P. and Lazdunski, M. (1986). Tetrodotoxin-sensitive and tetrodotoxin-resistant Na$^+$ channels differ in their sensitivity to Cd^{2+} and Zn^{2+}. *Eur. J. Pharmacol.*, **122**, 245–250

Furuya, S., Ohmori, H., Shigemoto, T. and Sugiyama, H. (1989). Intracellular calcium mobilization triggered by a glutamate receptor in rat cultured hippocampal cells. *J. Physiol. (Lond.)*, **414**, 539–548

Gallo, V., Ciotti, M. T., Coletti, A., Aloisi, F. and Levi, G. (1982). Selective release of glutamate from cerebellar granule cells differentiating in culture. *Proc. Natl Acad. Sci. USA*, **79**, 7919–7923

Gallo, V., Suergiu, R., Giovannini, C. and Levi, G. (1987). Glutamate receptor subtypes in cultured cerebellar neurons: modulation of glutamate and γ-aminobutyric acid release. *J. Neurochem.*, **49**, 1801–1809

Garthwaite, J., Charles, S. L. and Chess-Williams, R. (1988). Endothelium-derived relaxing factor release on activation of NMDA receptors suggests role as intercellular messenger in the brain. *Nature*, **336**, 385–388

Garthwaite, G. and Garthwaite, J. (1989a). Differential dependence on Ca^{2+} of N-methyl-D-aspartate and quisqualate neurotoxicity in young rat hippocampal slices. *Neurosci. Lett.*, **97**, 316–322

Garthwaite, G. and Garthwaite, J. (1989b). Quisqualate neurotoxicity: a delayed, CNQX-sensitive process triggered by a CNQX-insensitive mechanism in young rat hippocampal slices. *Neurosci. Lett.*, **99**, 113–118

Gay, V. L. and Plant, T. M. (1987). N-Methyl-D,L-aspartate elicits hypothalamic gonadotropin-releasing hormone release in prepubertal male rhesus monkeys (*Macaca mulatta*). *Endocrinology*, **120**, 2289–2296

Gilbert, M. E. (1988). The NMDA-receptor antagonist, MK-801, suppresses limbic kindling and kindled seizures. *Brain Res.*, **463**, 90–99

Gilman, A. G. (1987). G proteins: transducers of receptor-generated signals. *Ann. Rev. Biochem.*, **56**, 615–649

Goddard, G. V., McIntyre, D. C. and Leech, C. K. (1969). A permanent change in brain function resulting from daily electrical stimulation. *Exp. Neurol.*, **25**, 295–330

Godfrey, P. P., Wilkins, C. J. Tyler, W. and Watson, S. P. (1988). Stimulatory and inhibitory actions of excitatory amino acids on inositol phospholipid metabolism in rat cerebral cortex. *Br. J. Pharmacol.*, **95**, 131–138

Goh, J. W. and Pennefather, P. S. (1989). A pertussis toxin-sensitive G protein in hippocampal long-term potentiation. *Science, N.Y.*, **244**, 980–983

Gomperts, B. D. (1983). Involvement of guanine nucleotide binding protein in the gating of Ca^{2+} by receptors. *Nature*, **306**, 64–66

Gonzales, R. A. and Moerschbaecher, J. M. (1989). A phencyclidine recognition site is associated with N-methyl-D-aspartate inhibition of carbachol-stimulated phosphoinositide hydrolysis in rat cortical slices. *Molec. Pharmacol.*, **35**, 787–794

Gonzales, R. A., Greger, P. H. Jr, Baker, S. P., Ganz, N. I., Bolden, C., Raizada, M. H. and Crews, F. T. (1987). Phorbol esters inhibit agonist-stimulated phosphoinositide hydrolysis in neuronal primary cultures. *Dev. Brain Res.*, **37**, 59–66

Greenamyre, J. T., Maragos, W. F., Albin, R. L., Penney, J. B. and Young, A. B. (1988). Glutamate transmission and toxicity in Alzheimer disease. *Prog. Neuro-Psychopharmacol. Biol. Psychiat.*, **12**, 421–430

Guiramand, J., Nourigat, A., Sassetti, I. and Récasens, M. (1989a). K^+ differentially affects the excitatory amino acids- and carbachol-elicited inositol phosphate formation in rat brain synaptoneurosomes. *Neurosci. Lett.*, **98**, 222–228

Guiramand, J., Sassetti, I. and Récasens, M. (1989b). Developmental changes in the chemo-sensitivity of rat brain synaptoneurosomes to excitatory amino acids, estimated by inositol phosphate formation. *Int. J. Dev. Neurosci.*, **7**, 257–266

Gusovsky, F., Hollingsworth, E. B. and Daly, J. W. (1986). Regulation of phosphatidylinositol turnover in brain synaptoneurosomes: stimulatory effects of agents that enhance influx of sodium ions. *Proc. Natl Acad. Sci. USA*, **83**, 3003–3007

Gusovsky, F., McNeal, E. T. and Daly, J. W. (1987). Stimulation of phosphoinositide breakdown in brain synaptoneurosomes by agents that activate sodium influx: antagonism by tetrodotoxin, saxitoxin, and cadmium. *Molec. Pharmacol.*, **32**, 479–487

Gusovsky, F. and Daly, J. W. (1988a). Formation of inositol phosphates in synaptoneurosomes of guinea pig brain: stimulatory effects of receptor agonists, sodium channel agents and sodium and calcium ionophores. *Neuropharmacology*, **27**, 95–105

Gusovsky, F. and Daly, J. W. (1988b). Formation of second messengers in response to activation of ion channels in excitable cells. *Cell. Molec. Neurobiol.*, **8**, 157–169

Hamon, B. and Heinemann, U. (1988). Developmental changes in neuronal sensitivity to excitatory amino acids in area CA1 of the rat hippocampus. *Dev. Brain Res.*, **38**, 286–290

Harris, K. M. and Miller, R. J. (1989). CNQX (6-cyano-7-nitroquinoxaline-2,3-dione) antago-nizes NMDA-evoked [^{3}H]GABA release from cultured cortical neurons via an inhibitory action at the strychnine-insensitive glycine site. *Brain Res.*, **489**, 185–189

Harris, E. W. and Cotman, C. W. (1986). Long-term potentiation of guinea pig mossy fiber responses is not blocked by N-methyl-D-aspartate antagonists. *Neurosci. Lett.*, **70**, 132–137

Henn, F. A., Goldstein, M. N. and Hamberger, A. (1974). Uptake of the neurotransmitter glutamate by glia. *Nature*, **249**, 663–664

Hertz, L., Schousboe, A., Boechler, N., Mukerji, S. and Fedoroff, S. (1978). Kinetic characteristics of glutamate uptake into normal astrocytes in cultures. *Neurochem. Res.*, **3**, 1–14

Heuschneider, G. and Schwartz, R. D. (1989). cAMP and forskolin decrease gamma-aminobutyric acid-gated chloride flux in rat brain synaptoneurosomes. *Proc. Natl Acad. Sci. USA*, **86**, 2938–2942

Hoehn, K. and White, T. D. (1990). Role of excitatory amino acid receptors in K^+- and glutamate-evoked release of endogenous adenosine from rat cortical slices. *J. Neurochem.*, **54**, 256–265

Hokin, L. E. (1985) Receptors and phosphoinositide-generated second messengers. *Ann. Rev. Biochem.*, **54**, 205–235

Hokin, M. R. and Hokin, L. E. (1953). Enzyme secretion and the incorporation of ^{32}P into phospholipids of pancreas slices. *J. Biol. Chem.*, **203**, 967–977

Hollingsworth, E. B., McNeal, E. T., Burtyon, J. L., Williams, R. J., Daly, J. W. and Crevelling, C. R. (1985). Biochemical characterization of a filtered synaptoneurosomes preparation from guinea pig cerebral cortex: cyclic adenosine 3′:5′-monophosphate-generating systems, receptors, and enzymes. *J. Neurosci.*, **5**, 2240–2253

Hollingsworth, E. B., Sears, E. B., de la Cruz, R. A., Gusovsky, F. and Daly, J. W. (1986). Accumulations of cyclic AMP and inositol phosphates in guinea pig cerebral cortical synaptoneurosomes: enhancement by agents acting at sodium channels. *Biochim. Biophys. Acta*, **883**, 15–25

Honoré, T., Davies, S. N., Drejer, J., Fletcher, E. J., Jacobsen, P., Lodge, D. and Nielsen, F. E.

(1988). Quinoxalinediones: potent competitive non-NMDA glutamate receptor antagonists. *Science, N.Y.*, **241**, 701–703

Hood, W. F., Compton, R. P. and Monahan, J. B. (1989a). D-Cycloserine: a ligand for the *N*-methyl-D-aspartate coupled glycine receptor has partial agonist characteristics. *Neurosci. Lett.*, **98**, 91–95

Hood, W. F., Sun, E. T., Compton, R. P. and Monahan, J. B. (1989b). 1-aminocyclobutane-1-carboxylate (ACBC): a specific antagonist of the *N*-methyl-D-aspartate receptor coupled glycine receptor. *Eur. J. Pharmacol.*, **161**, 281–282

Huettner, J. E. (1989). Indole-2-carboxylic acid: a competitive antagonist of potentiation by glycine at the NMDA receptor. *Science, N.Y.*, **243**, 1611–1613

Iadarola, M. J., Nicoletti, F., Naranjo, J. R., Putman, F. and Costa, E. (1986). Kindling enhances the stimulation of inositol phospholipid hydrolysis elicited by ibotenic acid in rat hippocampal slices. *Brain Res.*, **374**, 174–178

Ito, I., Hirono, C., Yamagishi, S., Nomura, Y., Kaneko, S. and Sugiyama, H. (1988a). Roles of protein kinases in neurotransmitter responses in *Xenopus* oocytes injected with rat brain mRNA. *J. Cell. Physiol.*, **134**, 155–160

Ito, I., Okada, D. and Sugiyama, H. (1988b). Pertussis toxin suppresses long-term potentiation of hippocampal mossy fiber synapses. *Neurosci. Lett.*, **90**, 181–185

Jackson, H. and Parks, T. N. (1982). Functional synapse elimination in the developing avian cochlear nerve axon branching. *J. Neurosci.*, **2**, 1736–1743

Jackson, P. C. (1983). Reduced activity during development delays the normal rearrangement of synapses in the rabbit ciliary ganglion. *J. Physiol. (Lond.)*, **345**, 319–327

Jibiki, L., Ohtani, T., Kubota, T. and Yamaguchi, N. (1981). Development of kindling in acute experiments and serial changes of field excitatory and inhibitory post-synaptic potentials during the 'acute kindling'. *Brain Res.*, **209**, 210–215

Johnson, J. W. and Ascher, P. (1987). Glycine potentiates the NMDA response in cultured mouse brain neurons. *Nature*, **325**, 529–531

Jones, S. M., Snell, L. D. and Johnson, K. D. (1987). Phencyclidine selectively inhibits *N*-methyl-D-aspartate-induced hippocampal (^{3}H)noradrenaline release. *J. Pharmacol. Exp. Ther.*, **240**, 492–497

Jope, R. S. and Li, X. (1989). Inhibition of inositol phospholipid synthesis and norepinephrine-stimulated hydrolysis in rat brain slices by excitatory amino acids. *Biochem. Pharmacol.*, **38**, 589–596

Katan, M. and Parker, P. J. (1987). Purification of phosphoinositide-specific phospholipase C from a particulate fraction of bovine brain. *Eur. J. Biochem.*, **168**, 413–418

Katan, M., Kriz, R. W., Totty, N., Philp, R., Meldrum, E., Aldape, R. A., Knopf, J. L. and Parker, P. J. (1988). Determination of the primary structure of PLC-154 demonstrates diversity of phosphoinositide-specific phospholipase C activities. *Cell*, **54**, 171–177

Kawai, N., Saito, M. and Ohsako, S. (1988). Differential expression of glutamate receptors in *Xenopus* oocytes injected with messenger RNA from lobster muscle. *Neurosci. Lett.*, **95**, 203–207

Kawai, N., Miwa, A. and Abe, T. (1982). Spider venom contains specific receptor blocker of glutaminergic synapses. *Brain Res.*, **247**, 169–171

Kemp, J. A., Foster, A. C., Leeson, P. D. Priestley, T., Tridgett, R. and Iversen, L. L. (1988). 7-Chlorokynurenic acid is a selective antagonist at the glycine modulatory site of the *N*-methyl-D-aspartate receptor complex. *Proc. Natl Acad. Sci. USA*, **85**, 6547–6550

Kessler, M., Baudry, M. and Lynch, G. (1987). Use of cystine to distinguish glutamate binding from glutamate sequestration. *Neurosci. Lett.*, **81**, 221–226

Kikkawa, U. and Nishizuka, H. (1986). The role of protein kinase C in transmembrane signalling. *Ann. Rev. Cell Biol.*, **2**, 149–178

Krishtal, O. A., Petov, A. V., Smirnov, S. V. and Nowycky, M. C. (1989). Hippocampal synaptic plasticity induced by excitatory amino acids includes changes in sensitivity to the calcium channel blocker, ω-conotoxin. *Neurosci. Lett.*, **102**, 197–204

Labarca, R., Janowsky, A., Patel, J. and Paul, S. M. (1984). Phorbol esters inhibit agonist-induced [^{3}H]inositol-1-phosphate accumulation in rat hippocampal slices. *Biochem. Biophys. Res. Commun.*, **123**, 703–709

Lanthorn, T. H., Ganong, A. H. and Cotman, C. W. (1984). 2-Amino-4-phosphonobutyrate selectively blocks mossy fiber-CA3 responses in guinea pig but not rat hippocampus. *Brain Res.*, **290**, 174–178

Laroche, S., Errington, M. L., Lynch, M. A. and Bliss, T. V. P. (1987). Increase in [^{3}H]glutamate release from slices of dentate gyrus and hippocampus following classical conditioning in the rat. *Behav. Brain Res.*, **25**, 23–29

Lassing, I. and Lindberg, U. (1985). Specific interaction between phosphatidylinositol-4,5-bisphosphate and profilactin. *Nature*, **314**, 472–474

Lassing, I. and Lindberg, U. (1988). Evidence that the phosphatidylinositol cycle is linked to cell motility. *Exp. Cell Res.*, **174**, 1–15

Leach, M. J., Marden, C. M., Miller, A. A., O'Donnel, R. A. and Weston, S. B. (1985). Changes in cortical amino acids during electrical kindling in rats. *Neuropharmacology*, **24**, 937–940

Leach, M. J., O'Donnel, R. A., Collins, K. J., Marden, C. M. and Miller, A. A. (1987). Effect of cortical kindling on [³H]D-aspartate uptake and glutamate metabolism in rats. *Epilepsy Res.*, **1**, 145–148

Leeb-Lundberg, L. M. F., Cotecchia, S., Lomasney, J. W., DeBarnadis, J. F., Lefkowitz, R. J. and Caron, M. G. (1985). Phorbol esters promote alpha-1-adrenergic receptor phosphorylation and receptor uncoupling from inositol phospholipid metabolism. *Proc. Natl Acad. Sci. USA*, **82**, 5651–5655.

Lehman, J. and Scatton, B. (1982). Characterization of the excitatory amino acid receptor-mediated release of [³H]acetylcholine from rat striatal slices. *Brain Res.*, **252**, 77–89

Lehman, J., Tsai, C. and Wood, P. L. (1988). Homocysteic acid as a putative excitatory amino acid neurotransmitter. I. Postsynaptic characteristics at N-methyl-D-aspartate-type receptors on striatal cholinergic interneurons. *J. Neurochem.*, **51**, 1765–1770

Lenox, R. H., Hendley, D. and Ellis, J. (1988). Desensitization of muscarinic receptor-coupled phosphoinositide hydrolysis in rat hippocampus: comparisons with the α1 adrenergic response. *J. Neurochem.*, **50**, 558–564

Li, X. and Jope, R. S. (1989). Inhibition of receptor-coupled phosphoinositide hydrolysis by sulfur-containing amino acids in rat brain slices. *Biochem. Pharmacol.*, **38**, 2781–2787

Linden, D. J. and Routtenberg, A. (1989). The role of protein kinase C in long-term potentiation: a testable model. *Brain Res. Rev.*, **14**, 279–296

Linden, J. and Delahunty, T. M. (1989). Receptors that inhibit phosphoinositide breakdown. *Trends Pharmacol. Sci.*, **10**, 114–120

Lochrie, M. A. and Simon, M. I. (1988). G protein multiplicity in eukaryotic signal transduction systems. *Biochemistry*, **27**, 4957–4965

Lomo, T. (1966). Frequency potentiation of excitatory synaptic activity in the dentate area of the hippocampal formation. *Acta Physiol. Scand.*, **68** (Suppl. 277), 128–133

Lomo, T. (1971). Patterns of activation in a monosynaptic cortical pathway: the perforant path input to the dentate area of the hippocampal formation. *Exp. Brain Res.*, **12**, 18–45

Lopez-Colomé, A. M. and Roberts, P. J. (1987). Effect of excitatory amino acid analogues on the release of D-[³H]aspartate from chick retina. *Eur. J. Pharmacol.*, **142**, 409–417

Lovinger, D. M., Colley, P. A., Akers, R. F., Nelson, R. B. and Routtenberg, A. (1986). Direct relation of long-term synaptic potentiation to phosphorylation of membrane protein F_1, a substrate for membrane protein kinase C. *Brain Res.*, **399**, 205–211

Lovinger, D. M., Wong, Ka L., Murakami, K. and Routtenberg, A. (1987). Protein kinase C inhibitors eliminate hippocampal long-term potentiation. *Brain Res.*, **436**, 177–183

Luini, A., Goldberg, O. and Teichberg, V. I. (1981). Distinct pharmacological properties of excitatory amino acid receptors in the rat striatum: Study by Na^+ efflux assay. *Proc. Natl Acad. Sci. USA*, **78**, 3250–3254

Lynch, G. and Baudry, M. (1987). Brain spectrin, calpain and long-term changes in synaptic efficacy. *Brain Res. Bull.*, **18**, 809–815

Lynch, G., Larson, J., Kelso, S., Barrionuevo, G. and Schottler, F. (1983). Intracellular injections of EGTA block the induction of hippocampal long-term potentiation. *Nature*, **305**, 719–721

MacDermott, A. B., Mayer, M. L., Westbrook, G. L., Smith, S. J. and Barker, J. L. (1986). NMDA-receptor activation increases cytoplasmic calcium concentration in cultured spinal cord neurones. *Nature*, **321**, 519–522

McLennan, H. (1983). Receptors for the excitatory amino acids in the mammalian central nervous system. *Prog. Neurobiol.*, **20**, 251–271

Majerus, P. W., Connoly, T. M., Bansal, V. S., Inhorn, R. C., Ross, T. S. and Lips, D. L. (1988). Inositol phosphates: Synthesis and degradation. *J. Biol. Chem.*, **263**, 3051–3054

Malenka, R. C., Madison, D. V. and Nicoll, R. A. (1986). Potentiation of synaptic transmission in the hippocampus by phorbol esters. *Nature*, **321**, 175–177

Malenka, R. C., Kauer, J. A., Perkel, D. J. and Nicoll, R. A. (1989a). The impact of postsynaptic calcium on synaptic transmission: its role in long-term potentiation. *Trends Neurosci.*, **12**, 444–450

Malenka, R. C., Kauer, J. A., Perkel, D. J., Mauk, M. D., Kelly, P. T., Nicoll, R. A. and Waxham, M. N. (1989b). An essential role for postsynaptic calmodulin and protein kinase activity in long-term potentiation. *Nature*, **340**, 554–557

Malinow, R., Madison, D. V. and Tsien, R. W. (1988). Persistent protein kinase activity underlying long-term potentiation. *Nature*, **335**, 820–824

Manzoni, O. J. J., Finiels-Marlier, F., Sassetti, I., Bockaert, J., le Peuch, C. and Sladeczek, F. A. J. (1990). The glutamate receptor of the Q_p-type activates protein kinase C and is regulated by protein kinase C. *Neurosci. Lett.* (in press)

Mariani, J. (1983). Elimination of synapses during the development of the central nervous system. *Prog. Brain Res.*, **58**, 383–392

Marvizon, J.-C., Lewin, A. H. and Skolnick, P. (1989). 1-Aminocyclopropane carboxylic acid: a potent and selective ligand for the glycine modulatory site of the *N*-methyl-D-aspartate receptor complex. *J. Neurochem.*, **52**, 992–994

Mattson, M. P., Dou, P., Kater, S. B. (1988a). Outgrowth-regulating actions of glutamate in isolated hippocampal pyramidal neurons. *J. Neurosci.*, **8**, 2087–2100

Mattson, M. P., Guthrie, P. B. and Kater, S. B. (1988b). Intracellular messengers in the generation and degeneration of hippocampal neuroarchitecture. *J. Neurosci. Res.*, **21**, 447–464

Mayer, M. L., MacDermott, A. B., Westbrook, G. L., Smith, S. and Barker, J. L. (1987). Agonist and voltage-gated calcium entry in cultured mouse spinal cord neurons under voltage clamp measured using arsenazo III. *J. Neurosci.*, **7**, 3230–3244

Mayer, M. L. and Westbrook, G. L. (1985). The action of *N*-methyl-D-aspartic acid on mouse spinal neurones in culture. *J. Physiol. (Lond.)*, **361**, 65–90

Mayer, M., Westbrook, G. L. and Guthrie, P. B. (1984). Voltage-dependent block by Mg^{2+} of NMDA responses in spinal cord neurones. *Nature*, **309**, 261–263

Meldrum, B. S., Croucher, M. J., Badman, G. and Collins, J. F. (1983). Antiepileptic action of excitatory amino acid antagonists in the photosensitive baboon, *Papio papio. Neurosci. Lett.*, **39**, 101–104

Meldrum, E., Katan, M. and Parker, P. (1989). A novel inositol-phospholipid-specific phospholipase C. *Eur. J. Biochem.*, **182**, 673–677

Menéndez, N., Herreras, O., Solis, J. M., Herrantz, A. S. and Martin del Rio, R. (1989). Extracellular taurine increase in rat hippocampus evoked by specific glutamate receptor activation is related to the excitatory potency of glutamate agonists. *Neurosci. Lett.*, **102**, 64–69

Michell, R. H. (1975). Inositol phospholipids and cell surface receptor function. *Biochim. Biophys. Acta*, **415**, 81–147

Michell, R. H. (1980). Muscarinic acetylcholine receptors. In *Cellular Receptors for Hormones and Neurotransmitters* (ed. D. Schulster and A. Levitzki). Wiley, London, pp. 353–368

Milani, D., Facci, L., Guidolin, D., Leon, A. and Skaper, S. D. (1989). Activation of polyphosphoinositide metabolism as a signal-transducing system coupled to excitatory amino acid receptors in astroglial cells. *Glia*, **2**, 161–169

Miles, R. and Wong, R. K. S. (1987). Latent synaptic pathways revealed after tetanic stimulation in the hippocampus. *Nature*, **329**, 724–726

Monaghan, D. T., Holets, V. R., Toy, D. W. and Cotman, C. W. (1983a). Anatomical distributions of four pharmacologically distinct ³H-L-glutamate binding sites. *Nature*, **306**, 176–178

Monaghan, D. T., McMills, M. C., Chamberlin, A. R. and Cotman, C. W. (1983b). Synthesis of [3H]2-amino-4-phosphonobutyric acid and characterization of its binding to rat brain membranes: a selective ligand for the chloride/calcium-dependent class of L-glutamate binding sites. *Brain Res.*, **278**, 137–144

Moroni, F., Lombardi, G., Moneti, G. and Cortesini, C. (1983). The release and neosynthesis of glutamic acid are increased in experimental models of hepatic encephalopathy. *J. Neurochem.*, **40**, 850–855

Muller, D., Joly, M. and Lynch, G. (1988). Contributions of quisqualate and NMDA receptors to the induction and expression of LTP. *Science, N.Y.*, **242**, 1694–1697

Murphy, D. E., Hitchinson, A. J., Hurt, S. D., Williams, M. and Sills, M. A. (1988). Characterization of the binding of [3H]-CGS 19755: a novel *N*-methyl-D-aspartate antagonist with nanomolar affinity in rat brain. *Br. J. Pharmacol.*, **95**, 932–938

Murphy, S. N. and Miller, R. J. (1988). A glutamate receptor regulates Ca^{2+} mobilization in hippocampal neurons. *Proc. Natl Acad. Sci. USA*, **85**, 8737–8741

Nadler, V., Kloog, Y. and Sokolovsky, M. (1988). 1-Aminocyclopropane-1-carboxylic acid (ACC) mimics the effects of glycine on the NMDA receptor ion channel. *Eur. J. Pharmacol.*, **157**, 115–116

Nakanishi, O., Homma, Y., Kawasaki, H., Emori, Y., Suzuki, K. and Takenawa, T. (1988). Purification of two distinct types of phosphoinositide-specific phospholipase C from rat liver. *Biochem. J.*, **256**, 453–459

Nathanson, N. M. (1987). Molecular properties of the muscarinic acetylcholine receptor. *Ann. Rev. Neurosci.*, **10**, 195–236

Nawy, S. and Copenhagen, D. R. (1987). Multiple classes of glutamate receptor on depolarizing bipolar cells in retina. *Nature*, **325**, 56–58

Nicoletti, F. and Canonico, P. L. (1989). Glycine potentiates the stimulation of inositol phospholipid hydrolysis by excitatory amino acids in primary cultures of cerebellar neurons. *J. Neurochem.*, **53**, 724–727

Nicoletti, F., Iadarola, M. J., Wroblewski, J. T., and Costa, E. (1986a). Excitatory amino acid recognition sites coupled with inositol phospholipid metabolism: Developmental changes and interaction with alpha 1-adrenoceptors. *Proc. Natl Acad. Sci. USA*, **83**, 1931–1935

Nicoletti, F., Meek, J. L., Iadarola, M. J., Chuang, D. M., Roth, B. L. and Costa, E. (1986b). Coupling of inositol phospholipid metabolism with excitatory amino acid recognition sites in rat hippocampus. *J. Neurochem.*, **46**, 40–46

Nicoletti, F., Valerio, C., Pellegrino, C., Drago, F., Scapagnini, U. and Canonico, P. L. (1988). Spatial learning potentiates the stimulation of phosphoinositide hydrolysis by excitatory amino acids in rat hippocampal slices. *J. Neurochem.*, **51**, 725–729

Nicoletti, F., Wroblewski, J. T., Alho, H., Eva, C., Fadda, E. and Costa, E. (1987a). Lesions of putative glutamatergic pathways potentiate the increase of inositol phospholipid hydrolysis elicited by excitatory amino acids. *Brain Res.*, **436**, 103–112

Nicoletti, F., Wroblewski, J. T. and Costa, E. (1987b). Magnesium ions inhibit the stimulation of inositol phospholipid hydrolysis by endogenous excitatory amino acids in primary cultures of cerebellar granule cells. *J. Neurochem.*, **48**, 967–973

Nicoletti, F., Wroblewski, J. T., Iadarola, M. J. and Costa, E. (1986c). Serine-O-phosphate, an endogenous metabolite, inhibits the stimulation of inositol phospholipid hydrolysis elicited by ibotenic acid in rat hippocampal slices. *Neuropharmacology*, **25**, 335–338

Nicoletti, F., Wroblewski, J. T., Novelli, A., Alho, H., Guidotti, A. and Costa, E. (1986d). The activation of inositol phospholipid metabolism as a signal-transducing system for excitatory amino acids in primary cultures of cerebellar granule cells. *J. Neurosci.*, **6**, 1905–1911

Nishizuka, Y. (1984a). Turnover of inositol phospholipids and signal transduction. *Science, N. Y.*, **233**, 305–312

Nishizuka, Y. (1984b). The role of protein kinase C in cell surface signal transduction and tumour promotion. *Nature*, **308**, 693–698

Nishizuka, Y. (1988). The molecular heterogeneity of protein kinase C and its implications for cellular regulation. *Nature*, **334**, 661–665

Noble, E. P., Sincini, E., Bergman, D. and Bruggencate, G. T. (1989). Excitatory amino acids inhibit stimulated phosphoinositide hydrolysis in the rat prefrontal cortex. *Life Sci.*, **44**, 19–26

Nowak, L., Bregestovski, P., Ascher, P., Herbert, A. and Prochiantz, A. (1984). Magnesium gates glutamate-activated channels in mouse central neurones. *Nature*, **307**, 462–465

Nowycky, M. C., Fox, A. P. and Tsien, R. W. (1985). Three types of neuronal calcium channel with different calcium agonist sensitivity. *Nature*, **316**, 440–443

Oosawa, Y. and Yamagishi, S. (1989). Rat brain glutamate receptors activate chloride channels in *Xenopus* oocytes coupled by inositol trisphosphate and Ca^{2+}. *J. Physiol. (Lond.)*, **408**, 223–232

Osborne, N. N. (1990). Stimulatory and inhibitory actions of excitatory amino acids on inositol phospholipid metabolism in rabbit retina. Evidence for a specific quisqualate receptor subtype associated with neurones. *Exp. Eye Res.*, **50**, 397–405

Palmer, E., Monaghan, D. T. and Cotman, C. W. (1988). Glutamate receptors and phosphoinositide metabolism: stimulation via quisqualate receptors is inhibited by *N*-methyl-D-aspartate receptor activation. *Molec. Brain Res.*, **4**, 161–165

Palmer, E., Monaghan, D. T. and Cotman, C. W. (1989). Trans-ACPD, a selective agonist of the phosphoinositide-coupled excitatory amino acid receptor. *Eur. J. Pharmacol.*, **166**, 585–587

Pardee, A. B. (1989). G1 events and regulation of cell proliferation. *Science, N. Y.*, **246**, 603–608

Pearce, B., Albrecht, J., Morrow, C. and Murphy, S. (1986). Astrocyte glutamate receptor activation promotes inositol phospholipid turnover and calcium flux. *Neurosci. Lett.*, **72**, 335–340

Pearce, I. A., Cambrey-Deakin, M. A. and Burgoyne, R. D. (1987). Glutamate acting on NMDA receptors stimulates neurite outgrowth from cerebellar granule cells. *FEBS Lett.*, **223**, 143–147

Peterson, D. W., Collins, J. F. and Bradford, H. F. (1983). The kindled amygdala model of epilepsy: anticonvulsant action of amino acid antagonists. *Brain Res.*, **275**, 169–172

Pin, J.-P., Bockaert, J. and Récasens, M. (1984a). The Ca^{2+}/Cl^- dependent L-[3H]glutamate binding: a new receptor or a particular transport process? *FEBS Lett.*, **175**, 31–36

Pin, J.-P., Rumigny, J.-F., Bockaert, J. and Récasens, M. (1984b). Multiple Cl-independent binding sites for the excitatory amino-acids: glutamate, aspartate and cysteine sulfinate in rat brain membranes. *Brain Res.*, **402**, 11–20

Pin, J.-P., Van-Vliet, B. J. and Bockaert, J. (1988). NMDA- and kainate-evoked GABA release from striatal neurones differentiated in primary culture: differential blocking by phencyclidine. *Neurosci. Lett.*, **87**, 87–92

Purves, D. and Lichtman, J. W. (1980). Elimination of synapses in the developing nervous system. *Science, N.Y.*, **210**, 153–157

Ransom, R. W. and Deschenes, N. L. (1988). NMDA-induced [³H]norepinephrine release is modulated by glycine. *Eur. J. Pharmacol.*, **156**, 149–155

Récasens, M., Guiramand, J., Mayat, E., Saffiedine, S. and Sassetti, I. (1988a). Na$^+$ ions are a prerequisite for the enhanced formation of inositol phosphates via the activation of the new quisqualate receptor (sAA2). *8th European Winter Conference on Brain Research, Tignes, France*, p. 55 (Abstract)

Récasens, M., Guiramand, J., Nourigat, A., Sassetti, I. and Devilliers, G. (1988b). A new quisqualate receptor subtype (sAA$_2$) responsible for the glutamate-induced inositol phosphate formation in rat brain synaptoneurosomes. *Neurochem. Int.*, **13**, 463–467

Récasens, M., Pin, J.-P. and Bockaert, J. (1987a). Chloride transport blockers inhibit the chloride-dependent glutamate binding to rat brain membranes. *Neurosci. Lett.*, **74**, 211–216

Récasens, M., Sassetti, I., Nourigat, A., Sladeczek, F. and Bockaert, J. (1987b). Characterization of subtypes of excitatory amino acid receptors involved in the stimulation of inositol phosphate synthesis in rat brain synaptoneurosomes. *Eur. J. Pharmacol.*, **141**, 87–93

Récasens, M., Varga, V., Nanopoulos, D., Saadoun, F., Vincendon, G. and Benavides, J. (1982). Evidence for cysteine sulfinate as a neurotransmitter. *Brain Res.*, **239**, 153–173

Renard, D., Poggioli, J., Berthon, B. and Claret, M. (1987). How far does phospholipase C activity depend on the cell calcium concentration? *Biochem. J.*, **243**, 391–398

Renaud, J.-F., Kazazoglou, T., Lombet, A., Chicheportiche, R., Jaimovitch, E., Romey, G. and Lazdunski, M. (1983). The Na$^+$ channel in mammalian cardiac cells. Two kinds of tetrodotoxin receptors in rat heart membranes. *J. Biol. Chem.*, **258**, 8799–8805

Roberts, P. J. and Anderson, S. D. (1979). Stimulatory effect of L-glutamate and related amino acids on [3H]dopamine release from rat striatum: an *in vitro* model for glutamate actions. *J. Neurochem.*, **32**, 1539–1545

Rothman, S. M. (1985). The neurotoxicity of excitatory amino acids is produced by passive chloride influx. *J. Neurosci.*, **5**, 1483–1489

Savage, D. D., Werling, L. L., Nadler, J. V. and McNamara, J. O. (1982). Selective increase in L-[³H]glutamate binding to a quisqualate-sensitive site on hippocampal synaptic membrane after angular bundle kindling. *Eur. J. Pharmacol.*, **85**, 255–256

Schmidt, B. H., Weiss, S., Sebben, M., Kemp, D. E., Bockaert, J. and Sladeczek, F. (1987). Dual action of excitatory amino acids on the metabolism of inositol phosphates in striatal neurons. *Molec. Pharmacol.*, **32**, 364–368

Schmidt, C. J. and Taylor, V. L. (1988). Release of [³H]norepinephrine from rat hippocampal slices by N-methyl-D-aspartate: comparison of the inhibitory effect of Mg^{2+} and MK-801. *Eur. J. Pharmacol.*, **156**, 111–120

Schoepp, D. D. (1989). Protein kinase C-mediated inhibition of excitatory amino acid-stimulated phosphoinositide hydrolysis in the neonatal rat hippocampus. *Neurochem. Int.*, **15**, 131–136

Schoepp, D. D. and Hillman, C. C. (1990). Developmental and pharmacological characterization of quisqualate, ibotenate, and trans-1-amino-1,3-cyclopentanedicarboxylic acid stimulations of phosphoinositide hydrolysis in rat cortical brain slices. *Biogenic Amines* (in press)

Schoepp, D. D. and Johnson, B. G. (1988a). Excitatory amino acid agonist–antagonist interactions at 2-amino-4-phosphonobutyric acid-sensitive quisqualate receptors coupled to phosphoinositide hydrolysis in slices of rat hippocampus. *J. Neurochem.*, **50**, 1605–1613

Schoepp, D. D. and Johnson, B. G. (1988b). Selective inhibition of excitatory amino acid-stimulated phosphoinositide hydrolysis in the rat hippocampus by activation of protein kinase C. *Biochem. Pharmacol.*, **37**, 4299–4305

Schoepp, D. D. and Johnson, B. G. (1989a). Comparison of excitatory amino acid-stimulated phosphoinositide hydrolysis and *N*-[³H]acetylaspartylglutamate binding in rat brain: selective inhibition of phosphoinositide hydrolysis by 2-amino-3-phosphonopropionate. *J. Neurochem.*, **53**, 273–278

Schoepp, D. D. and Johnson, B. G. (1989b). Inhibition of excitatory amino acid-stimulated phosphoinositide hydrolysis in the neonatal rat hippocampus by 2-amino-3-phosphonopropionate. *J. Neurochem.*, **53**, 1865–1870

Seren, M. S., Aldinio, C., Zanoni, R., Leon, A. and Nicoletti, F. (1989). Stimulation of inositol phospholipid hydrolysis by excitatory amino acids is enhanced in brain slices from vulnerable regions after transient global ischemia. *J. Neurochem.*, **53**, 1700–1705

Shapira, R., Silberberg, S. D., Ginsburg, S. and Rahamimoff, R. (1987). Activation of protein kinase C augments evoked transmitter release. *Nature*, **325**, 58–60

Shears, S. B. (1989). Metabolism of the inositol phosphates produced upon receptor activation. *Biochem. J.*, **260**, 313–324

Shuntoh, H., Taniyama, K. and Tanaka, C. (1989). Involvement of protein kinase C in the Ca²⁺-dependent vesicular release of GABA from central and enteric neurons of the guinea pig. *Brain Res.*, **483**, 384–388

Simon, R. P., Swan, J. H., Griffiths, T. and Meldrum, B. S. (1984). Blockade of *N*-methyl-D-aspartate receptors may protect against ischemic brain damage in the brain. *Science, N.Y.*, **226**, 850–852

Sladeczek, F., Pin, J.-P., Récasens, M., Bockaert, J. and Weiss, S. (1985). Glutamate stimulates inositol phosphate formation in striatal neurons. *Nature*, **317**, 717–719

Sladeczek, F., Récasens, M. and Bockaert, J. (1988). A new mechanism for glutamate receptor action: phosphoinositide hydrolysis. *Trends Neurosci.*, **11**, 545–549

Slaughter, M. M. and Miller, R. F. (1981). 2-Amino-4-phosphonobutyric acid: a new pharmacological tool for retina research. *Science, N.Y.*, **211**, 182–184

Smart, T. G. (1989). Excitatory amino acids: the involvement of second messengers in signal transduction process. *Cell. Molec. Neurobiol.*, **9**, 193–206

Snell, L. D. and Johnson, K. M. (1988). Cycloleucine competitively antagonizes the strychnine-insensitive glycine receptor. *Eur. J. Pharmacol.*, **151**, 165–166

Snell, L. D. and Johnson, K. M. (1986). Characterization of the inhibition of excitatory amino acid-induced neurotransmitter release in the rat striatum by phencyclidine-like drugs. *J. Pharmacol. Exp. Ther.*, **238**, 938–946

Stone, T. W. and Burton, N. R. (1988). NMDA receptors and ligands in the vertebrate CNS. *Prog. Neurobiol.*, **30**, 333–368

Sugiyama, H., Ito, I. and Hirono, C. (1987). A new type of glutamate receptor linked to inositol phospholipid metabolism. *Nature*, **325**, 531–533

Sugiyama, H., Ito, I. and Watanabe, M. (1989). Glutamate receptor subtypes may be classified into two major categories: a study on *Xenopus* oocytes injected with rat brain mRNA. *Neuron*, **3**, 129–132

Suh, P.-G., Ryu, S. H., Moon, K. H., Suh, H. W. and Rhee, S. G. (1988). Cloning and sequence of multiple forms of phospholipase C. *Cell*, **54**, 161–169

Swanson, L., Teyler, T. and Thompson, R. F. (1982). Hippocampal long-term potentiation mechanisms and implications for memory based on a NRP worksession. *Neurosci. Res. Prog. Bull.*, **20**, 613–769

Szekely, A. M., Barbaccia, M. L., Alho, H. and Costa, E. (1989). In primary cultures of cerebellar granule cells the activation of *N*-methyl-D-aspartate-sensitive glutamate receptors induces c-fos mRNA expression. *Molec. Pharmacol.*, **35**, 401–408

Tapia-Arancibia, L. and Astier, H. (1989). Actions of excitatory amino acids on somatostatin release from cortical neurons in primary cultures. *J. Neurochem.*, **53**, 1134–1141

Thompson, W. (1983). Synapse elimination in neonatal rat muscle is sensitive to pattern of muscle use. *Nature*, **302**, 614–616

Tremblay, E., Roisin, M. P., Represa, A., Charriaut-Marlangue, C. and Ben-Ari, Y. (1988). Transient increased density of NMDA binding sites in the developing rat hippocampus. *Brain Res.*, **461**, 393–396

Tuff, L. P., Racine, R. J. and Adamac, R. (1983). The effect of kindling on GABA mediated inhibition in the dentate gyrus of the rat. I. Paired pulse depression. *Brain Res.*, **277**, 79–90

Wakade, A. R., Malhotra, R. K. and Wakade, T. D. (1985). Phorbol ester, an activator of protein kinase C, enhances calcium-dependent release of sympathetic neurotransmitter. *Naunyn-Schmiedebergs Arch. Pathol. Exp. Pharmacol.*, **331**, 122–124

Watkins, J. C. and Evans, R. H. (1981). Excitatory amino acid transmitters. *Ann. Rev. Pharmacol. Toxicol.*, **21**, 165–204

Watkins, J. C. and Olvermann, H. J. (1987). Agonists and antagonists for excitatory amino acid receptors. *Trends Neurosci.*, **10**, 265–272

Weiss, S. (1988). Excitatory amino acid-evoked release of gamma-[³H]aminobutyric acid from striatal neurons in primary culture. *J. Neurochem.*, **51**, 435–411

Weiss, S. (1989). Two distinct quisqualate receptor systems are present on striatal neurons. *Brain Res.*, **491**, 189–193

Weiss, S., Ellis, J., Hendley, D. D. and Lenox, R. H. (1989). Translocation and activation of protein kinase C in striatal neurons in primary culture: relationship to phorbol dibutyrate actions on the inositol phosphate generating system and neurotransmitter release. *J. Neurochem.*, **52**, 530–536

Wieloch, T. (1985). Hypoglycemia-induced neuronal damage prevented by an *N*-methyl-D-aspartate antagonist. *Science, N.Y.*, **230**, 681–683

Williams, J. H., Errington, M. L., Lynch, M. A. and Bliss, T. V. P. (1989). Arachidonic acid induces a long-term activity-dependent enhancement of synaptic transmission in the hippocampus. *Nature*, **341**, 739–742

Williams, K., Romano, C. and Molinoff, P. B. (1989). Effects of polyamines on the binding of [³H]MK-801 to the *N*-methyl-D-aspartate receptor: pharmacological evidence for the existence of a polyamine recognition site. *Molec. Pharmacol.*, **36**, 575–581

Wroblewski, J. T., Nicoletti, F., Fadda, E. and Costa, E. (1987). Phencyclidine is a negative allosteric modulator of signal transduction at two subclasses of excitatory amino acid receptors. *Proc. Natl Acad. Sci. USA*, **84**, 5068–5072

Yamada, N., Akiyama, K. and Otsuki, S. (1989). Hippocampal kindling enhances excitatory amino acid receptor-mediated polyphosphoinositide hydrolysis in the hippocampus and amygdala/pyriform cortex. *Brain Res.*, **490**, 126–132

Yamamoto, C., Sawada, S. and Takada, S. (1983). Suppressing action of 2-amino-4-phosphonobutyric acid on mossy fiber-induced excitation in the guinea pig hippocampus. *Exp. Brain Res.*, **51**, 128–134

Yaksh, T. L., Furui, T., Kanawati, I. S. and Go, V. L. W. (1987). Release of cholecystokinin from rat cerebral cortex *in vivo*: role of GABA and glutamate receptor systems. *Brain Res.*, **406**, 207–214

Young, A. M. J., Crowder, J. M. and Bradford, H. F. (1988). Potentiation by kainate of excitatory amino acid release in striatum: complementary *in vivo* and *in vitro* experiments. *J. Neurochem.*, **50**, 337–345

Zurgil, N., Yarom, M. and Zisapel, N. (1986). Concerted enhancement of calcium influx, neurotransmitter release and protein phosphorylation by a phorbol ester in cultured brain neurons. *Neuroscience*, **19**, 1255–1264

5

The GABA$_A$ Receptors: Structure and Function

F. ANNE STEPHENSON

Department of Pharmaceutical Chemistry, School of Pharmacy, 29/39 Brunswick Square, London WC1N 1AX, UK

Contents

Current Aspects of the Neurosciences, Vol. 3. Edited by N. N. Osborne. © The Macmillan Press Ltd 1991

1. Introduction

In recent years considerable attention has been given to the study of the GABA$_A$ receptors. This is because GABA is the major inhibitory neurotransmitter in the mammalian central nervous system, where the GABA receptors are ubiquitous, playing an important role in the control of neuronal excitability. There are two pharmacological subclasses of GABA receptors. These are the GABA$_A$ receptor, a ligand-gated chloride ion channel, whose pharmacology is defined by the competitive antagonism by the plant alkaloid bicuculline; and the GABA$_B$ receptor which is bicuculline-insensitive and (-)baclofen-sensitive and the activation of which results in the production of second messengers via interaction with an as yet unknown G protein (for a review see Bowery, 1989; Stephenson and Dolphin, 1989). The GABA$_A$ receptor is the most characterized of the two receptor types. This is because it is the site of action of several groups of therapeutically important drugs, such as the benzodiazepines, the barbiturates and some steroids (reviewed in Olsen and Venter, 1986), each of which allosterically modulate GABA$_A$ receptor function at distinct binding sites within the receptor protein.

In early 1987 it was thought that the elucidation of the structure of the GABA$_A$ receptor was well advanced. The fortuitous coexistence of the binding site for the anxiolytic benzodiazepines on the GABA$_A$ receptor oligomer had enabled the purification of the protein by benzodiazepine affinity chromatography (reviewed in Stephenson, 1988). The isolated receptor possessed all the distinct ligand binding sites and the allosteric interactions between them that were known to occur in the membrane-bound form of the receptor (Sigel et al., 1983; Sigel and Barnard, 1984). The protein was shown to have a molecular size of 240–250 kD (Mamalaki et al., 1989); it was a glycoprotein, apparently homogeneous as analysed by one-dimensional isoelectric focusing, and the GABA$_A$ receptor purified from several vertebrate species was shown to consist of two subunit types—namely, the α subunit with M_r 53 000 and the β subunit with M_r 57 000–58 000 (reviewed in Stephenson, 1988). It was proposed that the receptor was a heterologous tetramer, $\alpha_2\beta_2$, which was consistent with both the molecular weight determination of the native protein and densitometric scans of SDS–PAGE of the isolated protein (Mamalaki et al., 1987). The ligand binding sites were mapped by photoaffinity labelling experiments which showed that the α subunit was specifically photoaffinity labelled by the agonist benzodiazepine [^{3}H]flunitrazepam, whereas the β subunit was predominantly photoaffinity labelled by the high-affinity GABA$_A$ receptor agonist [^{3}H]muscimol (Casalotti et al., 1986). Antibodies were raised against the purified receptor and these were shown to be either α-subunit- or β-subunit-specific and had been employed to map the distribution of the GABA$_A$ receptor in the brain (e.g. Richards et al., 1987). Later that year the cDNAs encoding the bovine GABA$_A$ receptor α and β subunits were identified and the corresponding primary structures of the polypeptides were deduced (Schofield et al., 1987).

The availablity of these new tools with which to study the structure of the GABA$_A$ receptor led rapidly to discoveries which have necessitated a complete re-evaluation of all the previous biochemical investigations into the structure of the GABA$_A$ receptor. Most notably, it is now clear that there is not a GABA$_A$ receptor but that there exists a multiplicity of structurally related GABA$_A$ receptors. This chapter will discuss recent developments in the elucidation of the structures and functions of this family of receptor proteins.

2. *Molecular Cloning of GABA$_A$ Receptor Polypeptides*

In the original work on the cloning of the GABA$_A$ receptor, the classical methodology was followed. Thus, the receptor was purified from bovine brain; the isolated native receptor and the gel-purified α subunit were subjected to cyanogen bromide cleavage, peptide purification and amino acid sequencing. Oligonucleotide probes were constructed from the resultant amino acid sequences, bovine brain cDNA libraries were screened with these probes and two different cDNAs were identified which contained these oligonucleotide probe sequences (Schofield *et al.*, 1987). The cDNA encoding the α subunit was identified, because the deduced primary structure contained an amino acid sequence which was derived from the gel-purified α subunit band. The cDNA encoding the β subunit was identified by default, because, although the deduced primary structure of this was homologous with that of the α subunit, it did not contain the α-subunit-specific sequence and the deduced molecular weight of the mature polypeptide was larger than that deduced from the α subunit cDNA (Schofield *et al.*, 1987). Subsequently, cDNAs encoding other GABA$_A$ receptor subunits were discovered by cDNA homology hybridization under low stringency conditions and these include isoforms of each of the α and β subunits—namely the α1 (original), α2, α3, α4, α5 and α6 (Levitan *et al.*, 1988; Pritchett *et al.*, 1988a; Khrestchatisky *et al.*, 1989; Ymer *et al.*, 1989b); β1 (original), β2 and β3 polypeptides (Ymer *et al.*, 1989a); and additionally two novel GABA$_A$ receptor subunit types, γ1 and γ2 (Pritchett *et al.*, 1989c) and δ (Shivers *et al.*, 1989). The nomenclature of the α and β subunits is based on the order of discovery; and γ and δ polypeptides are each distinct subunit types and are named following the nomenclature of the nicotinic acetylcholine receptor. Additional chemically determined amino acid sequences from the purified receptor were found within the deduced primary structures of the α2 and β2 polypeptides only (Levitan *et al.*, 1988; Ymer *et al.*, 1989a).

The deduced primary structures of all the GABA$_A$ receptor subunits are similar. The 12 GABA$_A$ receptor subunit amino acid sequences which have been described to date range in length from 424 to 521 amino acids, with corresponding deduced molecular weights in the range M_r 48 000–64 000 (Table 1). Each polypeptide type has a similar hydrophobicity profile with a large presumed extracellular N-terminal hydrophilic domain of ~220 amino acids in length which contains putative sites for N-glycosylation; four putative transmembrane spanning domains M1–M4, each of ~22 amino acids in length which are thought to form the chloride ion channel; and an intracellular hydrophilic cytoplasmic loop region (Figure 1). The different subunit types also share a degree of amino acid sequence identity. Overall, the different

Table 1   Summary of known GABA$_A$ receptor subunits

Subunit type	No. of amino acid residues[a]	Molecular weight[b]
α1	429	48 800
α2	423	48 000
α3	464	52 000
α4[c]	521	64 000
α5	433	48 400
α6[c]		
β1	449	51 400
β2	450	52 000
β3	447	52 000
γ1[c]		
γ2	428	49 800
δ	433	48 500

[a] The number of amino acids in the respective mature polypeptides; α1, α2, α3, β1, β2, β3 are bovine sequences; α4, γ2 and δ are rat sequences. For the other species, whose corresponding amino acid sequences have been published, only the rat α1 differs, in that it has 428 residues.
[b] The molecular weight of each polypeptide deduced from the cDNA sequence, which does not take account of a molecular mass contribution by N-linked carbohydrate.
[c] The cDNA and amino acid sequences for these subunits have not yet been published.

Figure 1   Proposed structure of the GABA$_A$ receptor. A is the transmembrane topology of the mature α1 subunit of the GABA$_A$ receptor, showing the complete primary structure of the polypeptide as deduced from the corresponding cDNA sequence. The four clusters of hydrophobic amino acids are the putative membrane-spanning domains, M1–M4, and the arrowheads show the potential sites of N-glycosylation in the extracellular domain. Note also the putative cys loop in the extracellular domain. The bovine α1 GABA$_A$ receptor subunit sequence was aligned with the bovine GABA$_A$ receptor β1 subunit and the rat glycine receptor α subunit as in Barnard *et al.* (1987). The amino acids that are identical in all three polypeptides are shown grey, and the cross-hatched ones show the amino acids in the alignment which represent conservative substitutions. Overall, the three polypeptides share 35–40% amino acid sequence identity and 55–60% amino acid sequence similarity in pairwise combinations. B is a schematic representation of the postulated pentameric GABA$_A$ receptor as viewed perpendicular to the plane of the membrane. It shows five subunits of the receptor and the central ion channel. Within each polypeptide can be seen the four transmembrane regions M1–M4, with the M2 helix lining the wall of the channel. The ordering of the subunits around the central pore is arbitrary. Reprinted from Stephenson and Dolphin (1989), with the kind permission of Saunders Scientific Publications, Philadelphia, USA

subunit types have 35–40% amino acid sequence identity and ~55% amino acid sequence similarity, with the most conserved regions found within the transmembrane regions and the N-terminal extracellular domains. Isoforms of one subunit type have 70–80% amino acid sequence identity, with the divergent regions between these being found in the predicted cytoplasmic

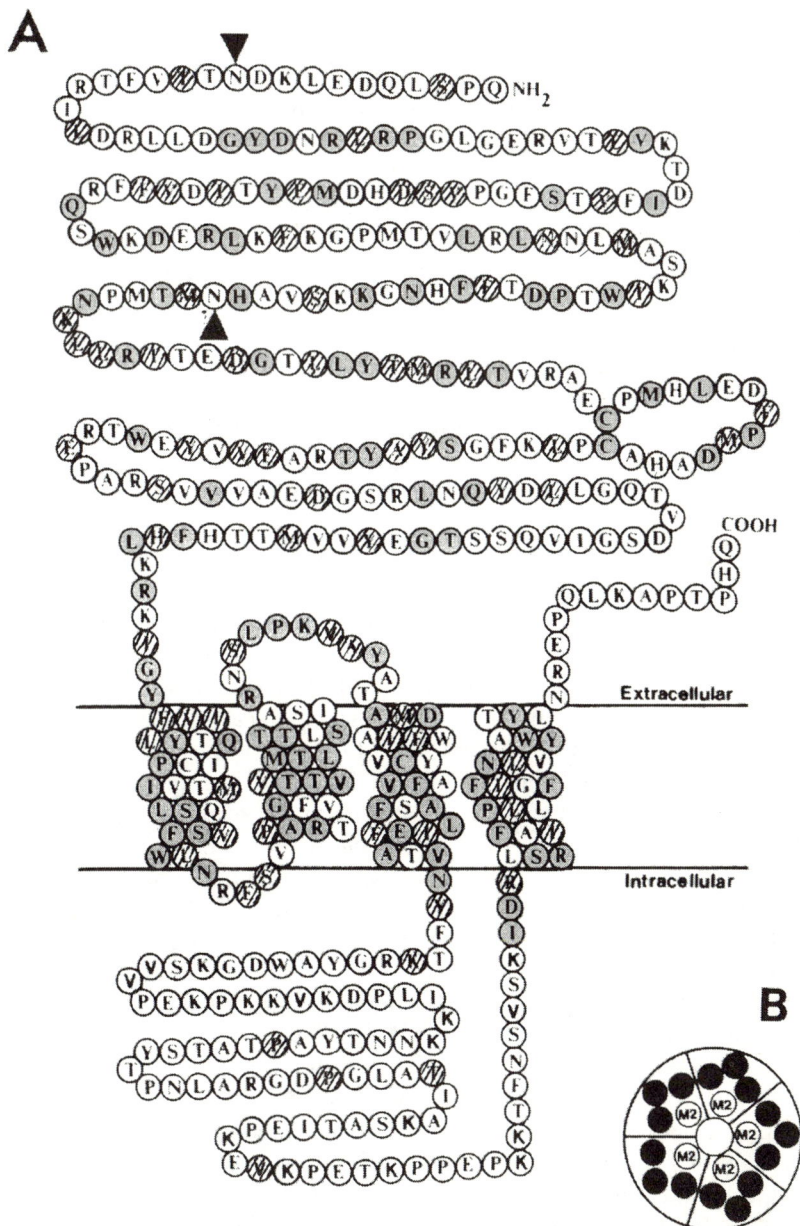

loop domains (e.g. Levitan *et al.*, 1988). Various rat and human GABA$_A$ receptor subunit amino acid sequences are now known (e.g. Garrett *et al.*, 1988; Lolait *et al.*, 1989; Schofield *et al.*, 1989); they have 98–99% amino acid sequence identity with the corresponding bovine sequences, indicating a high degree of conservation of structure between species.

3.   *The Structure of the GABA$_A$ Receptors*

The predicted transmembrane topology of the GABA$_A$ receptor polypeptides (Figure 1) is similar to that of other ligand-gated ion channels— namely the nicotinic acetylcholine receptor (e.g. Numa, 1986), the glycine receptor (Grenningloh *et al.*, 1987) and the kainate subclass of excitatory amino acid receptor (e.g. Hollmann *et al.*, 1989). Indeed, specific domains within the nicotinic acetylcholine receptor, the glycine receptor and the GABA$_A$ receptor are conserved at the amino acid level, most notably again the transmembrane regions and the disulphide-bonded loop in the hydrophi- lic N-terminal region. These findings led to the discovery of the ligand-gated ion channel superfamily (Schofield *et al.*, 1987; Grenningloh *et al.*, 1987). This immediately raised several questions concerning the structure of the GABA$_A$ receptor. If all the ligand-gated ion channels belong to the same family of proteins as the conservation in amino acid sequence suggests, then it is a reasonable assumption that the structural features of all the members of the family are conserved. Elegant three-dimensional image reconstruction has shown that the peripheral nicotinic acetylcholine receptor has a pentameric structure $\alpha2\beta\gamma\delta$ (Brisson and Unwin, 1985) and cross-linking experiments showed that the glycine receptor also has the quaternary structure of a pentamer (Langosch *et al.*, 1988). Early biochemical studies had suggested that the GABA$_A$ receptor was a tetramer (Mamalaki *et al.*, 1987). This model was based on the molecular weight determination of the native receptor by hydrodynamic methods (Mamalaki *et al.*, 1989) and the densitometric scan- ning of Coomassie blue stained SDS–PAGE of the purified receptor, which showed that the apparent α and β subunits were present in a 1:1 ratio. Following the discovery of the multiple isoforms of the subunits by molecular cloning, additional polypeptides have been found to be present in purified receptor preparations. For example, Kirkness and Turner (1988) made an antibody to the amino acid sequence $\alpha1$ 101–109. In immunoblots using receptors purified from porcine cerebral cortex this antibody recognized two bands. These were a band with M_r 51 kD which was coincident with the major band that was photoaffinity-labelled with [^{3}H]flunitrazepam and thus iden- tified as the α subunit, and a band with M_r 58 kD which was of higher molecular weight than the subunit irreversibly labelled with [^{3}H]muscimol (i.e. β subunit) and therefore named α-like. Resolution of these now three polypeptides was obtained and they were shown to be present in a ratio of $2(\alpha)$: $1(\beta)$: $1(\alpha$-like) by densitometric scanning. Using an antibody directed against the sequence Cys α3 454–467, this band was identified as the α3 polypeptide and the higher molecule weight found agreed with that predicted from the respective cDNA (Stephenson *et al.*, 1989). These results demonstrated that the methods which were employed for the determination of the quaternary structure of the GABA_A receptor as described above were inadequate, since in one-dimensional SDS–PAGE, as indicated, the β (isoform not known) and α3 polypeptides comigrate, and indeed it is now known, again using subunit-specific antibodies, that the α1, the α2 and the γ2 polypeptides comigrate (Stephenson *et al.*, 1990). Thus, the quaternary structures of the GABA_A receptors are still not known, although it is generally assumed that, in common with the other members of the ligand-gated ion channel superfamily, they are pentamers. However, it should be noted that a combination of densitometric scanning of SDS–PAGE, N-terminal amino acid sequence determination and quantitative radioiodination has shown that the neuronal nicotinic acetylcholine receptor of chick brain is composed of two α and two β subunits (Whiting *et al.*, 1989). Negative staining of purified GABA_A receptors with uranyl acetate has shown that the

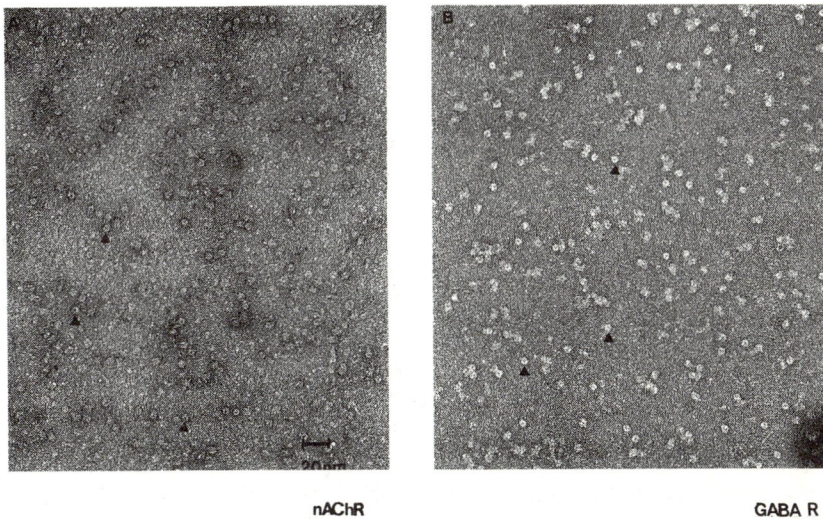

nAChR   GABA R

Figure 2   A comparison of nicotinic acetylcholine receptors and GABA_A receptors as seen in the electron microscope under negative stain. A is a photograph of the negative stain of the nicotinic acetylcholine receptor purified from *Torpedo californica* and B is a photograph of the negative stain of the GABA_A purified from bovine cerebral cortex. Both protein preparations were treated with uranyl acetate and the material was viewed by standard electron microscopy techniques. Note that both preparations appear similar and consist of an array of homogeneous round structures with dark centres which in each case are thought to be the mouths of the respective ion channels. Arrowheads indicate typical structures. The negative staining and photography was carried out by Nigel Unwin of the MRC Laboratory of Molecular Biology in Cambridge, England

general architecture of the receptor is similar to that of the peripheral nicotinic acetylcholine receptor, but the resolution obtained with these images does not yet permit a distinction between an axis of four- or fivefold symmetry around the central pit which is assumed to be the mouth of the ion channel (Figure 2).

The multiplicity of the GABA$_A$ receptor polypeptides described would predict a large number of different receptor proteins if every permutation of subunits were employed for either a tetrameric or a pentameric structure. Although the subunit compositions of the GABA$_A$ receptor oligomers are not known, some clues as to the subunit complements have been obtained by *in situ* hybridization and the use of isoform-specific antibodies. For example, both Northern blots and *in situ* hybridization using $\alpha 1$, $\alpha 2$ and $\alpha 3$ subunit-specific oligonucleotide probes found a differential brain-regional distribution and abundance for each of the α subunit isoforms (Levitan *et al.*, 1988; Wisden *et al.*, 1988, 1989b). The $\alpha 1$ mRNA is the most abundant of the three in all bovine brain areas, compared with the $\alpha 2$ and $\alpha 3$ transcripts, which are of low abundance but are enriched in the hippocampus and layers V and VI of the frontal cerebral cortex, respectively (Wisden *et al.*, 1988). Although the abundance of the mRNA does not necessarily correlate with the concentration of the respective polypeptides, immunoprecipitation of benzodiazepine binding sites from detergent extracts of bovine brain with anti-α-subunit isoform-specific antibodies demonstrated a brain-regional distribution of the $\alpha 1$, $\alpha 2$ and $\alpha 3$ polypeptides (Duggan and Stephenson, 1989, 1990). In three brain regions studied, the $\alpha 1$ subunit was the most abundant in cerebral cortex and, notably, in cerebellum immunoprecipitated $\geqslant 80\%$ of the benzodiazepine binding sites; the $\alpha 3$ subunit was detectable in cerebral cortex and hippocampus, where it was present at approximately equal concentration, whereas the $\alpha 2$ subunit was the most abundant isoform in the hippocampus (Figure 3; Duggan and Stephenson, 1990). Furthermore, addition of two or three different anti-α-subunit isoform-specific antibodies to the immunoprecipitation assay (i.e. anti-$\alpha 1$- + anti-$\alpha 2$- + anti-$\alpha 3$-subunit antibodies) resulted in an additive increase in the percentage of the benzodiazepine binding sites pelleted compared with the immunoprecipitation with the individual anti-α-subunit isoform-specific antibody alone (Duggan and Stephenson, 1990). These results support the conclusions reached from the *in situ* hybridization studies that the different α subunits are part of functionally distinct GABA$_A$ receptors and that only one type of α subunit is found within a single GABA$_A$ receptor oligomer.

The remaining subunit complement has still to be determined. *In situ* hybridization studies have shown that the pattern of distribution of $\gamma 2$ mRNA resembles that of the $\alpha 1$ subunit mRNA and, indeed, in many neurons a codistribution of $\alpha 1$, $\beta 2$ (the most abundant isoform of the β subunit mRNAs) and $\gamma 2$ exists (Shivers *et al.*, 1989). In contrast, δ mRNA is found in a subset of neurons distinct from those containing $\gamma 2$ mRNA, and the pattern of distribution of the δ mRNA in these neurons does not match the

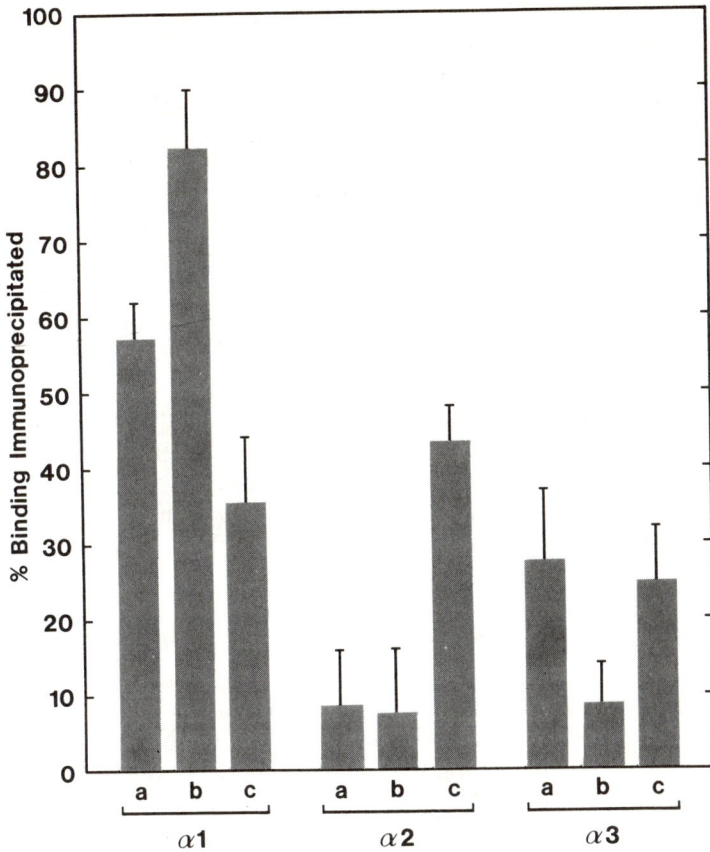

Figure 3 Demonstration of brain-regional distribution of α subunit isoforms of GABA_A receptor by immunoprecipitation with anti-α1 324–341, anti-Cys α2 414–424 and anti-Cys α3 454–467 antibodies. The amino acid sequences α1 324–341, Cys α2 414–424 and Cys α3 454–467 of the bovine GABA_A receptor subunits were synthesized and coupled to keyhole limpet haemocyanin and the resultant conjugate was used for the production of polyclonal antibodies. Each peptide was from a region unique to the α subunit isoform—i.e. α1 324–341 is from the cytoplasmic loop; Cys α2 414–424 and Cys α3 454–467 are the C-terminal sequences of the α2 and α3 polypeptides, respectively (see Figure 1). Na⁺ deoxycholate extracts were prepared from adult bovine cerebral cortex, cerebellum and hippocampus. An immunoprecipitation assay was carried out as described in Duggan and Stephenson (1989, 1990), using the respective affinity-purified antibodies, for each soluble extract. Following immunoprecipitation, the specific benzodiazepine binding sites remaining in the supernatant or present in the pellet were measured by radioligand binding assay. The figure shows the maximum percentage of [³H]flunitrazepam binding sites immunoprecipitated for each brain region for each antibody, and the results are expressed as the percentage of sites immunoprecipitated with respect to control samples which contained normal IgG only. a is immunoprecipitation from Na⁺ deoxycholate extracts from adult bovine cerebral cortex, b is from cerebellum and c is from hippocampus. α1 is immunoprecipitation with anti-α1 324–341 antibodies, α2 is immunoprecipitation with anti-Cys α2 414–424 antibodies and α3 is immunoprecipitation with anti-Cys α3 454–467 antibodies

distribution of any of the known GABA$_A$ receptor subunit mRNAs (Shivers *et al.* 1989). On the basis of this, Shivers *et al.*, (1989) suggest that one version of the receptor may be composed of α1, β2 and γ2 subunits but with unknown stoichiometry. However, they acknowledge that their observations are of the abundance of the respective mRNAs and, as pointed out before, these may not necessarily be cognate with the abundance of the respective subunits. There is a possibility also that some GABA$_A$ receptors exist as homo-oligomers. The feasibility of this arose from the finding that each of the α, β, γ and δ subunits when expressed singly in either *Xenopus* oocytes (Blair *et al.*, 1988) or human embryonic kidney 293 cells transfected with the respective subunit-encoding cDNAs, form GABA-gated chloride ion channels (Pritch-ett *et al.*, 1989c).

In the end, the issue can only be resolved by the development of antibodies specific for each of the isoforms and then the use of these antibodies either for isoform-immunoaffinity purification and characteriza-tion *or* for the immunocytochemical distribution of each isoform in adjacent brain sections.

4. *Expression of Recombinant GABA$_A$ Receptors*

While the polypeptide compositions of the GABA$_A$ receptor *in vivo* remain unknown, it must be recognized that the study of the properties of the recombinant GABA$_A$ receptors, whether expressed in *Xenopus* oocytes or in cells, is limited, since it is not known how these relate to the native receptor. Furthermore, it should also be recognized that until more information is available regarding the control of the biogenesis of the receptor, extrapola-tions from what combination of subunit RNAs are injected into *Xenopus* oocytes or subunit cDNAs transfected into cells to what type of recombinant receptor is made should be made with caution, particularly with respect to the final stoichiometry of receptor subunits in one oligomeric structure. How-ever, despite these caveats the study of expressed GABA$_A$ receptors has yielded important information. The first and initially most pertinent finding was that when bovine α1 subunit and β1 subunit RNAs were coinjected into *Xenopus* oocytes, GABA-gated chloride ion channels were formed and this was the definitive proof that the cDNAs that had been identified did indeed encode GABA$_A$ receptor polypeptides (Schofield *et al.*, 1987). In this first report it was shown that these channels had the expected pharmacology of a GABA$_A$ receptor—i.e. they were bicuculline- and picrotoxin-sensitive and they were potentiated both by barbiturates and a benzodiazepine, clorazepate (Schofield *et al.*, 1987).

Further studies found that the benzodiazepine facilitation of the GABA-gated chloride ion conductance was variable in the α1 + β1 receptors ex-pressed in oocytes. Coexpression of the human α1 + β1 + γ2 subunits in human embryonic kidney 293 cells formed GABA-gated channels which showed a large reproducible benzodiazepine response (Pritchett *et al.*, 1989c). The benzodiazepine response had the same pharmacology as that found for native receptors in that it was blocked by the benzodiazepine antagonist Ro 15-1788 and methyl-4-ethyl-6,7-dimethoxy-carboline-3-carboxylate (DMCM), a benzodiazepine inverse agonist, reduced the GABA-induced chloride current. Furthermore, specific benzodiazepine radioligand binding activity was present in the cells transfected with all the three $\alpha1 + \beta1 + \gamma2$ subunits (Pritchett *et al.*, 1989c). However, the group of Mohler found that expression of rat $\alpha1 + \beta1$ subunits only, either in oocytes or in cells, gave a weak benzodiazepine facilitation (Mohler *et al.*, 1989). However, in these receptors inverse agonists acted as potentiators of the conductance increase, which is at variance with the properties of these compounds *in vivo* (Mohler *et al.*, 1989). Following the discovery of the $\gamma2$ polypeptide by molecular cloning, it was proposed that the $\gamma2$ polypeptide migrated with the α subunit in SDS–PAGE of the purified receptor and that the site of the agonist benzodiazepine photoaffinity labelling site was actually on the $\gamma2$ polypeptide rather than the $\alpha1$ subunit (Pritchett *et al.*, 1989c). Indeed, the α and γ polypeptides have been shown to comigrate in SDS–PAGE but, although the $\gamma2$ subunit is an integral component of some GABA$_A$ receptors, the use of subunit-specific antibodies has demonstrated that it is the α subunit that is the principal site for the agonist benzodiazepine photoaffinity labelling reaction (Stephenson *et al.*, 1990). The current hypothesis now is that either the binding site is shared between the α and $\gamma2$ subunits or the $\gamma2$ polypeptide stabilizes the benzodiazepine binding site within a GABA$_A$ receptor oligomer. Note also in this context that, although it is the $\gamma2$ subunit that confers the large benzodiazepine response, it is the α subunit isoform that confers the subclass of benzodiazepine receptor pharmacology in the recombinant GABA$_A$ receptors (Pritchett *et al.*, 1989a; see next section).

In contrast to the benzodiazepine response in expressed GABA$_A$ receptors, which requires at least three subunit types, as mentioned earlier, GABA-gated channels can be recorded following expression of a single subunit type only. GABA$_A$ receptor homo-oligomers can be formed by the expression of either the α, β, $\gamma2$ or δ subunits alone, albeit at a reduced efficiency compared with when combinations of subunits are expressed (Blair *et al.*, 1988; Pritchett *et al.*, 1988b, 1989c). Bovine GABA$_A$ receptor $\alpha1$ or $\beta1$ homo-oligomers have the same multiple conductance states as are found for native receptors. However, the main conductance state in the expressed receptors was the 19 pS state, which compares with a main conductance state of 27–30 pS in GABA$_A$ receptor channels recorded from spinal cord neurons (Blair *et al.*, 1988; Moss *et al.*, 1990). This suggests that the multiple conductance states are a property of the chloride ion channel but that the main state must be dependent on the complement of subunits present in a receptor. All homo-oligomers are also potentiated by barbiturates. These observations must imply that all GABA$_A$ receptor subunits carry the binding sites for both GABA and the barbiturates. Again there is a discrepancy between the biochemical studies and those derived from the study of the recombinant receptors. It was shown initially that the GABA agonist [^{3}H]muscimol specifically photoaffinity labelled the β subunit of the purified GABA$_A$ receptor (Casalotti *et al.*, 1986), although later reports showed that there was also some minor specific incorporation of radioactivity into the α subunit region in SDS–PAGE of purified receptor preparations (Bureau and Olsen, 1988). The agonist site that is photoaffinity labelled is a high-affinity site which may be a densitized state of the receptor. For the nicotinic acetylcholine receptor, it was suggested that a physiologically important low-affinity binding site for acetylcholine, which is detectable by rapid flux determinations but not by standard radioligand binding assays, is present on all these receptor subunits, whereas affinity labelling studies showed that a high-affinity acetylcholine binding site was present on the α subunit only (Dunn *et al.*, 1983). Such must also be the case for the GABA$_A$ receptors.

α variant (i.e. α1 + β1, α2 + β1, etc.) and β variant expressed GABA$_A$ receptors (i.e. α1 + β1, α1 + β2, etc.) do show a differential sensitivity to agonist activation and different degrees of desensitization (Levitan *et al.*, 1988; Ymer *et al.*, 1989a). This has been reported fully for the α1 + β1, α2 + β1 and α3 + β1 receptors, where a thirtyfold difference in sensitivity to agonists is found between the α2/β1 receptor which is the most sensitive, with a half-maximal response elicited by 1.3 μM GABA concentration, and the α3/β1, which is the least sensitive, with a value of 42 μM (Levitan *et al.*, 1988). The differences found may not necessarily be a direct result of subtle differences in the binding site between the agonist and receptor for the various α isoforms but may reflect differences in the conformational coupling between ligand binding and channel opening. Nevertheless, it is interesting to speculate on the location of the GABA binding site. It must be within the extracellular domain of the receptor, since GABA is impermeable to membranes and trypsin treatment of intact embryonic chick brain cells in culture results in the specific loss of GABA binding activity (Czajkowski *et al.*, 1989). A favoured candidate region for the agonist binding site is the 'cys' loop (Figure 1)—a domain that is highly conserved not only between all GABA$_A$ receptor subunit types, but also between other members of the ligand-gated ion channel superfamily. Indeed, there is some evidence for its participation in the binding of acetylcholine in the peripheral nicotinic acetylcholine receptor (summarized in Cockcroft *et al.*, 1990), but its role in the binding of agonists in the GABA$_A$ receptors is so far not substantiated by experimental evidence.

5.   *Functions of the GABA$_A$ Receptors*

With such a potential diversity in GABA$_A$ receptor structure, the question immediately arises as to what the physiological functions of the various subtypes are. Receptor subtype heterogeneity is a general feature of the neuroreceptors and voltage-gated ion channels, and has been recently discussed in general terms by Schofield *et al.* (1990).

The question of the significance of functional diversity can be considered at different levels. At the most fundamental level, it is now recognized that GABA$_A$ receptors are found in both neuronal and glial cells. In neuronal cells the GABA$_A$ receptors have their classical role of hyperpolarization and inhibition of the conductance of the nerve impulse, whereas in glial cells a role for GABA$_A$ receptors in the buffering of chloride ions has been suggested (Bormann and Kettenmann, 1988). The α2 mRNA has been localized to the Bergmann glial cells layer of the cerebellum (Wisden *et al.*, 1989a).

Within the neuronal population of cells, it is not clear whether only one subtype of receptors exists within a single cell type or whether multiple receptors are present within a single neuron. Whatever the case, there are important differences between the putative subtypes which could have differential consequences, whether present on a single cell or on a population of adjacent neurons. For example, the study of the α and β variant GABA$_A$ receptor subtypes showed that each differed in its sensitivity to agonist activation (Levitan *et al.*, 1988; see previous section). Thus, the activation of a particular receptor subtype and, hence, neuronal pathway will be dependent upon the concentration of GABA released from the input neuron. This may be pertinent to the development of the synaptic connections within the nervous system. It has been suggested that some of the GABA$_A$ receptor polypeptides are developmentally regulated—in particular, α3 subunit mRNA, which, of the α variant receptors, shows the least sensitivity to agonist activation, was shown to be elevated in 12 day calf brain compared with adult bovine brain (Levitan *et al.*, 1988).

There is also the possibility of pharmacological differences between the GABA$_A$ receptor subtypes, which has important implications for the manipulation of the specific pathways. So far, no differences have been found in the pharmacological profiles of the GABA recognition site in the recombinant receptors, but exhaustive structure–activity studies have not yet been carried out. More attention has focused on the pharmacology of the benzodiazepine recognition site. Again studies of expressed receptors have demonstrated clearly that there is a structural basis for the type I and type II benzodiazepine receptor subtypes (Pritchett *et al.*, 1989a). (The existence of these subtypes was predicted by radioligand binding studies and the use of selective drugs—e.g. the β carboline series of compounds, which inhibited benzodiazepine binding activity with a shallow displacement curve: Nielsen and Braestrup (1980).) Coexpression of α variant (α + β1 + γ2) GABA$_A$ receptors demonstrated that the α1 subunit conferred type I benzodiazepine receptor subtype pharmacology, whereas α2- or α3-containing oligomers conferred type II pharmacology (Pritchett *et al.*, 1989b). This agrees well with the distribution of these receptor subclasses by the initial radioligand binding studies (Nielsen and Braestrup, 1980) and the distribution of the α1, α2 and α3 subunits, using α subunit isoform-specific antibodies (Duggan and

Stephenson, 1990). With the discovery of the other α subunit isoforms, $\alpha4$, $\alpha5$ and $\alpha6$, it is now known that there is an additional pharmacological subclass of benzodiazepine binding site. The $\alpha5$ subunit was shown to be of the type II class, but with differential behaviour of the compound zolpidem compared with the $\alpha2$ and $\alpha3$ variant receptors (Pritchett *et al.*, 1989b).

It has always been an issue as to whether there exists a GABA receptor with A-type pharmacology which is insensitive to benzodiazepines, as indirect observations in the literature suggest (reviewed in Stephenson, 1988). It has been shown recently that antibodies directed specifically at the $\alpha6$ polypeptide immunoprecipitate [^{3}H]muscimol but not [^{3}H]flunitrazepam binding sites from solution. This is the first positive proof that such a receptor subclass does exist (Pritchett *et al.*, 1989b). With respect to the different functions of the GABA$_A$ receptors, this reopens the question of the endogenous ligand for the benzodiazepine recognition site, and if it does indeed exist, it must then modulate subpopulations of GABA$_A$ receptors.

Finally, in this discussion it is necessary to consider the importance of intracellular regulation of GABA$_A$ receptor function. It is notable that, for all the GABA$_A$ receptor polypeptides, the most divergent regions in amino acid sequences, whether between subunit types or isoforms of one subunit type, are found in the predicted cytoplasmic hydrophilic loops of the polypeptides. These regions, therefore, are available for isoform-specific intracellular regulation by second messengers, and, indeed, a consensus amino acid sequence for cAMP-dependent protein kinase for all the β subunits and a consensus amino acid sequence for tyrosine kinase for the $\gamma2$ polypeptide are both located here (Schofield *et al.*, 1987; Pritchett *et al.*, 1989c; Ymer *et al.*, 1989a). The GABA$_A$ receptor is phosphorylated *in vitro* by protein kinase A (Kirkness *et al.*, 1989) and several groups have shown that the run-down of the GABA-activated conductance is prevented by magnesium-ATP, implying that phosphorylation of the receptor is required to maintain function (Gyenes *et al.*, 1988; Stelzer *et al.*, 1988). Therefore, the presence of different isoforms of subunits within one receptor or between two receptors within a single neuronal cell permits selective intracellular regulation.

6. *Future Trends*

In this chapter, I have summarized the recent developments in the study of the GABA$_A$ receptors. In so doing, I have tried to reconcile the early GABA$_A$ receptor purification work, where the emphasis was on fitting experimental observations to a model of *the* GABA$_A$ receptor structure, with the recent findings of multiple, closely related GABA$_A$ receptor polypeptides by recombinant DNA methodology. (It should be noted that the elegant work of Sieghart and colleagues on the membrane-bound form of the receptor had suggested the existence of multiple α subunits before the cloning work had succeeded: summarized in Sieghart (1989).) Yet despite the wealth of information that has been forthcoming from the application of molecular biological techniques to the study of this family of proteins, important fundamental questions remain. The most notable of these are: what are the polypeptide compositions of the GABA$_A$ receptors in the brain? How may these be related to their different functional properties? What controls the differential expression of the various subtypes within particular neuronal or glial cell populations? An integrated approach involving molecular biology, the development and use of antibodies directed at each of the subtypes of receptor polypeptides, and electrophysiological studies is needed to answer these questions.

Acknowledgements

F.A.S. is a Royal Society University Research Fellow. I thank Gill Patterson for secretarial assistance in the preparation of the manuscript.

References

Barnard, E. A., Darlison, M. G. and Seeburg, P. H. (1987). Molecular biology of the GABA$_A$ receptor; the receptor/channel superfamily. *Trends Neurosci.*, **12**, 502–509

Blair, L. A. C., Levitan, E. S., Marshall, J., Dionne, V. E. and Barnard, E. A. (1988). Single subunits of the GABA$_A$ receptor form ion channels with properties of the native receptor. *Science, N.Y.*, **242**, 577–579

Bormann, J. and Kettenmann, H. (1988). Patch clamp study of γ-aminobutyric acid receptor Cl$^-$ channels in cultured astrocytes. *Proc. Natl Acad. Sci. USA*, **85**, 9336–9340

Bowery, N. G. (1989). GABA$_B$ receptors and their significance in mammalian pharmacology. *Trends Pharmacol. Sci.*, **10**, 401–407

Brisson, A. and Unwin, P. N. T. (1985). Quaternary structure of the acetylcholine receptor. *Nature*, **315**, 474–477

Bureau, M. and Olsen, R. W. (1988). GABA/benzodiazepine receptor protein carries binding sites for both ligands on both of two major peptide subunits. *Biochem. Biophys. Res. Commun.*, **153**, 1006–1011

Casalotti, S. O., Stephenson, F. A. and Barnard, E. A. (1986). Separate subunits for agonist and benzodiazepine binding in the γ-aminobutyric acid$_A$ receptor oligomer. *J. Biol. Chem.*, **261**, 15013–15016

Cockcroft, V. B., Osguthorpe, D., Barnard, E. A. and Lunt, G. G. (1990). Modelling of agonist binding to the ligand-gated ion channel super-family of receptors. *Proteins*, in press.

Czajkowski, C., Gibbs, T. T. and Farb, D. H. (1989). Transmembrane topology of the γ-aminobutyric acid$_A$/benzodiazepine receptors subcellular distribution and allosteric coupling determined *in situ*. *Molec. Pharmacol.*, **35**, 75–84

Duggan, M. J. and Stephenson, F. A. (1989). Bovine γ-aminobutyric acid$_A$ receptor sequence-specific antibodies; identification of two epitopes which are recognised in both native and denatured γ-aminobutyric acid$_A$ receptors. *J. Neurochem.*, **53**, 132–139

Duggan, M. J. and Stephenson, F. A. (1990). Biochemical evidence for the existence of γ-aminobutyric acid$_A$ receptor iso-oligomers. *J. Biol. Chem.*, **265**, 3831–3835

Dunn, S. M. J., Conti-Tronconi, B. M. and Raftery, M. A. (1983). Separate sites of low and high affinity for agonists on *Torpedo californica* acetylcholine receptor. *Biochemistry*, **22**, 2512–2518

Garrett, K. M., Duman, R. S., Saito, N., Blume, A. J., Vitek, M. P. and Tallman, J. F. (1988). Isolation of a cDNA clone for the alpha subunit of the human GABA receptor. *Biochem. Biophys. Res. Commun.*, **156**, 1039–1045

Greeningloh, G., Rienitz, A., Schmitt, B., Methfessel, C., Zensen, M., Beyreuther, K.,

Gundelfinger, E. D. and Betz, H. (1987). The strychnine-binding subunit of the glycine receptor shows homology with nicotinic acetylcholine receptors. *Nature*, **328**, 215–220

Gyenes, M., Farrant, M. and Farb, D. H. (1988). Run-down of γ-aminobutyric acid$_A$ receptor function during whole-cell recording; a possible role for phosphorylation. *Molec. Pharmacol.*, **34**, 719–723

Hollmann, M., O'Shea-Greenfeld, A., Rogers, S. W. and Heinemann, S. (1989). Cloning by functional expression of a member of the glutamate receptor family. *Nature*, **342**, 643–648

Khrestchatisky, M., MacLennan, A. J., Chiang, M.-Y., Xu, W., Jackson, M. B., Brecha, N., Sternini, C., Olsen, R. W. and Tobin, A. J. (1989). A novel α subunit in rat brain GABA$_A$ receptors. *Neuron*, **3**, 745–753

Kirkness, E. F., Bovenkirk, C. F., Ueda, T. and Turner, A. J. (1989). Phosphorylation of γ-aminobutyrate (GABA)/benzodiazepine receptors by cyclic AMP-dependent protein kinase. *Biochem. J.*, **259**, 613–616

Kirkness, E. F. and Turner, A. J. (1988). Antibodies directed against a nonapeptide sequence of the γ-aminobutyrate (GABA) benzodiazepine receptor α subunit. *Biochem. J.*, **256**, 291–294

Langosch, D, Thomas, L. and Betz, H. (1988). Conserved quaternary structure of ligand-gated ion channels: the postsynaptic glycine receptor is a pentamer. *Proc. Natl Acad. Sci. USA*, **85**, 7394–7398

Levitan, E. S., Schofield, P. R., Burt, D. R., Rhee, L. M., Wisden, W., Kohler, M., Rodriguez, H., Stephenson, F. A., Darlison, M. G., Barnard, E. A. and Seeburg, P. H. (1988). Structural and functional basis for GABA$_A$ receptor heterogeneity. *Nature*, **335**, 76–79

Lolait, S. J., O'Carroll, A.-M., Kusano, K., Muller, J. M., Brownstein, M. J. and Mahan, L. C. (1989). Cloning and expression of a novel rat GABA$_A$ receptor. *FEBS Lett.*, **246**, 145–148

Mamalaki, C., Barnard, E. A. and Stephenson, F. A. (1989). Molecular size of the γ-aminobutyric acid$_A$ receptor purified from mammalian cerebral cortex. *J. Neurochem.*, **52**, 124–134

Mamalaki, C., Stephenson, F. A. and Barnard, E. A. (1987). The GABA$_A$/benzodiazepine receptor is a heterotetramer of homologous α and β subunits. *EMBO Jl*, **6**, 561–565

Mohler, H., Malherbe, P. and Draghun, A. (1989). GABA$_A$ receptors expressed from rat α- and β-subunits in *Xenopus* oocytes are modulated by benzodiazepine receptor ligands. *Soc. Neurosci. Abstr.*, **15**, 997

Moss, S. J., Smart, T., Porter, N. M., Naushaba, N., Devine, J., Stephenson, F. A., Mcdonald, R. L. and Barnard, E. A. (1990). Cloned GABA receptors are maintained in a stable cell line: allosteric and channel properties. *Eur. J. Pharmacol.*, in press

Nielsen, M. and Braestrup, C. (1980). Ethyl-β-carboline-3-carboxylate shows differential benzodiazepine receptor interactions. *Nature*, **286**, 606–607

Numa, S. (1986). Molecular basis for the function of ionic channels. *Biochem. Soc. Symp.*, **52**, 119–143

Olsen, R. W. and Venter, J. C. (Eds) (1986). *Benzodiazepine/GABA Receptors and Chloride Channels: Structure and Functional Properties*. Alan R. Liss, New York

Pritchett, D. B., Luddens, H. and Seeburg, P. H. (1989a). Type I and type II GABA$_A$-benzodiazepine receptors produced in transfected cells. *Science, N.Y.*, **245**, 1389–1392

Pritchett, D. B., Luddens, H. and Seeburg, P. H. (1989b). Structural basis of type I and type II GABA$_A$/benzodiazepine receptors. *Soc. Neurosci. Abstr.*, **15**, 641

Pritchett, D. B., Schofield, P. R., Sontheimer, H., Ymer, S., Kettenmann, H. and Seeburg, P. H. (1988a). GABA$_A$ receptor cDNAs expressed in transfected cells and studied by path-clamp and binding assay. *Soc. Neurosci. Abstr.*, **14**, 641

Pritchett, D. B., Sontheimer, H., Gorman, C. M., Kettenmann, H., Seeburg, P. H. and Schofield, P. R. (1988b). Transient expression shows ligand gating and allosteric potentiation of GABA$_A$ receptor subunits. *Science, N.Y.*, **242**, 1306–1308

Pritchett, D. B., Sontheimer, H., Shivers, B. D., Ymer, S., Kettenmann, H., Schofield, P. R. and Seeburg, P. H. (1989c). Importance of a novel GABA$_A$ receptor subunit for benzodiazepine pharmacology. *Nature*, **338**, 582–585

Richards, J. G., Schoch, P., Haring, P., Takacs, B. and Mohler, H. (1987). Resolving GABA$_A$/benzodiazepine receptors; cellular and subcellular localisation in the CNS with monoclonal antibodies. *J. Neurosci.*, **7**, 1866–1886

Schofield, P. R., Darlison, M. G., Fujita, N., Burt, D. R., Stephenson, F. A., Rodriguez, H., Rhee, L. M., Ramachandran, J., Reale, V., Glencorse, T. A., Seeburg, P. H. and Barnard, E. A. (1987). Sequence and functional expression of the GABA$_A$ receptor shows a ligand-gated receptor super-family. *Nature*, **323**, 221–227

Schofield, P. R., Pritchett, D. B., Sontheimer, H., Kettenmann, H. and Seeburg, P. H. (1989). Sequence and expression of human GABA$_A$ receptor α1 and β1 subunits. *FEBS Lett.*, **244**, 361–364

Schofield, P. R., Shivers, B. D. and Seeburg, P. H. (1990). The role of receptor subtype diversity in the CNS. *Trends Neurosci.*, **13**, 8–11

Shivers, B. D., Killisch, I., Sprengel, R., Sontheimer, H., Kohler, M., Schofield, P. R. and Seeburg, P. H. (1989). Two novel GABA$_A$ receptor subunits exist in distinct neuronal populations. *Neuron*, **3**, 327–337

Sieghart, W. (1989). Multiplicity GABA$_A$-benzodiazepine receptors. *Trends Pharmacol. Sci.*, **10**, 407–411

Sigel, E., and Barnard, E. A. (1984). A γ-aminobutyric acid/benzodiazepine receptor complex from bovine cerebral cortex. Improved purification with preservation of regulatory sites and their interactions. *J. Biol. Chem.*, **259**, 7219–7223

Sigel, E., Stephenson, F. A., Mamalaki, C. and Barnard, E. A. (1983). A γ-aminobutyric acid/benzodiazepine receptor complex of bovine cerebral cortex. *J. Biol. Chem.*, **258**, 6965–6971

Stelzer, A., Kay, A. R. and Wong, R. K. S. (1988). GABA$_A$ receptor function in hippocampal cells is maintained by phosphorylation factors. *Science, N.Y.*, **241**, 339–341

Stephenson, F. A. (1988). Understanding the GABA$_A$ receptor: a chemically-gated ion channel. *Biochem. J.*, **249**, 21–32

Stephenson, F. A. and Dolphin, A. C. (1989). GABA and glycine neutotransmission. *Seminars Neurosci.*, **1**, 115–123

Stephenson, F. A., Duggan, M. J. and Casalotti, S. O. (1989). Identification of the α3 subunit in the GABA$_A$ receptor purified from bovine brain. *FEBS Lett.*, **243**, 358–362

Stephenson, F. A., Duggan, M. J. and Vollard, S. (1990). The γ2 subunit is an integral component of the γ-aminobutyric$_A$ receptor but the α1 polypeptide is the principal site of the agonist benzodiazepine photoaffinity labelling reaction. *J. Biol. Chem.*, in press

Whiting, P., Cooper, J., Conroy, W. G. and Lindstrom, J. (1989). Subunit stoichometry of neuronal nicotinic acetylcholine receptors. *Soc. Neurosci. Abstr.*, **15**, 496

Wisden, W., McNaughton, L. A., Darlison, M. G., Hunt, S. P. and Barnard, E. A. (1989a). Differential distribution of GABA$_A$ receptor mRNAs in bovine cerebellum—localisation of α2 mRNA in Bergmann glia layer. *Neurosci. Lett.*, **106**, 7–12

Wisden, W., Morris, B. J., Darlison, M. G., Hunt, S. P. and Barnard, E. A. (1988). Distinct GABA$_A$ receptor α subunit mRNAs show differential patterns of expression in bovine brain. *Neuron*, **1**, 937–947

Wisden, W., Morris, B. J., Darlison, M. G., Hunt, S. P. and Barnard, E. A. (1989b). Localisation of GABA$_A$ receptor α subunit mRNAs in relation to receptor subtypes. *Molec. Brain Res.*, **5**, 305–310

Ymer, S., Schofield, P. R., Draguhn, A., Werner, P., Kohler, M. and Seeburg, P. H. (1989a). GABA$_A$ receptor β subunit heterogeneity; functional expression of cloned cDNAs. *EMBO Jl*, **8**, 1665–1670

Ymer, S., Draguhn, A., Kohler, M., Schofield, P. R. and Seeburg, P. H. (1989b). Sequence and expression of a novel GABA$_A$ receptor α subunit. *FEBS Lett.*, **258**, 119–122

6

Studying the Acetylcholine Receptor with Monoclonal Antibodies

SOCRATES J. TZARTOS

Hellenic Pasteur Institute, 127 Vas. Sofias Ave., Athens 11521, Greece

Contents

Current Aspects of the Neurosciences, Vol. 3. Edited by N. N. Osborne. © The Macmillan Press Ltd 1991

1. Introduction

Although not all expectations for the use of monoclonal antibodies (mAbs) have been satisfied, undoubtedly they have proved an invaluable set of tools in biomedical research. The early availability of purified acetylcholine receptor (AChR) in significant amounts and the involvement of anti-AChR antibodies in the disease myasthenia gravis (MG) were adequate motives for anti-AChR mAbs to be prepared by several groups from the first years of the mAb era. As was the case with mAbs raised against many other antigens, some of these mAbs have been used extensively, thus significantly contributing to the advancement of AChR and MG research, whereas others proved much less valuable tools.

This chapter presents a summary of the current knowledge on the AChR and MG, followed by some of the approaches that have been used for the detailed characterization of the binding sites—of anti-protein mAbs in general and, more specifically, anti-AChR mAbs. Finally, a subjective overview of the progress achieved using these mAbs as tools for the study of the AChR and the disease will be presented. Unavoidably, some important data have been omitted, whereas some other less critical data may have been overpresented. The use of mAbs for the study of various aspects of AChRs and MG has been reviewed (Lindstrom, 1986; Lindstrom et al., 1987; Tzartos, 1988; Tzartos et al., 1990a).

2. Acetylcholine Receptor

AChR is an integral glycoprotein of the postsynaptic membrane, composed of five homologous subunits with the stoichiometry $\alpha_2\beta\gamma\delta$ and a total molecular weight of about 290 000 (Changeux and Revah, 1987; Numa, 1987; Maelicke, 1988). The molecule, approximately 110 Å long and 80 Å wide, extends on both sides of the membrane (Brisson and Unwin, 1985; Mitra et al., 1989). The complete amino acid sequences of Torpedo electric organ and mammalian muscle AChR subunits are known. The four subunits within the same species have an approximately 40% homology among themselves, while the α subunits of Torpedo electric organ and human muscle AChR are 80% homologous (McCarthy et al., 1986; Numa, 1987). Each subunit is thought to transverse the membrane four times through four hydrophobic α helices, M1–M4 (reviewed in Changeux and Revah, 1987; Numa, 1987). Additional transmembrane helices have been proposed in the past (McCarthy et al., 1986; Ratnam et al., 1986a).

There is a general consensus that the N terminal of each subunit is located extracellularly, but there are conflicting models and data concerning the location of the C terminal (McCarthy et al., 1986; Dipaola et al., 1989). If four transmembrane helices amend to exist, the C end must be extracellular; in fact, this theory is supported by recent convincing data concerning the

C-terminal end of the δ subunit (Dipaola *et al.*, 1989).

Acetylcholine released from the nerve terminal binds to the AChR and causes opening of the cation channel which allows Na^+ to enter the muscle cell or electroplaque (Changeux and Revah, 1987; Maelicke, 1988). The cation channel is an integral part of the AChR molecule. All four kinds of subunit are required for the assembly of a fully functional AChR (Mishina *et al.*, 1984). The M2 helices from each subunit contribute to the formation of the cation channel (Hucho *et al.*, 1986; Giraudat *et al.*, 1987). Snake venom α toxins, a group of small proteins of approximate molecular weight 7500–8000, such as α-bungarotoxin, bind with high affinity to the two α subunits (K_d approximately 2×10^{-11}M), at or near the acetylcholine binding sites, competitively blocking AChR function (Changeux and Revah, 1987; Maelicke, 1988). Another group of molecules, including local anaesthetics, non-competitively block AChR function; these appear to bind at or near the ion channel (Changeux and Revah, 1987; Giraudat *et al.*, 1987).

3. *Myasthenia Gravis*

Myasthenia gravis (MG) is characterized by weakness and fatigability of the skeletal muscles. The disease occurs in about 1 out of 20 000 persons. The target of the spontaneously induced autoantibodies in MG patients is their own AChR (Oosterhuis, 1984; Drachman, 1987; Lindstrom *et al.*, 1988).

Anti-AChR antibodies are detected by radioimmunoassay in about 85% of MG patients. Such antibodies are essentially absent in healthy humans, though with a few characteristic exceptions: (1) most newborn infants of MG mothers do not show MG symptoms, although they carry their mothers' antibodies (Morel *et al.*, 1988a); (2) MG patients in remission usually continue having anti-AChR antibodies in their blood; and (3) healthy relatives of MG patients have been reported to have anti-AChR mAbs (Lefvert *et al.*, 1985).

Variations in anti-AChR antibody titre in a particular patient's sera correlate well with clinical improvement. In contrast, studies of populations of MG patients show only a weak correlation between absolute anti-AChR antibody concentration and severity of the disease (Lindstrom *et al.*, 1976). It is uncertain whether some antibody specificities are more potent than others in causing impairment of neuromuscular transmission (Drachman *et al.*, 1982; Tzartos *et al.*, 1986b). A large fraction of the anti-AChR antibodies bind to a region on the α subunit, named the main immunogenic region (MIR) (Tzartos and Lindstrom, 1980).

Loss of AChRs seems to be the main effect of the antibodies in MG, which in turn impairs neuromuscular transmission. AChR loss is caused by at least two mechanisms: (1) bivalent and polyvalent antibodies crosslink membrane-bound AChRs, resulting in an increase in their internalization and degradation rate (antigenic modulation); (2) complement binds to those antibodies which are bound on the membrane AChRs and mediates lysis of the AChR-containing membranes (Engel, 1984). Direct blockage of AChR function by antibodies to the acetylcholine binding site might be an additional cause of impairment of the neuromuscular transmission (Harvey *et al.*, 1978; Drachman *et al.*, 1982; Gomez and Richman, 1983; Morel *et al.*, 1988b).

4. *Monoclonal Antibodies*

Since the classical work of Kohler and Milstein (1975), in which they immortalized antibody-producing lymphocytes by fusing them with immortal myelomas, numerous reports have presented various improvements in the methodology of mAb production. Important steps include the following:

1. The introduction of polyethylene glycol, instead of virus, for fusing the lymphocytes with myelomas (Kohler and Milstein, 1976); this made the methodology applicable to a broader range of laboratories.

2. The use of myelomas which have lost the ability to synthesize their own immunoglobulin chains (Milstein, 1986); therefore, the hybrid cells produce only the immunoglobulin chains of the lymphocyte—i.e. the mAb is a real monoclonal rather than a hybrid molecule.

3. The introduction of *in vitro* immunization, which allows the use of minute amounts of immunogen (Luben and Mohler, 1980).

4. Several modifications designed to increase the yield, such as electrically induced fusion (electrofusion) (Lo *et al.*, 1984).

5. The use of human myelomas for the production of human mAbs (Olsson and Kaplan, 1980); there are still several difficulties with this much-needed technology.

6. Hybrid mAbs with two specificities.

7. Abzymes—i.e. mAbs with enzymatic activity (Lerner and Tramontano, 1987).

8. Improved antigen binding affinity and specificity by site-directed mutagenesis (Roberts *et al.*, 1987).

9. Humanized mAbs: these are hybrid molecules formed by the antigen binding segments of the animal mAb (essentially the hypervariable regions) while the rest of the molecule is substituted by the corresponding parts of a human myeloma protein (Riechmann *et al.*, 1988).

10. Single domain antibodies (dAbs); these form a promising new generation of mAbs which does not involve cell fusion or eucaryotic cell cultures but exclusively genetic engineering techniques (Ward *et al.*, 1989).

In order to produce a large number of anti-AChR mAbs, we devised a modification of the classical technique, named 'direct cloning', which has facilitated and accelerated the production of about 150 mAbs (Tzartos and Lindstrom, 1980). The main modification of this technique is that the

PEG-treated lymphocyte–myeloma hybrids are mixed immediately with agar and are then dispensed into 24-well plates. The solidified agar is overlaid with culture medium, which allows for subsequent screening assays, whereas the agar keeps the various clones separate as distinct colonies. Each colony of the antibody-positive wells is then transferred into a new well in order to identify later the antibody-positive colonies. This technique saves considerable time and effort.

Several laboratories have obtained anti-AChR mAbs. Monoclonals to AChR from *Torpedo* electric organ or animal muscles were followed by mAbs to AChR from sparser sources, including human muscles (Tzartos *et al.*, 1983; Whiting *et al.*, 1986) and neuronal sources (Whiting *et al.*, 1987), or even human mAbs from MG origin (Kamo *et al.*, 1982; Blair *et al.*, 1986). mAbs to various sites of the AChR have been obtained, including the MIR, the toxin and acetylcholine binding sites, other extracellular sites and many cytoplasmic sites of all four subunits.

5. *Epitope Localization*

The remarkable specificity of the mAbs makes them unparalleled probes for studying several aspects of the corresponding biomolecules. It is obvious, however, that this high specificity has to be determined. Nevertheless, quite often this requirement is not adequately appreciated, resulting in a waste of efforts to produce mAbs which are set aside after a first account of their availability and preliminary use. In order to make the best use of a mAb, an extensive characterization of its various parameters has first to be performed. This includes validation of its homogeneity; determination of its immunoglobulin class and subclass, affinity for the immunogen, and crossreactivity with antigens related or not with the immunogen; and, perhaps most important (and usually most difficult), localization of the corresponding epitope on the immunogen. Only methods for the latter will be discussed in this review.

Numerous approaches have been reported for mapping mAbs against various antigens. These can be classified into several groups that in turn fall into two major sections: indirect and direct mAb mapping. All have disadvantages and advantages. Essentially, none of the approaches is sufficient by itself but a combination of them must be tested for any single mAb in order to attain satisfactory and reliable epitope localization. Rather than give technical details, I shall mainly concentrate on the feasibility, advantages and disadvantages of the approaches, and give examples from anti-AChR mAb mapping.

Indirect mAb Mapping Techniques

mAb Binding to Antigen Variants Derived from Different Sources

Monoclonal antibodies have proved useful in determining the phylogenetic stability of several antigens. Conversely, when the detailed structure of an antigen in several species is known (the amino acid sequence and, if possible, the three-dimensional structure), this knowledge may be used for mapping the mAb epitopes. A prerequisite for such mapping techniques is that the used variants differ only by very few residues and that the epitopes of the test mAbs include some of these substituted residues. Therefore, the technique is best for rather small antigens, such as, for example, myoglobin (Berzofsky, 1984). An example of how it may be applied is the following. The immunogen differs from variant 1 at sites a,b,c, from variant 2 at sites a,b,d, and from variant 3 at sites a,d,e. If mAb I cross-reacts with variants 1 and 2, whereas mAb II crossreacts with variants 2 and 3, the epitope for the first mAb includes site e, whereas that for the second mAb includes site c.

Such conclusions are usually correct; however, one should be cautious, since even single substitutions may cause gross alterations of the conformation of the antigen, resulting in misleading interpretations. In cases where the mAbs bind also to the denatured antigen, interference of allosteric effects can be essentially excluded.

Largely because of the multiple substitutions which occur among AChRs, and the large size of this molecule, this kind of mapping has not been used on its own for anti-AChR mAb mapping. However, it has been proved valuable in confirming the results of other mapping techniques (Tzartos *et al.*, 1990c).

Use of Modified Antigens

These techniques are based on the same principle as that described above, but instead of relying on natural tools (the variants), the experimenter himself designs his tools. Protein modifications can be obtained by genetic engineering techniques (site-directed mutagenesis) by which we can test the exact sites that we suspect for contributing to the epitopes (Cunningham *et al.*, 1989). Alternatively, several biochemical modifications may be induced, such as removing or modifying the polysaccharide moieties, chemically modifying certain amino acids, etc. (Syu and Kahan, 1989; Van Regenmortel, 1989). Of course, the problems of allosteric effects mentioned above also apply here. So far there has been limited use of this approach on the anti-AChR mAbs. De Baets *et al.* (1988) studied the effect of proteolysis on the various AChR epitopes; they showed that the MIR is very resistant to proteolysis, in contrast to the majority of epitopes on the cytoplasmic side of the AChR, which are very sensitive to such treatment.

Binding Efficiency to Various Forms of the Antigen

Comparison of mAb binding to the antigen in different forms, such as embedded in the membranes of intact cells, in closed membrane vesicles, in permeabilized membranes, native and solubilized in non-denaturing detergent, SDS-denatured, etc., produces substantial information for the location of the epitopes. Thus, anti-AChR mAbs which bind only to intact muscle cells or to closed right-side-out *Torpedo* membrane vesicles are directed to the extracellular side, whereas mAbs which require permeabilization of the membranes in order to bind are assumed to bind to the cytoplasmic side (Froehner *et al.*, 1983; Ratnam *et al.*, 1986a). A few mAbs bind only to the solubilized AChR, suggesting that their epitopes are within very near the part of the AChR embedded in the membrane lipids (Gullick *et al.*, 1981).

Competition of mAbs with Ligands and Effect on Antigen Function

Testing competition between mAbs and ligands of the antigen is usually a critical kind of mapping, since such competing mAbs are likely to have a functional role or at least will be valuable tools for elucidating the mechanisms of protein function. Several anti-AChR mAbs have been found to inhibit toxin and acetylcholine binding and block channel opening. The mAbs of our library do not bind to the toxin binding sites, mainly as a result of the system used for their initial selection: the toxin binding sites of the AChR used in the mAb screening RIAs were saturated with ^{125}I-labelled toxin. However, a few mAbs inhibited channel function by binding to other sites, possibly located near the ion channel (described below).

Other functional effects of the mAbs could also be included within this mapping group. For example, the capacity of some anti-AChR mAbs to cause MG in experimental animals and antigenic modulation of the AChR in cell cultures strongly suggests that these mAbs bind to the extracellular side of the AChR (Tzartos *et al.*, 1985, 1987).

Competition between mAbs for Binding to the Antigen

This technique, despite several disadvantages, is valuable because it can be applied to practically any antigen and any mAb. Each mAb is tested with, if possible, each of the others, in independent experiments, for binding to the antigen. There are a number of alternative techniques that can be used. In general, among the three interacting molecules (the antigen and the two competing mAbs) one is labelled (e.g. by ^{125}I or peroxidase). In some cases the antigen is insoluble or has been insolubilized (e.g. attached to plastic or bound to Sepharose beads); excess of a first 'protecting' mAb is added to saturate the corresponding epitope on the antigen and then a labelled second 'test' mAb is added in order to determine its ability to bind to the protected antigen. Detection of bound radioactivity (or enzymic activity) on the insoluble antigen denotes that the two mAbs bind to distinct epitopes, whereas absence of bound activity denotes that the two mAbs bind to the same, to overlapping or to neighbouring epitopes. Alternatively, instead of using insoluble antigen, one of the mAbs may be immobilized, having either the other mAb or the antigen labelled. We (Tzartos and Lindstrom, 1980; Kordossi and Tzartos, 1987, 1989) and others (Whiting *et al.*, 1986; Heidenreich *et al.*, 1988a) have made extensive use of this approach.

The technique requires that at least the approximate location of some of the used mAbs be known from other approaches. As with all other indirect techniques, false conclusions due to allosteric effects are possible and these must be taken into consideration.

The validity of this technique was tested by applying it to a group of mAbs of known sequential epitopes on the cytoplasmic side of the AChR (determined according to techniques described below). The knowledge of the exact epitopes of these mAbs, several of which were overlapping (Ratnam *et al.*, 1986a,b; Tzartos *et al.*, 1988a) allowed a detailed investigation of the sensitivity and limits of the competition technique (Kordossi and Tzartos, 1987). Taking into account mainly mutual binding inhibitions of ≥50%, within each tested pair of mAbs, it was shown that, despite the large size of antibody molecules, the competition technique is very sensitive. mAbs to epitopes separated by only about seven residues did not exclude each other, and mAbs to overlapping epitopes exhibited differential competition with other mAbs. The location of the unknown epitope of a mAb was correctly estimated, on the basis of its competitions with mAbs to known epitopes (Tzartos *et al.*, 1988b, 1990c). Nevertheless, the excellent correlation observed in this system does not preclude the involvement of allosteric effects in other cases.

Direct mAb Mapping Techniques

Use of Antigenic Fragments

When large antigenic molecules are studied, such as AChR, this approach may involve several steps: use of intact subunits, large proteolytic fragments, medium-size recombinant fragments and, finally, small synthetic peptides. Recently, interesting modifications of the classical peptide synthesis techniques have been invented by which tens (Houghten, 1985) or hundreds (Geysen *et al.*, 1984) of peptides are synthesized in parallel in a few days (though with some loss of quantity and quality). In this way the whole sequence of the antigen can be analysed by overlapping peptides. The principle of the mapping assay is simple: in one of the alternative techniques the peptides are bound to an insoluble material and are incubated with the test mAb. A labelled anti-antibody is added in order to identify the mAb-binding peptide (Tzartos *et al.*, 1988c).

This group of techniques is powerful so long as the mAbs bind detectably to the antigenic fragments, which requires that their epitopes be sequential— i.e. formed by a single segment of the amino acid chain. Furthermore, even the conformation of a sequential epitope may be dramatically different in the fragment as compared with the intact molecule, resulting in very weak or undetectable mAb binding. Very often epitopes are discontinuous—i.e. a single epitope is formed by two or more short-sequence segments from remote sites of the primary amino acid sequence of the antigen (Amit *et al.*, 1986). Concerning the anti-AChR mAbs, several of them have been found to bind well to the denatured fragments, while others bind very weakly or not at all (see next section).

Even for mAbs the binding of which can be clearly localized by synthetic peptides, this mapping technique also is usually incomplete, for several reasons. Some of these are as follows. First, binding of a mAb to a certain sequence of a delineated chain or to a synthetic peptide does not guarantee that this mAb will bind exclusively at the same segment on the intact AChR: the apparently multiple foldings of the AChR chains may bring in contact certain distant amino acids with the potential to mimic sequential epitopes located on other, perhaps internal, sites. Second, the identified sequence may form only part of a discontinuous epitope, whereas the other smaller parts may remain undetectable by this technique. Third, for molecules such as the AChR, whose detailed three-dimensional structure is unknown, knowledge of the exact location of the epitopes on the amino acid sequence is not sufficient to locate these sites on the intact molecule. Thus, mapping techniques, indirect or direct, using the intact antigen must be performed in parallel in order to confirm and complement the peptide studies.

Visualization of mAb Binding by Electron Microscopy
Despite the fact that electron microscopy does not allow the determination of the exact epitope, because of limits of sensitivity, it is very useful, as it allows the unequivocal approximate localization of the bound mAb on the intact antigen. By electron microscopy, the transmembrane orientation of epitopes for many anti-AChR mAbs has been determined (Sargent *et al.*, 1984; Ratnam *et al.*, 1986a) and this proved valuable for the structural analysis of the AChR (Ratnam *et al.*, 1986a). Binding of many anti-AChR mAbs has been determined by several such studies. By electron image analysis of two-dimensional AChR crystals with bound Fab of mAbs, a finer localization of the mAb binding sites can be obtained (Kubalek *et al.*, 1987); binding of two anti-AChR mAbs was localized on the AChR surface, at approximately 17 Å resolution. This information was also used for the determination of the relative location of the subunits on the AChR molecule.

Mapping of the Epitopes by X-ray Crystallography
This is perhaps the ultimate mAb mapping approach, although arguments concerning the possible effects of the crystallization may be raised. Unfortunately, this technique is far from trivial, especially for large membrane antigens such as AChR, for which, only very recently, small crystals of the antigen alone have been obtained (Hertling-Jaweed *et al.*, 1988). Nevertheless, even the very few known examples of the structure of antigen–antibody complexes at around 2.8 Å resolution have been invaluable in helping us to understand the details of the antigen–antibody interaction (Amit *et al.*, 1986; Colman *et al.*, 1987).

Anti-AChR mAbs have been used in various aspects of AChR research. I shall describe some of their applications for the elucidation of the synthesis, structure and function of the muscle and electric organ AChR, then the use of mAbs in the study of MG and finally, very briefly, their use for the neuronal nicotinic AChR.

6. Studying Electric Organ and Muscle AChR by Monoclonal Antibodies

AChR Synthesis and Acquisition of Conformation

mAbs served as valuable tools in an extensive series of studies on the synthesis of muscle AChR by Merlie and co-workers (Merlie and Smith, 1986). mAbs to both conformation-independent and conformation-dependent epitopes were used. Using the first group, synthesis of the α subunit could be monitored from the beginning, before it assembles into the pentamer or acquires the toxin binding conformation. Comparing binding of the two kinds of mAbs and of α-bungarotoxin, it was shown that, after synthesis, the α subunit undergoes a series of conformational transitions as it gradually acquires its native conformation. Subunit assembly was assayed by testing the ability of a mAb to a single subunit to coprecipitate all other subunits (Merlie et al., 1982; Merlie and Lindstrom, 1983; Merlie and Smith, 1986).

cDNA of AChR subunits can be stably expressed in eukaryotic cells (Fujita et al., 1986; Claudio et al., 1987; Blount and Merlie, 1988). Binding of mAbs to α subunit expressed in yeast cells (Fujita et al., 1986) showed that both extracellular and normally cytoplasmic epitopes were located on the extracellular surface of the yeast; this conformation of α subunit may represent an intermediate conformation attained during its synthesis and maturation process. α subunit expressed in a quail fibroblast cell line was inserted in the correct orientation in intracellular membranes, although it was not transported to the plasma membrane. This protein acquired high affinity for anti-MIR mAbs and an affinity for α-bungarotoxin as high as that of the intact AChR, yet its affinity for small ligands was low (Blount and Merlie, 1988).

The process of renaturation of the denatured α subunit was also monitored as well as enhanced by anti-AChR mAbs (Tzartos and Changeux, 1983, 1984). Dissociation of the intact AChR into its subunits requires SDS denaturation. After this treatment, α-bungarotoxin and anti-MIR antibody binding affinity of the α subunit decreases dramatically. Two distinct conditions were established by which partial recovery of these binding sites was attained. The first, involving the use of certain low concentrations of SDS (~0.015%), achieved high affinity for α-bungarotoxin ($K_d \sim 3$ nM) but no significant enhancement of anti-MIR mAb binding. A similar SDS improvement of toxin binding was also observed for 27 kD proteolytic peptide of α subunit (Tzartos and Changeux, 1983) as well as for synthetic peptides carrying the α-bungarotoxin binding site (Wilson and Lentz, 1988). The second renaturation condition, which involved the addition of lipids (asolectin), reached a higher affinity of the α subunit for α-bungarotoxin and its 27 kD peptide ($K_d \sim 0.5$ nM) and also a dramatic recovery, though partial, of the MIR conformation. Furthermore, an anti-MIR mAb was capable of further enhancing the α-bungarotoxin binding activity of the α subunit (Tzartos and Changeux, 1984).

AChR Purification

mAbs are generally very good tools for the purification of the corresponding antigen by affinity chromatography. However, in contrast to their extensive use for purifying neuronal AChR, purification procedures for electric organ and muscle AChR had been well established before the advent of mAbs, mainly by the use of α neurotoxins (Maelicke, 1988). Nevertheless, AChR of *Torpedo* or human origin was successfully purified by the use of mAbs (Momoy and Lennon, 1982). Such an approach may be useful in separating antigenically distinct AChR subpopulations such as those of innervated and non-innervated muscle.

AChR Structure

Before the amino acid sequence of the AChR subunits was known, mAbs to the *Torpedo* AChR showed that its subunits present similarities among themselves, because single mAbs crossreacted with more than one subunit. On the basis of these data it was suggested that the AChR subunit genes derived from a common ancestral gene (Tzartos and Lindstrom, 1980). This was subsequently confirmed by amino acid and cDNA sequencing studies (Raftery *et al.*, 1980; Numa, 1987).

By testing the crossreactive capacity of mAbs it was shown that AChRs from fish electric organs and mammalian muscles are quite related molecules (Tzartos and Lindstrom, 1980; Tzartos *et al.*, 1981). Furthermore, homologous AChR subunits among species were identified in many studies.

The transmembrane orientation of several segments of the AChR subunits has been determined by the use of mAbs (Anderson *et al.*, 1983; La Rochelle *et al.*, 1985; Ratnam *et al.*, 1986a; Maelicke *et al.*, 1989). In fact, this is nothing more than a proper localization of mAb epitopes. A combination of two mapping procedures is required—one to determine the epitope on the primary structure (best by synthetic peptides) and one to determine the transmembrane location of the bound mAb (best but not necessarily by electron microscopy). When specific sequences are to be localized, antibodies can be raised by immunizing animals against the specific peptides. Nevertheless, even in this case, the epitopes have to be confirmed by testing the antibodies with several synthetic peptides, since often unexpected crossreactivities occur (Maelicke *et al.*, 1989).

The hydrophobicity profile of the AChR subunits has generated models according to which each subunit transverses the membrane about 4–5 times through equal hydrophobic helices. A five-transmembrane-helix model (M1–M5) of which the amphipathic M5 helix from each subunit assembles the ion channel had been popular for some time (McCarthy *et al.*, 1986). However, the epitopes of several mAbs, capable of binding well to the intact AChR, were localized within the α-subunit segment corresponding to M5 (Ratnam *et al.*, 1986a,b; Kordossi and Tzartos, 1987). These results strongly suggested that M5 is not transmembrane but rather lies on the cytoplasmic surface. That M5 is not part of the channel has been subsequently further confirmed by various other approaches.

From electron image analysis of AChRs, with bound mAbs or other ligands, the relative location of the *Torpedo* subunits was estimated as being α,β,α,γ,δ (Kubalek *et al.*, 1987). Competition experiments between anti-subunit mAbs also led to the proposition of putative points of contact between γ and δ subunits (Tzartos and Kordossi, 1986).

Ligand Binding Sites on Ion Channel Function

The acetylcholine and toxin binding sites have been studied by specific mAbs capable of binding at or near these sites. Mochly-Rosen and Fuchs (1981) identified one mAb (the 5.5.G.12) out of 32 mAbs raised against *Torpedo* AChR which was directed to the cholinergic binding site. This mAb bound also to AChRs from various species, demonstrating the wide structural homology between the acetylcholine binding site of the various AChRs. Watters and Maelicke (1983) selectively produced a set of six mAbs competing with cholinergic ligands. They identified two structurally distinct ligand binding regions on the AChR, apparently on its two α subunits, each with three subsites of different specificity for carbamylcholine, decamethonium and tubocurarine. As in studies of other groups (Mihovilovic and Richman, 1984; Heidenreich *et al.*, 1988a), some mAbs bound to both sites, but most bound only to a single site. mAbs capable of blocking only half of the acetylcholine binding sites can completely block the acetylcholine-induced channel opening (Fels *et al.*, 1986). This observation confirmed that two acetylcholine molecules are required to activate the ion channel.

mAbs also helped to confirm studies on the location of the cholinergic binding sites on the α subunit primary structure. mAbs prepared against the segment α127–132, a site earlier proposed to be involved in the cholinergic ligand binding sites (McCormick and Atassi, 1984) were not inhibited from binding to the intact AChR by any tested ligand (α-cobratoxin, carbamylcholine, tubocurarine or decamethonium), suggesting that this segment is not involved in the ligand binding site (Plumer *et al.*, 1984). In contrast, three mAbs raised against *Torpedo* peptide α188–201 bound to the ^{125}I-labelled AChR but not to ^{125}I-AChR preincubated with α-bungarotoxin (Gotti *et al.*, 1988). Similarly, an anti-AChR mAb which blocks the agonist-induced ion flux and is inhibited from binding to the AChR by α-bungarotoxin or cholinergic agonists was mapped to residues α187–205 (Chinchetru *et al.*, 1989). In fact, synthetic peptides within the segment 180–205 were known to bind α-bungarotoxin (Wilson and Lentz, 1988), but a confirmation of the actual mode of binding on the intact AChR was essential and this was offered by the mAbs.

In addition to mAbs against the acetylcholine binding site, a few mAbs to other sites also have been observed to affect ion channel. Richman and co-workers identified a mAb, bound to the extracellular part of the α subunit but distinct from the ligand binding site(s), which blocks the agonist-induced channel opening (Donnelly *et al.*, 1984). Unfortunately, efforts to map the epitope for this mAb were unsuccessful, although it binds to the denatured α subunit (Chinchetru *et al.*, 1989). None of the many tested anti-MIR mAbs affected channel opening (Lindstrom *et al.*, 1981). Four mAbs to the cytoplasmic side of the α, β and γ subunits were capable of inhibiting channel function (Lindstrom *et al.*, 1981; Wan and Lindstrom, 1985). Fab fragments of at least two of these mAbs were inactive, despite binding to the AChR; this suggests that the intact mAbs distort the AChR conformation by crosslinking rather than by binding to critical sites.

7. *Studying Myasthenia Gravis by Monoclonal Antibodies*

Analysis of the Antigenic Structure of AChR

Since anti-AChR antibodies are pathogenic, causing MG, anti-AChR mAbs were obviously expected to help in analysing the antigenic structure of the molecule. Two different approaches have been used.

One involves simply mapping the epitopes of the produced mAbs and drawing conclusions about the antigenic regions of the AChR. However, in this case the immunization procedure may play a critical role, and this should be taken seriously into account.

It has already been mentioned that animal anti-AChR sera and mAbs bind to several sites of the different subunits of the molecule, both cytoplasmic and extracellular, near the toxin binding site as well as away from it. Immunization with intact AChR induces antibodies mainly to the extracellular side. Some bind to the toxin binding site, although the majority bind to other sites. The majority of the rat antibodies, both from polyclonal sera and from the available rat mAbs against intact AChR, bind to the MIR (to be described below).

Immunization with denatured AChR subunits induces mAbs mainly to the cytoplasmic side (Froehner *et al.*, 1983; Swanson *et al.*, 1983). These are directed to several sites, but highly immunogenic areas have been identified near the C-terminal end of the α subunit, between residues α330 and α380 (Ratnam *et al.*, 1986a), as well as to corresponding sequences of the β, γ and δ subunits (La Rochelle *et al.*, 1985; Ratnam *et al.*, 1986b).

In the second mapping approach, mAbs of identified epitopes are used as tools to indirectly probe the antibody repertoire in the human sera. Here competition experiments between mAbs and MG sera for binding to the intact human muscle AChR are involved. This kind of study, although indirect and raising ambiguities concerning its accuracy, is valuable, since direct determination of the epitopes for serum anti-AChR antibodies by the use of peptides would produce false conclusions. This is because the majority of the serum antibodies do not bind or bind with very low affinity to the denatured peptides; at the same time an antibody minority may bind to certain peptides with high affinity, leading to an overestimation of the importance of this population.

By such competition experiments it was found that the human MG antibody specificities are significantly similar to those of the anti-AChR antibodies in experimental rats (Tzartos *et al.*, 1982) and in the sera of the spontaneous autoimmune myasthenic dogs (Shelton *et al.*, 1988).

There is considerable variation in the fine antigenic specificities of the anti-AChR antibodies among MG patients, but in most cases anti-MIR mAbs inhibited the binding of the majority of the human antibodies. mAbs to other regions on the α as well as on the β and γ subunits also exerted considerable inhibition (Tzartos *et al.*, 1982; Heidenreich *et al.*, 1988a). Within a single patient the antibody repertoire seemed quite stable with time despite various treatments (including thymectomy) and variations in the overall anti-AChR titre (Tzartos *et al.*, 1982; Heidenreich *et al.*, 1988b).

The antibody repertoires in the sera of infants from MG mothers were very similar to those of their mothers' sera. Also, no characteristic differences were detected between the antibody repertoires of mothers who transferred the disease to their infants and those who did not transfer it (Tzartos *et al.*, 1990b).

The MIR

Among 66 mAbs raised in rats against intact AChR from several species (from *Torpedo* electric organ to human muscle), 41 (i.e. 62%) competed with each other for binding to the MIR (Tzartos and Lindstrom, 1980; Tzartos *et al.*, 1981, 1983). About half of those anti-MIR mAbs bound detectably to the α subunit, while the rest were unable to bind to any subunit; this suggested that the MIR is on the α subunits of the AChR. mAb 35 exhibited very good crossreactivity with AChRs from almost all tested species and thus became the reference anti-MIR mAb. The hybridomas producing this mAb are now available from the American Type Culture Collection.

Several lines of evidence proved that antibodies to the MIR are heterogeneous and that the MIR is at best a group of mutually and intimately overlapping epitopes. First, their crossreactivity with AChR from various species varies widely (Tzartos and Lindstrom, 1980; Swanson *et al.*, 1983; Tzartos *et al.*, 1983; Sargent *et al.*, 1984). Second, some anti-MIR mAbs are capable of crosslinking the AChR molecules; others form only 1:1 complexes with AChR (Conti-Tronconi *et al.*, 1981; Tzartos *et al.*, 1986a). This implies that at least the orientation of the bound mAb differs between the two groups of mAbs. Third, binding efficiency of the anti-MIR mAbs to the intact AChR as well as to its fragments varies dramatically (Tzartos *et al.*, 1981, 1988c; Barkas *et al.*, 1987). Fourth, although anti-idiotypic sera against the antigen binding site (paratope-related) of a single anti-MIR mAb partially crossreacted with other anti-MIR mAbs (Verschuuren, 1989), similar sera against other anti-MIR mAbs were not crossreactive (Killen *et al.*, 1985; Verschuuren, 1989).

The MIR is clearly on the extracellular side of the AChR. This is evident from the fact that anti-MIR mAbs induce experimental MG when injected into rats (Tzartos and Lindstrom, 1980; Tzartos *et al.*, 1987) and antigenic modulation of AChR on cell cultures (Tzartos *et al.*, 1985; Sophianos and Tzartos, 1989), as well as from their direct visualization in several electron microscopy studies (Swanson *et al.*, 1983; Kubalek *et al.*, 1987).

The MIR is independent of the acetylcholine and toxin binding sites, since none of the anti-MIR mAbs competes with toxin for binding to the AChR or affects ion channel function (Tzartos and Lindstrom, 1980; Lindstrom *et al.*, 1981; Tzartos *et al.*, 1981; Heidenreich *et al.*, 1988a). However, mAbs have been reported which partially compete with both toxin and anti-MIR mAbs (Heidenreich *et al.*, 1988a; Xu *et al.*, 1988), suggesting that the two sites are not distantly located in the intact AChR. Electron image analysis of AChR with bound toxin or Fab of the anti-MIR mAb 35 showed that on each α subunit the toxin and mAb 35 binding sites are distinct, separated by angles of approximately 45° (Kubalek *et al.*, 1987). Figure 1 shows a model of the AChR with approximate location of the MIR.

Other laboratories have also identified the relative location of their rat and mouse mAbs to the MIR. Four out of five rat anti-AChR mAbs of Lennon and co-workers (Lennon and Lambert, 1981; Lennon and Griesmann, 1989) appear to bind to the MIR, as judged from competition experiments with mAb 35 and from the crossreactivity of anti-idiotypic sera. The anti-AChR repertoire in mice seems to be somewhat different from that in rats and humans. Mice seem not to be as good models for experimental MG as are the rats and this is in accordance with the observation that, in sera from mice immunized with intact AChR, only about one-third of their antibodies compete with anti-MIR mAbs from binding to the AChR (Tzartos, unpublished). Nevertheless, several anti-MIR mAbs have also been

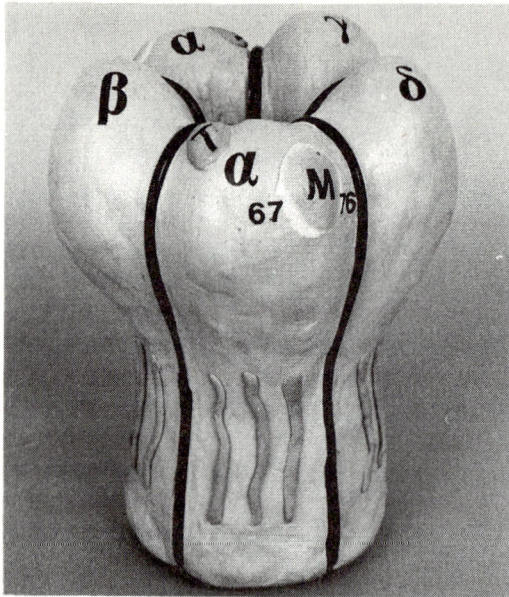

Figure 1 A model of the AChR based on numerous studies and earlier models (Brisson and Unwin, 1985; Kubalek *et al.*, 1987; Mitra *et al.*, 1989). T, α-bungarotoxin binding site; M, MIR (main immunogenic region). 67 and 76 denote the N- and C-terminal residues of the segment containing the main loop of the epitope(s) for the anti-MIR mAbs. (Tzartos *et al.* 1988a)

obtained from immunized mice. Two of the five anti-*Torpedo* AChR mAbs of Chase *et al.* (1987) competed with mAb 35, suggesting that they bind to the MIR. Heidenreich *et al.*, (1988a), using mouse anti-human AChR mAbs, identified five immunogenic regions: the MIR, a region overlapping with the MIR, and three regions near on either of the two toxin binding sites.

Considerable efforts have been devoted to the localization of the MIR on the primary structure of the AChR. The low affinity of the anti-MIR mAbs for AChR fragments delayed but did not stop progress. Using α-subunit proteolytic peptides, anti-MIR mAb binding was restricted between α1–161 (Barkas *et al.*, 1986) and α46–120 (Ratnam *et al.*, 1986b). Recombinant proteins containing α-subunit segments narrowed down the binding of three anti-MIR mAbs to α37–85 (Barkas *et al.*, 1987). Finally, synthetic peptides allowed the fine localization of the epitopes for several anti-MIR mAbs. Barkas *et al.* (1988) detected anti-MIR mAb binding between α61 and α76 of *Torpedo* and mouse AChR. Tzartos *et al.* (1988a, 1990c) screened 26 overlapping synthetic peptides covering most of the human α subunit and 31 peptides covering the whole *Torpedo* AChR α subunit. Using these peptides, the epitopes for eleven anti-MIR mAbs were localized between α67 and α76 of both human and *Torpedo* AChR. Several other anti-MIR mAbs did not bind to any peptide but none bound predominantly to any other sequence. Wood *et al.* (1989) also localized binding of a mouse anti-MIR mAb within α65 and α78.

Torpedo and human α67–76 (WNPADYGGIK and WNPDDYGGVK, respectively) differ on residues α70 and α75, which result in significantly different binding behaviour of the anti-*Torpedo* and anti-human mAbs to the peptides. The relative binding of these mAbs to the *Torpedo* and human α67–76 decapeptides perfectly correlated with their relative binding to the corresponding intact AChRs. This strongly suggested that indeed peptide mapping uncovered the actual epitopes on the intact AChR (Tzartos *et al.*, 1990c).

The antigenic role of each residue within α67–76 was then tested by the use of peptide analogues of the α67–76, in each of which one residue was substituted by alanine. The segment α68–71 was found to be the most critical. Residues α68 and α71 were indispensable for binding of any of the six tested mAbs, other residues were critical only for some of the mAbs, whereas some were not important. Some analogues exhibited higher binding capacity than the original decapeptide (Tzartos *et al.*, 1989; Papadouli *et al.*, 1990). This observation may lead to the construction of a modified MIR peptide with high affinity for the serum antibodies.

The conformation of the *Torpedo* α67–76 and its analogues was studied by two-dimensional NMR spectroscopy. In DMSO, α67–76 acquired a folded conformation stabilized by three interactions involving the D71, G74 and K76 amide protons. Alanine substitutions significantly affected this conformation (Cung *et al.*, 1989).

Smaller peptides within α67–76 also have anti-MIR binding activity. Das and Lindstrom (1989) detected binding of an anti-MIR mAb to the nonapeptide α68–76 and we detected anti-MIR mAb binding to peptides as small as pentapeptides (Papadouli *et al.*, unpublished).

As mentioned above, anti-MIR mAbs are also very potent in inhibiting human MG antibodies from binding to the human AChR. In fact, a single mAb inhibits binding of two-thirds (on average) of the MG antibodies (Tzartos *et al.*, 1982). From this it can be inferred that the two-thirds of the MG antibodies are directed against the MIR. Nevertheless, the actual size of this region in human MG is uncertain, as it cannot yet be tested by other means. Peptide mapping would not give reliable results, as explained above.

Since identification of the anti-MIR antibodies in human sera is so far based solely on competition experiments with anti-MIR mAbs, the possibility has been considered that the anti-MIR human antibodies may bind to a group of epitopes located on various distant sites, broadly sterically or allosterically interacting with each other (Tzartos *et al.*, 1981; Lennon and Griesmann, 1989). This possibility cannot be excluded. However, the fine correlation between antibody competition and peptide mapping which was shown with mAbs both to cytoplasmic regions and to the MIR (Kordossi and Tzartos, 1987, 1989; Tzartos *et al.*, 1988a) strongly suggests that a similar correlation should be expected with the MG antibodies. The segment $\alpha 125–147$, which induces antibodies that are also significant inhibitors of the MG antibodies (Lennon and Griesmann, 1989), may be located near $\alpha 67–76$ in the folded conformation of the intact molecule.

The pathogenic role of the anti-MIR mAbs and of the anti-MIR antibody fraction in MG sera has been studied in experimental animals and cell cultures. It will be shown below that this region appears to play an important role in MG. The current status of our knowledge on the MIR has been recently reviewed in more detail (Tzartos *et al.*, 1990a).

Anti-AChR mAbs in Search for the Immunogen in MG

Although MG is probably the best-studied autoimmune disease, it is not yet known what triggers the autoimmune response in MG. AChR on the surface of myoid cells of the thymus is thought, by several investigators, to be the immunogen. On the other hand, non-AChR exogenous or endogenous crossreactive molecules could also be implicated in the triggering of the disease (Stefansson *et al.*, 1987; Marx *et al.*, 1989; Schwimmbeck *et al.*, 1989).

Stefansson *et al.* detected shared epitopes between bacterial antigens and AChR. They tested binding of 30 anti-AChR mAbs with bacteria and found that two mAbs crossreacted with two polypeptides of *E. coli* and *Klebsiella pneumoniae* and with one polypeptide of *Yersinia enterocolitica*. They also detected significantly higher binding of MG than normal human sera to bacterial polypeptides (Stefansson *et al.*, 1987). Such molecules could induce initiation of the response, leaving its maintenance to the responsibility of the 'damaged' AChRs.

Kirchner *et al.* (1988) and Marx *et al.* (1989) detected two proteins in epithelial cells of thymomas from MG patients (but not of thymomas from non-MG patients) having common epitopes with the human AChR α subunit. Cell lines derived from such epitheliomas of MG patients (but not of non-MG) also produced these molecules. The crossreactive molecules (45 kD and 155 kD) are clearly distinct from the AChR subunits, and probably they do not bear many other epitopes common to the AChR. More importantly, they do not carry the MIR. Actually the corresponding AChR epitopes are located on the cytoplasmic side of the AChR α subunit. Nevertheless, the nearly perfect correlation with the occurrence of MG in thymomatous patients raises the possibility that these proteins trigger the autoimmune process by expressing recognition sites for autoreactive T cells but not binding sites for antibodies (Kirchner *et al.*, 1988; Marx *et al.*, 1989). In fact, it has been shown that T and B epitopes are on distinct sites on the AChR molecule (see below).

MG symptoms and anti-AChR antibodies are occasionally induced in patients with rheumatoid arthritis or other diseases when treated with D-penicillamine. Both the symptoms and the antibodies remit after drug cessation (Oosterhuis, 1984). Should the anti-AChR antibody repertoire in D-penicillamine-induced MG be similar to that in the idiopathic MG, the former will be an excellent human model of MG. Indeed, competition experiments between patients' sera and mAbs showed that sera from both groups of MG patients have antibodies to similar AChR regions (Tzartos *et al.*, 1988c). Therefore, penicillamine-induced MG deserves extensive investigation in order to draw conclusions for the pathogenic mechanisms in idiopathic MG.

Anti-idiotypic routes have been also proposed as candidate mechanisms for the induction of MG. Anti-AChR and anti-idiotypic mAbs have been used as tools in such studies (Souroujon *et al.*, 1986; Dwyer *et al.*, 1987; Erlanger *et al.*, 1987; Agius *et al.*, 1988; De Baets *et al.*, 1988; Verschuuren, 1989).

T Cell Epitopes and B–T Cell Interactions

Synthesis of anti-AChR antibodies is, in part, regulated by AChR-specific helper T lymphocytes which have been isolated from several MG patients (Hohlfeld *et al.*, 1984, 1987).

The α subunit of the AChR, in addition to carrying the MIR also seems to be the predominant site of T cell epitopes (Hohlfeld *et al.*, 1987; Zhang *et al.*, 1988a). However, anti-MIR mAbs could not inhibit the AChR-induced stimulation of the specific T cells, suggesting that the majority of the AChR T-cell epitopes are distinct from its B-cell epitopes despite being on the same subunit (Hohlfeld *et al.*, 1987). Indeed α subunit segments other than the α67–76 (which participates in the MIR) were identified as carrying T-cell epitopes (Zhang *et al.*, 1988a; Newsom-Davis *et al.*, 1989).

Hybridomas producing anti-AChR antibodies were used as model B cells in cell culture experiments in order to study B–T cell interactions in experimental MG (Zhang *et al.*, 1988b). Several such hybridomas were able to present antigen to AChR-specific T cells in a privileged manner. Privileged presentation depended on the reactivity of the secreted antibodies with epitopes of the AChR α subunit and on the expression of MHC class II antigens on the hybridoma cell surface. However, neither fine specificity nor isotype of the mAbs was critical. It appears that the different hybridomas differ in their ability to process the antigen and that this ability determines their antigen-presenting efficiency.

Passive Transfer of Experimental MG in Animals by mAbs

Single anti-AChR mAbs are capable of inducing MG symptoms in experimental animals. This is an unequivocal proof that anti-AChR specificity, and not other serum contaminants, is capable of causing MG. MG has been induced by mAbs to two specified sites—the MIR and the toxin binding site—as well as to other yet unspecified sites.

Two groups reported MG symptoms in chickens after injection of mAbs to the acetylcholine binding sites (Gomez and Richman, 1983; Souroujon et al., 1986). In one of these studies muscular weakness was exhibited within only an hour from the injection. In contrast to MG induced by anti-sera, the AChR content of the chickens was not affected; muscular weakness was apparently induced by blockage of AChR function (Gomez and Richman, 1983). Electrophysiological studies suggested that a reduction of the neurally evoked release of acetylcholine from the nerve terminal may also have contributed to the acute effect (Maselli et al., 1989). However, in the other study weakness appeared only after 8–10 h from the injection of the mAb 5.5 (Souroujon et al., 1986). It appears that this mAb did not act only by blocking the channel.

Five anti-MIR mAbs, together with eight mAbs to other AChR sites (one to the extracellular side of the β subunit, three to the cytoplasmic side of various subunits, one binding only to the solubilized AChR and three to AChRs from species other than rats) were injected into rats. All five anti-MIR mAbs (three IgG1 and two IgG2a) caused severe MG symptoms in the rats and reduced their AChR content to about half of that of the controls. None of the other mAbs caused any symptoms of muscular weakness, nor did they reduce the AChR content of the animals, although the mAb to the extracellular side of the β subunit was found bound to the majority of the AChR molecules of the sacrificed rats (Tzartos and Lindstrom, 1980; Tzartos et al., 1987). These results suggest that the anti-MIR antibodies are very potent in passively transferring MG independently of their IgG subclass specificity. Since only a single mAb directed to non-MIR sites of the extracellular surface of the rat AChR has been tested, we cannot draw conclusions on the effect of mAbs to other than the MIR sites.

Antigenic Modulation of AChR by mAbs

It has been mentioned earlier that anti-AChR antibodies exert their pathogenic effect upon the AChR by at least three mechanisms. This complex effect has to be analysed in order to understand adequately the details of the MG mechanism. Muscle cell cultures provide the opportunity to analyse the pathogenic role of the anti-AChR antibodies. They are especially appropriate for studying AChR loss via antigenic modulation—i.e. the accelerated internalization and degradation rate of the AChR by antibody-crosslinking (Heinemann et al., 1977). An additional advantage of cell cultures over the animal experiments is the ability to test the effect of antibodies on human AChR.

Anti-AChR mAbs have been used with muscle cell cultures in two ways: first, to test directly the ability of the different antigenic specificities expressed by the mAbs in causing AChR loss, and, second, to indirectly test the effect of antigenic specificities present in the patients' sera.

Single mAbs caused antigenic modulation of the AChR in animal and human muscle cell cultures (Conti-Tronconi *et al.*, 1981; Souroujon *et al.*, 1983; Tzartos *et al.*, 1985; Sophianos and Tzartos, 1989). Anti-MIR mAbs were especially efficient in increasing AChR internalization rates (up to threefold). Univalent Fab fragments of the mAbs, as expected, lost their capacity to accelerate AChR internalization because they cannot crosslink it (Tzartos *et al.*, 1985). As a consequence of the MIR being on the α subunit, two copies of which are present in each AChR molecule, an anti-MIR mAb is capable of crosslinking many AChR molecules into large polymers. Formation of such polymers could be a prerequisite for antigenic modulation. Interestingly, an anti-β-subunit and an anti-γ-subunit mAb also caused antigenic modulation of AChR in human muscle cell cultures (Tzartos and Starzinski-Powitz, 1986). These antibodies can only form complexes of one antibody with two AChR molecules. Consequently, it was inferred that small complexes of only three molecules are adequate to accelerate AChR internalization.

The relative contribution of separate anti-AChR antibody fractions to the total antigenic modulation capacity of human MG sera was tested by using competition experiments between mAbs and human sera. Antigenic regions on the AChR of cultured muscle cells from mouse (Tzartos *et al.*, 1985) or human (Sophianos and Tzartos, 1989) origin were 'protected' by Fab fragments from specific anti-AChR mAbs. Upon addition of the test sera, only the antibodies directed against regions other than the 'protected' one could bind and cause antigenic modulation. By this approach it was estimated that anti-MIR antibodies are responsible for 70–80% of the total antigenic modulation capacity of the MG sera. Thus, the MIR may be the major pathogenic region of the AChR.

Souroujon *et al.* (1983) tested the modulating effect of four anti-AChR mAbs on primary chicken muscle cultures. All four mAbs bound well to the cultured cells; however, only two of them induced AChR loss. One of these mAbs (mAb 5.5) is directed against the acetylcholine binding site. Therefore, antibodies to this site can play a dual pathogenic role.

Potential Use of Anti-AChR mAbs for MG Therapy

On the basis of the fact that single anti-MIR mAbs inhibit the majority of the anti-AChR antibodies from binding to the AChR, a tentative therapeutic use of these mAbs could be envisaged, provided that the pathogenic (but not the binding) activity of the mAbs themselves could be neutralized. In fact, Fab fragments of the anti-MIR mAbs are expected to be pathogenically inactive, since Fab cannot crosslink AChRs; thus, they cannot induce antigenic modulation. Also, they do not bind complement; thus, they cannot induce complement-mediated lysis.

As mentioned above, protection of the MIR of the cell-bound AChR by Fab of single mAbs dramatically protects the AChR against the activity of the subsequently added MG sera. Although the degree of contribution of antigenic modulation to MG is still uncertain, it is reasonable to expect a similar protection against the complement-mediated AChR loss; in fact, protection against modulation simply correlates with protection against binding of the MG antibodies (Tzartos *et al.*, 1985; Sophianos and Tzartos, 1989).

Inhibition of two-thirds of the anti-AChR antibodies in a patient from binding to his AChR would be probably equivalent to a drop in his anti-AChR antibody titre by a similar extent. It is well known that such a drop in a patient's titre is followed by a dramatic improvement of his clinical condition (Oosterhuis, 1984; Lindstrom *et al.*, 1988). However, several steps have to be accomplished before establishing such a therapeutic approach. The Fab must bind with a high affinity to the human AChR; they should be modified in such a manner as to avoid fast clearance from the circulation; they should be either human or humanized (Riechmann *et al.*, 1988); or the recipient patient must be rendered tolerant. Finally, it must be proved that these Fabs can indeed be efficient *in vivo*.

Therapy with anti-idiotypic mAbs would be another interesting approach, although the polyclonality of the anti-AChR response, even within the MIR (Killen *et al.*, 1985; Verschuuren, 1989), makes the success of such an approach rather unlikely.

8. *Studying Neuronal Nicotinic AChR by Monoclonal Antibodies*

Neuronal nicotinic AChRs are the set of AchR molecules that have most profited from the use of anti-AChR mAbs. These studies have been reviewed in detail elsewhere (Lindstrom *et al.*, 1987); therefore, they will be outlined here only briefly.

Confusion has surrounded neuronal nicotinic AChRs and, as has recently been proved, for good reason. Earlier use of α-bungarotoxin to localize neuronal AChRs gave conflicting results, since α-bungarotoxin binding did not block cholinergic activity (Kouvelas *et al.*, 1978). Finally, a combination of data obtained from the use of a chain of anti-AChR mAbs, novel neurotoxins (such as k-bungarotoxin) and cDNAs suggests that the several subtypes of nicotinic AChRs on neurons identified to date are part of a gene superfamily which includes skeletal muscle AChRs, neuronal α-bungarotoxin binding proteins that usually do not have AChR activity, as well as receptors for glycine and GABA (Barnard *et al.*, 1987; Lindstrom *et al.*, 1987).

Sets of mAbs against *Torpedo* or muscle AChR were successfully used to identify neuronal nicotinic AChRs or AChR-like molecules from *Drosophila* (Chase *et al.*, 1987) and locust (Fels *et al.*, 1983). The α-bungarotoxin binding protein from chick neural tissues also crossreacts with mAbs to muscle AChR (Mehraban *et al.*, 1984).

Monoclonal antibodies to electric organ and muscle AChR (especially the anti-MIR ones) bound also to non-α-bungarotoxin binding chick brain and ganglionic molecules but not to mouse or rat brain molecules (Swanson *et al.*, 1983; Jacob and Berg, 1988). These molecules were subsequently isolated by affinity chromatography (using the same mAbs) and characterized as functional AChRs. Unlike muscle AChR, these AChRs consist of two kinds of subunits—α and β (Whiting and Lindstrom, 1986).

In addition to the chick, the anti-MIR mAbs also crossreacted with goldfish brain AChR (Henley *et al.*, 1988), bovine chromaffin cell AChR (Higgins and Berg, 1987) and frog retina and optic tectum molecules (Sargent *et al.*, 1989), and have been used in extensive studies of these molecules.

The inability of the then available mAbs to bind to mammalian brain AChR did not stop progress in this field. Instead an admirable chain of mAb steps led the way from fish electric organ to human brain (Lindstrom *et al.*, 1987)! mAbs prepared against the purified (by antimuscle AChR) chick brain AChR crossreacted with rat brain AChR and were used for its purification (Whiting *et al.*, 1987). In turn mAbs raised against the latter AChR crossreacted with human and bovine brain AChRs and were used for their purification and study as well (Whiting and Lindstrom, 1988).

The fact that anti-MIR mAbs bound to chick and goldfish neuronal AChRs but not to mammalian brain, which indeed delayed progress in this field, can now be explained. Antigenically critical residues (especially α68) within the MIR segment α67–76, have been conserved in known sequences of goldfish and chick brain AChRs but not in those of mammalian neuronal AChRs (Nef *et al.*, 1988; Wada *et al.*, 1988; Cauley *et al.*, 1989).

9. Future Trends

There is still much important work to be done with anti-AChR mAbs as tools. However, the anti-AChR mAbs available in the various laboratories must first be further characterized. In fact, with regard to several mAbs with interesting characteristics, we have no idea where they bind on the AChR. Co-operation among the relevant laboratories would accelerate progress in this respect. An easy and fruitful step will be to determine for each mAb its relative location to the MIR. Also, all mAbs which bind to denatured subunits must be mapped by synthetic peptides.

New techniques will have to be applied for the accurate mapping of mAbs to discontinuous epitopes but also to complement mapping of the mAbs to sequential epitopes. Cells expressing mutant AChRs, by site-directed mutagenesis, will be valuable for such mAb mapping. Electron microscopy combined with image analysis could map a number of mAbs to important sites. X-Ray crystallography of the AChR will apparently soon become a 'hot' subject; this may allow us to see all the details of the interaction of a membrane autoantigen with a few critical autoantibodies. When scanning tunnelling microscopy is introduced to the study of the AChR, hopefully in the near future, a detailed map of the binding sites for many mAbs may become feasible.

Study of muscle and electric organ AChR has still a lot to gain from the well-characterized mAbs. For example, we know very little about the structures which form the surface of the AChR. mAbs to known selected sequences would contribute much to the elucidation of the AChR structure in significant detail. A systematic study to obtain antipeptide mAbs with the capacity of non-competitively affecting ion channel will uncover the functional pathways on the AChR.

The role of the MIR in human MG will have to be clarified. While it is a fact that single mAbs to α67–76 inhibit the majority of the MG antibodies from binding to the AChR, the size of the AChR area(s) that contains the actual epitopes for the human anti-MIR antibodies is still uncertain. Different techniques will have to be employed. Mutated AChRs will be once more useful.

The α67–76 synthetic peptide has low affinity for the anti-MIR mAbs. Should the α67–76 region prove crucial for the human MG antibodies, construction of a modified α67–76 with high affinity for the anti-MIR antibodies will be valuable, both for the study of MG and for therapeutic strategies. Moreover, if α67–76 is important in MG, anti-idiotypic mAbs may be 'designed' with broad activity and, therefore, therapeutic significance.

Since anti-MIR mAbs are capable of protecting the AChR in cell cultures against MG sera, it is likely that such mAbs will be used in therapeutic approaches.

The use of anti-AChR mAbs in the search for endogenous and exogenous antigens that might play a role in triggering the disease will probably continue.

T–B cell interactions are crucial in MG. mAb-producing hybridomas could be valuable model B cells for analysing such interactions.

The study of neuronal AChRs will undoubtedly continue to profit highly from the use of mAbs. New AChR subtypes may be identified and purified by the mAbs. Also, these and new mAbs will be used for studies similar to those described on muscle and electric organ AChRs.

Although there have been at least two reports on the production of human anti-AChR mAbs, such a species is not yet in significant use. Techniques for the production of human mAbs are gradually improving; therefore, it is expected that such valuable tools will be adequately available. In parallel, currently available mAbs are expected to be engineered by molecular genetics in order to acquire higher affinity for human AChR and to become 'humanized', both factors useful for *in vivo* use.

10. *Summary*

Monoclonal antibodies against the nicotinic AChR have been used since 1979. They have proved valuable probes for studying AChR and the disease myasthenia gravis, which is caused by anti-AChR antibodies. For a mAb to be a useful tool its epitope must first be identified. Various techniques were applied for mAb mapping. Such techniques can be direct or indirect and can use either intact antigen or fragments of it. None is fully adequate on its own; therefore a combination of mapping techniques must be applied for each mAb.

mAbs have been used (a) for studying various aspects of synthesis, structure and function of AChR from electric organs and muscles; (b) for studying the antigenic structure of the animal and human AChR, including the identification of the MIR on the α subunit and evaluation of its pathogenic role; and (c) to identify, purify and study several neuronal nicotinic AChRs.

Acknowledgements

Part of the original work presented here was supported by grants from the Greek General Secretariat of Research and Technology, the Muscular Dystrophy Association of America and the Association Francaise contre les Myopathies. I am indebted to the many colleagues who participated in some of the studies described here. I thank Drs T. Barkas and R. Matsas for critical reading of the manuscript and valuable suggestions.

References

Agius, M. A., Geannopoulos, C. J., Fairclough, R. H. and Richmann, D. P. (1988). Monoclonal anti-idiotopic antibodies against myasthenia-inducing anti-acetylcholine receptor monoclonal antibodies. Preponderance of nonparatope-directed antibodies affecting antigen binding. *J. Immunol.*, **140**, 62–68

Amit, A. G., Mariuzza, R. A., Phillips, S. E. V. and Poljak, R. (1986). Three-dimensional structure of an antigen-antibody complex at 2.8 Å resolution. *Science, N.Y.*, **233**, 747–753

Anderson, D., Blobel, G., Tzartos, S. J., Gullick, W. and Lindstrom, J. (1983). Transmembrane orientation of an early biosynthetic form of acetylcholine receptor subunit determined by proteolytic dissection in conjunction with monoclonal antibodies. *J. Neurosci.*, **3**, 1773–1784

Barkas, T., Gabriel, J. M., Juillerat, M., Kokla, A. and Tzartos, S. J. (1986). Localization of the main immunogenic region of the nicotinic acetylcholine receptor. *FEBS Lett.*, **196**, 237–241

Barkas, T., Gabriel, J.-M., Mauron, A., Hughes, G. J., Roth, B., Alliod, C., Tzartos, S. J. and Ballivet, M. (1988). Fine localisation of the main immunogenic region of the nicotinic acetylcholine receptor to residues 61–76 of the α subunit. *J. Biol. Chem.*, **263**, 5916–5920

Barkas, T., Mauron, A., Roth, B., Alliod, C., Tzartos, S. J. and Ballivet, M. (1987). Mapping the main immunogenic region and toxin binding site of the nicotinic acetylcholine receptor. *Science, N.Y.*, **235**, 77–80

Barnard, E. A., Darlison, M. G. and Seeburg, P. (1987). Molecular biology of the GABA-A receptor: the receptor/channel superfamily. *Trends Neurosci.*, **10**, 502–509

Berzofsky, J. A. (1984). Monoclonal antibodies as probes of antigenic structure. In *Monoclonal and Anti-idiotypic Antibodies: Probes for Receptor Structure and Function* (ed. J. C. Venter,

C. M. Fraser and J. Lindstrom) Alan R. Liss, New York, pp. 1–19

Blair, D. A., Richman, D. P., Taves, C. J. and Koethe, S. (1986). Monoclonal antibodies to acetylcholine receptor secreted by human × human hybridomas derived from lymphocytes of a patient with myasthenia gravis. *Immunol. Invest.*, **15**, 351–364

Blount, P. and Merlie, J. P. (1988). Native folding of an acetylcholine receptor α subunit expressed in the absence of other receptor subunits. *J. Biol. Chem.*, **263**, 1072–1080

Brisson, A. and Unwin, P. (1985). Quaternary structure of the acetylcholine receptor. *Nature*, **315**, 474–477

Cauley, K., Agranoff, B. W. and Goldman, D. (1989). Identification of a novel nicotinic acetylcholine receptor structural subunit expressed in goldfish retina. *J. Cell Biol.*, **108**, 637–645

Changeux, J.-P. and Revah, F. (1987). The acetylcholine receptor molecule: allosteric sites and the ion channel. *TINS*, **10**, 245–250

Chase, B. A., Holliday, J., Reese, J. H., Chun, L. L. Y. and Hawrot, E. (1987). Monoclonal antibodies with defined specificities for *Torpedo* nicotinic acetylcholine receptor cross-react with *Drosophila* neural tissue. *Neuroscience*, **21**, 959–976

Chinchetru, M. A., Marquez, J., Garcia-Borron, J. C., Richman, D. P. and Martinez-Carrion, M. (1989). Interaction of nicotinic acetylcholine receptor with 2 monoclonal antibodies recognizing different epitopes. *Biochemistry*, **28**, 4222–4229

Claudio, T., Green, W. N., Hartman, D. S., Hayden, D., Paulson, H. L., Sigworth, F. J., Sine, S. M. and Swedlund, A. (1987). Genetic reconstitution of functional acetylcholine receptor channels in mouse fibroblasts. *Science, N.Y.*, **238**, 1688–1693

Colman, P. M., Laver, W. G., Varghese, J. N., Baker, A. T., Tulloch, P. A., Air, G. M. and Webster, R. G. (1987). Three-dimensional structure of a complex of antibody with influenza virus neuraminidase. *Nature*, **326**, 358–363

Conti-Tronconi, B., Tzartos, S. J. and Lindstrom, J. (1981). Monoclonal antibodies as probes of acetylcholine receptor structure. II. Binding to native receptor. *Biochemistry*, **20**, 2181–2191

Cung, M. T., Marraud, M., Hadjidakis, I., Bairaktari, H., Sakarellos, C., Kokla, A. and Tzartos, S. (1989). 2D-1H NMR study of a synthetic peptide containing the main immunogenic region of the *Torpedo* acetylcholine receptor. *Biopolymers*, **28**, 465–478

Cunningham, B. C., Jhurani, P., Ng, P. and Wells, J. A. (1989). Receptor and antibody epitopes in human growth hormone identified by homolog-scanning mutagenesis. *Science, N.Y.*, **243**, 1330–1336

Das, M. K. and Lindstrom, J. (1989). The main immunogenic region of the nicotinic acetylcholine receptor. Interaction of monoclonal antibodies with synthetic peptides. *Biochem. Biophys. Res. Commun.*, **165**, 865–871

De Baets, M. H., Verschuuren, J. and Van Brenda Vriesman, P. J. C. (1988). Experimental autoimmune myasthenia gravis. *Monogr. Allergy*, **25**, 1–11

Dipaola, M., Czajkowski, C. and Karlin, A. (1989). The sidedness of the COOH terminus of the acetylcholine receptor-delta-subunit, *J. Biol. Chem.*, **264**, 15457–15463

Donnelly, D., Mihovilovic, M., Gonzalez-Ros, J. M., Ferragut, J. A., Richman, D. and Martinez-Carrion, M. (1984). A noncholinergic site-directed monoclonal antibody can impair agonist-induced ion flux in *Torpedo californica* acetylcholine receptor. *Proc. Natl Acad. Sci. USA*, **81**, 7999–8003

Drachman, D. (Ed.) (1987). *Myasthenia Gravis. Ann. N.Y. Acad. Sci.*, **505**, 1–914

Drachman, D. B., Adams, R. N., Josifek, L. F. and Self, S. G. (1982). Functional activities of autoantibodies to acetylcholine receptors and the clinical severity of myasthenia gravis. *New Engl. J. Med.*, **307**, 769–775

Dwyer, D. S., Vakil, M., Bradley, R. J., Oh, S. J. and Kearney, J. F. (1987). A possible cause of myasthenia gravis: Idiotypic networks involving bacterial antigens. *Ann. N.Y. Acad. Sci.*, **505**, 461–471

Engel, A. G. (1984). Myasthenia gravis and myasthenic syndromes. *Ann. Neurol.*, **16**, 519–533

Erlanger, B. F., Cleveland, W. L., Wassermann, N. H., Ku, H. H., Hill, B. L., Sarangarajan, R. and Penn, A. S. (1987). Autoantibodies to receptors by an autoantiidiotypic route. *Ann. N.Y. Acad. Sci.*, **505**, 416–422

Fels, G., Breer, H. and Maelicke, A. (1983). Are there nicotinic acetylcholine receptors in invertebrate ganglionic tissue? In *Toxins as Tools in Neurochemistry* (ed. F. Huch and Y. A. Ovchinnikov). W. de Gruyter, Berlin, pp. 124–140

Fels, G., Plumer-Wilk, R., Schreiber, M. and Maelicke, A. (1986). A monoclonal antibody interfering with binding and response of the acetylcholine receptor. *J. Biol. Chem.*, **261**, 15746–15754

Froehner, S. C., Douville, K., Klink, S. and Culp, W. J. (1983). Monoclonal antibodies to cytoplasmic domains of the acetylcholine receptor. *J. Biol. Chem.*, **258**, 7112–7120

Fujita, N., Nelson, N., Fox, T. D., Claudio, T., Lindstrom, J., Riezman, H. and Hess, G. P. (1986). Biosynthesis of the *Torpedo californica* acetylcholine receptor α subunit in yeast. *Science, N.Y.*, **231**, 1284–1287

Geysen, H. M., Meloen, H. R. and Barteling, S. J. (1984). Use of peptide synthesis to probe viral antigens for epitopes to a resolution of a single amino acid. *Proc. Natl Acad. Sci. USA*, **81**, 3998–4002

Giraudat, J., Dennis, M., Heidmann, T., Haumont, P.-Y., Lederer, F. and Changeux, J.-P. (1987). Structure of the high-affinity binding site for noncompetitive blockers of the acetylcholine receptor: [3-H]chlorpromazine labels homologous residues in the β and δ chains. *Biochemistry*, **26**, 2410–2418

Gomez, C. M. and Richman, D. P. (1983). Anti-acetylcholine receptor antibodies directed against the α-bungarotoxin binding site induce a unique form of experimental myasthenia. *Proc. Natl Acad. Sci. USA*, **80**, 4089–4093

Gotti, C., Frigerio, F., Bolognesi, M., Longhi, R., Racchetti, G. and Clementi, F. (1988). Nicotinic acetylcholine receptor: a structural model for α subunit peptide 188–201, the putative binding site for cholinergic agents. *FEBS Lett.*, **228**, 118–122

Gullick, W. J., Tzartos, S. J. and Lindstrom, J. (1981). Monoclonal antibodies as probes of acetylcholine receptor structure. I. Peptide mapping. *Biochemistry*, **20**, 2173–2180

Harvey, A. L., Barkas, T., Harrison, R. and Lunt, G. G. (1978). Inhibition of receptor function in cultured chick myotubes by antiserum to purified *Torpedo* acetylcholine receptor and myasthenic sera. In *The Biochemistry of Myasthenia Gravis and Muscular Dystrophy* (ed. G. G. Lunt, and R. M. Marchbanks). Academic Press, London, pp. 167–175

Heidenreich, F., Vincent, A., Roberts, A. and Newsom-Davis, J. (1988a). Epitopes on human acetylcholine receptor defined by monoclonal antibodies and myasthenia gravis sera. *Autoimmunity*, **1**, 285–297

Heidenreich, F., Vincent, A., Willcox, N. and Newsom-Davis, J. (1988b). Anti-acetylcholine receptor antibody specificities in serum and in thymic cell culture supernatants from myasthenia gravis patients. *Neurology*, **38**, 1784–1788

Heinemann, S., Bevan, S., Kullberg, R., Lindstrom, J. and Rice, J. (1977). Modulation of the acetylcholine receptor by anti-receptor antibodies. *Proc. Natl Acad. Sci. USA*, **74**, 3090–3094

Henley, J. M., Lindstrom, J. M. and Oswald, R. E. (1988). Interaction of monoclonal antibodies with α-bungarotoxin and (−)-nicotine binding sites in goldfish brain. *J. Biol. Chem.*, **263**, 9686–9691

Hertling-Jaweed, S., Bandini, G., Muller-Fahrnow, A., Dommes, V. and Hucho, F. (1988). Rapid preparation of the nicotinic acetylcholine receptor for crystallization in detergent solution. *FEBS Lett.*, **241**, 29–32

Higgins, L. S. and Berg, D. K. (1987). Immunological identification of a nicotinic acetylcholine receptor on bovine chromaffin cells. *J. Neurosci.*, **7**, 1792–1798

Hohlfeld, R., Toyka, K. V., Heininger, K., Grosse-Wilde, H. and Kalies, I. (1984). Autoimmune human T lymphocytes specific for acetylcholine receptor. *Nature*, **310**, 244–246

Hohlfeld, R., Toyka, K., Tzartos, S. J., Carson, W. and Conti-Tronconi, B. (1987). Human T helper lymphocytes in myasthenia gravis recognize the nicotinic receptor α subunit. *Proc. Natl Acad. Sci. USA*, **84**, 5379–5383

Houghten, R. A. (1985). General method for the rapid solid-phase synthesis of large numbers of peptides: Specificity of antigen-antibody interaction at the level of individual amino acids. *Proc. Natl Acad. Sci. USA*, **82**, 5131–5135

Hucho, F., Oberthur, W. and Lottspeich, F. (1986). The ion channel of the nicotinic acetylcholine receptor is formed by the homologous helices M II of the receptor subunits. *FEBS Lett.*, **205**, 137–142

Jacob, M. H. and Berg, D. K. (1988). The distribution of acetylcholine receptors in chick ciliary ganglion neurons following disruption of ganglionic connections. *J. Neurosci.*, **8**, 3838–3849

Kamo, I., Furukawa, S., Tada, A., Mano, Y., Iwasaki, Y., Furuse, T., Ito, N., Hayashi, K. and Satoyoshi, E. (1982). Monoclonal antibody to acetylcholine receptor: cell line established from thymus of patient with myasthenia gravis. *Science, N.Y.*, **215**, 995–997

Killen, J., Hochschwender, S. and Lindstrom, J. (1985). The main immunogenic region of acetylcholine receptors does not provoke the formation of antibodies to a predominant idiotype. *J. Neuroimmunol.*, **9**, 229–241

Kirchner, T., Tzartos, S., Hoppe, F., Schalke, B., Wekerle, H. and Muller-Hermelink, H. K. (1988). Pathogenesis of myasthenia gravis. Acetylcholine receptor-related antigenic determinants in tumor-free thymuses and thymic epithelial tumors. *Am. J. Pathol.*, **130**, 268–279

Kohler, G. and Milstein, C. (1975). Continuous cultures of fused cells secreting antibody of predefined specificity. *Nature*, **256**, 495–497

Kohler, G. and Milstein, C. (1976). Derivation of specific antibody-producing tissue culture and tumor lines by cell fusion. *Eur. J. Immunol.*, **6**, 511–519

Kordossi, A. and Tzartos, S. J. (1987). Conformation of cytoplasmic segments of acetylcholine receptor α and β subunits probed by monoclonal antibodies. Sensitivity of the antibody competition approach. *EMBO Jl*, **6**, 1605–1610

Kordossi, A. A. and Tzartos, S. J. (1989). Monoclonal antibodies against the main immunogenic region of the acetylcholine receptor. Mapping on the intact molecule. *J. Neuroimmunol.*, **23**, 35–40

Kouvelas, E., Dichter, M. A. and Greene, L. A. (1978). Chick sympathetic neurons develop receptors for α-bungarotoxin *in vitro*, but the toxin does not block nicotinic receptors. *Brain Res.*, **154**, 83–93

Kubalek, E., Ralston, S., Lindstrom, J. and Unwin, N. (1987). Location of subunits within the acetylcholine receptor by electron image analysis of tubular crystals from *Torpedo marmorata*. *J. Cell Biol.*, **105**, 9–18

La Rochelle, W., Wray, B., Sealock, R. and Froehner, S. (1985). Immunochemical demonstration that amino acids 360–377 of the acetylcholine receptor γ subunit are cytoplasmic. *J. Cell Biol.*, **100**, 684–691

Lefvert, A. K., Pirskanen, R. and Svanborg, E. (1985). Anti-idiotypic antibodies, acetylcholine receptor antibodies and disturbed neuromuscular function in healthy relatives to patients with myasthenia gravis. *J. Neuroimmunol*, **9**, 41–53

Lennon, V. A. and Griesmann, G. E. (1989). Evidence against acetylcholine receptor having a main immunogenic region as target for autoantibodies in myasthenia gravis. *Neurology*, **39**, 1069–1076

Lennon, V. A. and Lambert, E. H. (1981). Monoclonal autoantibodies to acetylcholine receptors: evidence for a dominant idiotype and requirement of complement for pathogenicity. *Ann. N.Y. Acad. Sci.*, **377**, 77–96

Lerner, R. A. and Tramontano, A. (1987). Antibodies as enzymes. *TIBS*, **12**, 427–430

Lindstrom, J. (1986). Probing nicotinic acetylcholine receptors with monoclonal antibodies. *Trends Neurosci.*, **9**, 401–407

Lindstrom, J., Shoepfer, R. and Whiting, P. (1987). Molecular studies of the neuronal nicotinic acetylcholine receptor family. *Molec. Neurobiol.*, **1**, 281–337

Lindstrom, J., Shelton, D. and Fugii, Y. (1988). Myasthenia gravis. *Adv. Immunol.*, **42**, 233–284

Lindstrom, J., Tzartos, S. J. and Gullick, W. (1981). Structure and function of the acetylcholine receptor molecule studied using monoclonal antibodies. *Ann. N.Y. Acad. Sci.*, **377**, 1–19

Lindstrom, J. M., Seybold, M. E., Lennon, V. A., Whittingham, S. and Duane, D. (1976). Antibody to acetylcholine receptor in myasthenia gravis: Prevalence, clinical correlates and diagnostic value. *Neurology*, **26**, 1054–1059

Lo, M. S., Tsong, T. Y., Contad, M. K., Strittmatter, S. M., Hester, L. D. and Snyder, S. H. (1984). Monoclonal antibody production by receptor-mediated electrically induced cell fusion. *Nature*, **310**, 792–794

Luben, R. A. and Mohler, M. A. (1980). *In vitro* immunization as an adjunct to the production of hybridomas producing antibodies against the lymphokine osteoclast activating factor. *Molec. Immunol.*, **17**, 635–639

McCarthy, M. P., Earnest, J. P., Young, E. F., Choe, S. and Stroud, R. M. (1986). The molecular neurobiology of the aceteylcholine receptor. *Ann. Rev. Neurosci.*, **9**, 383–413

McCormick, D. J. and Atassi, M. Z. (1984). Localization and synthesis of the acetylcholine-binding site in the α-chain of the *Torpedo californica* acetylcholine receptor. *Biochem. J.*, **224**, 995–1000

Maelicke, A. (1988). Structure and function of the nicotinic acetylcholine receptor. In *Handbook of Experimental Pharmacology*, Vol. 86 (ed. V. P. Whittaker). Springer-Verlag, Berlin, pp. 267–313

Maelicke, A., Plumer-Wilk, R., Fels, G., Spencer, S. R., Engelhard, M., Veltel, D. and Conti-Tronconi, B. M. (1989). Epitope mapping employing antibodies raised against short synthetic peptides: A study of the nicotinic acetylcholine receptor. *Biochemistry*, **28**, 1396–1405

Marx, A., Kirchner, T., Hoppe, F., O'Connor, R., Schalke, B., Tzartos, S. and Muller-Hermelink, H. K. (1989). Proteins with epitopes of the acetylcholine receptor in epithelial cells of thymomas of patients with myasthenia gravis. *Am. J. Pathol.*, **134**, 865–877

Maselli, R. A., Nelson, D. J. and Richman, D. P. (1989). Effects of a monoclonal anti-acetylcholine receptor antibody on the avian end-plate. *J. Physiol. (Lond.)*, **411**, 271–283

Mehraban, F., Kemshead, J. T. and Dolly, J. O. (1984). Properties of monoclonal antibodies to nicotinic acetylcholine receptor from chick muscle. *Eur. J. Biochem.*, **138**, 53–61

Merlie, J. P. and Lindstrom, J. (1983). Assembly *in vivo* of mouse muscle acetylcholine receptor: Identification of an α-subunit species that may be an assembly intermediate. *Cell*, **34**, 747–757

Merlie, J. P., Sebbane, R., Tzartos, S. J. and Lindstrom, J. (1982). Inhibition of glycosylation with tunicamycin blocks assembly of newly synthesized acetylcholine receptor subunits in muscle cells. *J. Biol. Chem.*, **257**, 2694–2701

Merlie, J. P. and Smith, M. M. (1986). Synthesis and assembly of acetylcholine receptor, a multisubunit membrane glycoprotein. *J. Membr. Biol.*, **91**, 1–10

Mihovilovic, M. and Richman, D. P. (1984). Modification of α-bungarotoxin and cholinergic ligand-binding properties of *Torpedo* acetylcholine receptor by an anti-acetylcholine receptor monoclonal antibody. *J. Biol. Chem.*, **259**, 15051–15059

Milstein, C. (1986). From antibody structure to immunological diversification of immune response. *Science, N.Y.*, **231**, 1261–1268

Mishina, M. *et al.* (1984). Expression of functional acetylcholine receptor from cloned cDNAs. *Nature*, **307**, 604–608

Mitra, A. K., McCarthy, M. P. and Stroud, R. M. (1989). 3-Dimensional structure of the nicotinic acetylcholine receptor and location of the major associated 43-kd cytoskeletal protein, determined at 22-A by low dose electron microscopy and x-ray diffraction to 12.5-A. *J. Cell Biol.*, **109**, 755–774

Mochly-Rosen, C. and Fuchs, S. (1981). Monoclonal anti-acetylcholine receptor antibodies directed against the cholinergic binding site. *Biochemistry*, **20**, 5920–5924

Momoy, M. Y. and Lennon, V. A. (1982). Purification and biochemical characterization of nicotinic acetylcholine receptors of human muscle. *J. Biol. Chem.*, **257**, 12757–12764

Morel, E., Eymard, B., Vernet der Garabedian, B., Pannier, C., Dulac, O. and Bach, J. F. (1988a). Neonatal myasthenia gravis—A new clinical and immunologic appraisal on 30 cases. *Neurology*, **38**, 138–142

Morel, E., Vernet der Garabedian, B., Eymard, B., Raimond, F., Bustarret, F.-A. and Bach, J.-F. (1988b). Binding and blocking antibodies to the human acetylcholine receptor: are they selected in various myasthenia gravis forms. *Immunol. Res.*, **7**, 212–217

Nef, P., Oneyser, C., Alliod, C., Couturier, S. and Ballivet, M. (1988). Genes expressed in the brain define three distinct neuronal nicotinic acetylcholine receptors. *EMBO Jl*, **7**, 595–601

Newsom-Davis, J., Harcourt, G., Sommer, N., Beeson, D., Willcox, N. and Rothbard, J. B. (1989). T-cell reactivity in myasthenia gravis. *J. Autoimmun*, **2**, 101–108

Numa, S. (1987). Structure and function of ionic channels. In *Membrane Proteins: Structure, Function, Assembly* (ed. J. Rydstrom). *Chemica Scripta*, Vol. 27B, CUP, Cambridge, pp. 5–19

Olsson, L. and Kaplan, H. S. (1980). Human–human hybridomas producing monoclonal antibodies of predefined antigenic specificity. *Proc. Natl Acad. Sci. USA*, **77**, 5429–5431

Oosterhuis, H. I. G. H. (Ed.) (1984). *Myasthenia Gravis*. Churchill Livingstone. Edinburgh.

Papadouli, I., Potamianos, S., Hadjidakis, I., Bairaktari, E., Tsikaris, V., Sakarellos, C., Cung, M. T., Marraud, M. and Tzartos, S. J. (1990). Antigenic role of single residues within the main immunogenic region of the nicotinic acetylcholine receptor. *Biochem. J.*, **269**, 239–245

Plumer, R., Fels, G. and Maelicke, A. (1984). Antibodies against preselected peptides to map functional sites on the acetylcholine receptor. *FEBS Lett.*, **178**, 204–208

Raftery, M., Hunkapiller, M., Strader, C. and Hood, L. (1980). Acetylcholine receptor: Complex of homologous subunits. *Science, N.Y.*, **208**, 1454–1457

Ratnam, M., Le Nguyen, D., Rivier, J., Sargent, P. and Lindstrom, J. (1986a). Transmembrane topography of the nicotinic acetylcholine receptor: immunochemical tests contradict theoretical predictions based on hydrophobicity profile. *Biochemistry*, **25**, 2633–2643

Ratnam, M., Sargent, P., Sarin, V., Fox, J. L., Le Nguyen, D., Rivier, J., Criado, M. and Lindstrom, J. (1986b). Location of antigenic determinants on primary sequences of the subunits of the nicotinic acetylcholine receptor by peptide mapping. *Biochemistry*, **25**, 2621–2632

Riechmann, L., Clark, M., Waldmann, H. and Winter, G. (1988). Reshaping human antibodies for therapy. *Nature*, **332**, 323–327

Roberts, S., Cheetham, J. C. and Rees, A. R. (1987). Generation of an antibody with enhanced affinity and specificity for its antigen by protein engineering. *Nature*, **328**, 731–734

Sargent, P., Hedges, B., Tsavaler, L., Clemmons, L., Tzartos, S. J. and Lindstrom, J. (1984). The structure and transmembrane nature of the acetylcholine receptor in amphibian skeletal muscle as revealed by cross-reacting monoclonal antibodies. *J. Cell Biol.*, **98**, 609–618

Sargent, P. B., Pike, S. H., Nadel, D. B. and Lindstrom, J. M. (1989). Nicotinic acetylcholine receptor-like molecules in the retina, retinotectal pathway, and optic tectum of the frog. *J. Neurosci.*, **9**, 565–573

Schwimmbeck, P. L., Dyrberg, T., Drachman, D. B. and Oldstone, M. B. A. (1989). Molecular mimicry and myasthenia gravis—an autoantigenic site of the acetylcholine receptor alpha-subunit that has biologic activity and reacts immunochemically with herpes simplex virus. *J. Clin. Invest.*, **84**, 1174–1180

Shelton, G. D., Cardinet, G. H. III and Lindstrom, J. M. (1988). Canine and human myasthenia gravis autoantibodies recognize similar regions on the acetylcholine receptor. *Neurology*, **38**, 1417–1423

Sophianos, D. and Tzartos, S. J. (1989). Fab fragments of monoclonal antibodies protect the human acetylcholine receptor against degradation caused by myasthenic sera. *J. Autoimmun.*, **2**, 777–789

Souroujon, M. C., Mochly-Rosen, D., Gordon, A. S. and Fuchs, S. (1983). Interaction of monoclonal antibodies to *Torpedo* acetylcholine receptor with the receptor of skeletal muscle. *Muscle Nerve*, **6**, 303–311

Souroujon, M. C., Pachner, A. R. and Fuchs, S. (1986). The treatment of passively transferred experimental myasthenia with anti-idiotypic antibodies. *Neurology*, **36**, 622–625

Stefansson, K., Dieperink, M. E., Richman, D. P. and Marton, L. S. (1987). Sharing of epitopes by bacteria and the nicotinic acetylcholine receptor: A possible role in the pathogenesis of myasthenia gravis. *Ann. N.Y. Acad. Sci.*, **505**, 451–460

Swanson, L., Lindstrom, J., Tzartos, S. J., Schmued, L., O'Leary, D. D. and Cowan, W. M. (1983). Immunohistochemical localization of monoclonal antibodies to the nicotinic acetylcholine receptor in the midbrain of the chick. *Proc. Natl Acad. Sci. USA*, **80**, 4532–4536

Syu, W. J. and Kahan, L. (1989). Epitope characterization by modifications of antigens and by mapping on resin-bound peptides—discriminating epitopes near the C-terminus and N-terminus of *Escherichia coli* ribosomal protein-S13. *J. Immunol. Meth.*, **118**, 153–160

Tzartos, S. J. (1988). Myasthenia gravis studied by monoclonal antibodies to the acetylcholine receptor. *In Vivo*, **2**, 105–110

Tzartos, S. J., Barkas, T., Cung, M. T., Kordossi, A., Loutrari, E., Marraud, M., Papadouli, I., Sakarellos, C., Sophianos, D. and Tsikaris, V. (1990a). The main immunogenic region of the acetylcholine receptor, structure and role in myasthenia gravis. *Autoimmunity* (in press)

Tzartos, S. J. and Changeux, J.-P. (1983). High affinity binding of α-bungarotoxin to the purified α-subunit and its 27K proteolytic peptide from *Torpedo* acetylcholine receptor. Requirement for SDS. *EMBO Jl*, **2**, 381–387

Tzartos, S. J. and Changeux, J.-P. (1984). Lipid-dependent recovery of α-bungarotoxin and monoclonal antibody binding to the purified α-subunit from *Torpedo marmorata* acetylcholine receptor. *J. Biol. Chem.*, **259**, 11512–11519

Tzartos, S., Efthimiadis, A., Morel, E., Eymard, B. and Bach, J. F. (1990b). Neonatal myasthenia gravis: Antigenic specificities of antibodies in sera from mothers and their infants. *Clin. Exp. Immunol.*, **80**, 376–380

Tzartos, S. J., Hochschwender, S., Vasquez, P. and Lindstrom, J. (1987). Passive transfer of experimental autoimmune myasthenia gravis by monoclonal antibodies to the main immunogenic region of the acetylcholine receptor. *J. Neuroimmunol.*, **15**, 185–194

Tzartos, S. J., Kokla, A., Walgrave, S. and Conti-Tronconi, B. (1988a). Localization of the main immunogenic region of human muscle acetylcholine receptor to residues 67–76 of the α-subunit. *Proc. Natl Acad. Sci. USA*, **85**, 2899–2903

Tzartos, S. J. and Kordossi, A. (1986). Acetylcholine receptor conformation probed by subunit-specific monoclonal antibodies. In *Nicotinic Acetylcholine Receptor* (ed. A. Maelicke). NATO ASI series, Vol. H3, Springer-Verlag, Heidelberg, pp. 35–47

Tzartos, S. J., Kordossi, A., Walgrave, S. L., Kokla, A. and Conti-Tronconi, B. M. (1988b). Determination of antibody binding sites on the three-dimensional and primary structure of acetylcholine receptor. *Monogr. Allergy*, **25**, 20–32

Tzartos, S., Langeberg, L., Hochschwender, S. and Lindstrom, J. (1983). Demonstration of a main immunogenic region on acetylcholine receptors from human muscle using monoclonal antibodies to human receptor. *FEBS Lett*, **158**, 116–118

Tzartos, S., Langeberg, L., Hochschwender, S., Swanson, L. and Lindstrom, J. (1986a).

Characteristics of monoclonal antibodies to denatured *Torpedo* and to native calf acetylcholine receptors: species, subunit and region specificity. *J. Neuroimmunol.*, **10**, 235–253

Tzartos, S. J. and Lindstrom, J. L. (1980). Monoclonal antibodies to probe acetylcholine receptor structure: Localization of the main immunogenic region and detection of similarities between subunits. *Proc. Natl Acad. Sci. USA*, **77**, 755–759

Tzartos, S. J., Loutrari, H. V., Tang, F., Kokla, A., Walgrave, S. L., Milius, R. P. and Conti-Tronconi, B. M. (1990c). The main immunogenic region of *Torpedo electroplax* and human muscle acetylcholine receptor localization and micro-heterogeneity revealed by the use of synthetic peptides. *J. Neurochem.*, **54**, 51–61

Tzartos, S. J., Morel, E., Efthimiadis, A., Bustarret, A. F., D'Anglejan, J., Drosos, A. and Moutsopoulos, H. M. (1988c). Fine antigenic specificities of antibodies in sera from patients with D-penicillamine-induced myasthenia gravis. *Clin. Exp. Immunol.*, **74**, 80–86

Tzartos, S., Papadouli, I., Potamianos, S., Hadjidakis, I., Bairaktari, H., Tsikaris, V., Sakarellos, C., Cung, M. T. and Marraud, M. (1989). Fine structural characterization of the main immunogenic region of the nicotinic acetylcholine receptor. In *Molecular Biology of Neuroreceptors and Ion Channels* (ed. A. Maelicke). NATO ASI series, Vol. H32, Springer, Berlin, pp. 361–371

Tzartos, S. J., Rand, D. E., Einarson, B. E. and Lindstrom, J. M. (1981). Mapping of surface structures of *Electrophorus* acetylcholine receptor using monoclonal antibodies. *J. Biol. Chem.*, **256**, 8635–8645

Tzartos, S. J., Seybold, M. and Lindstrom, J. (1982). Specificities of antibodies to acetylcholine receptors in sera from myasthenia gravis patients measured by monoclonal antibodies. *Proc. Natl Acad. Sci. USA*, **79**, 188–192

Tzartos, S. J., Sophianos, D. and Efthimiadis, A. (1985). Role of the main immunogenic region of acetylcholine receptor in myasthenia gravis. An Fab monoclonal antibody protects against antigenic modulation by human sera. *J. Immunol.*, **134**, 2343–2349

Tzartos, S. J., Sophianos, D., Zimmermann, K. and Starzinski-Powitz, A. (1986b). Antigenic modulation of human muscle acetylcholine receptor by myasthenic sera. Serum titer determines receptor internalization. *J. Immunol.*, **136**, 3231–3237

Tzartos, S. J. and Starzinski-Powitz, A. (1986). Decrease in acetylcholine receptor content of human myotube cultures mediated by monoclonal antibodies to α, β and γ subunits. *FEBS Lett*, **196**, 91–95

Van Regenmortel, M. H. V. (1989). Structural and functional approaches to the study of protein antigenicity. *Immunol. Today*, **10**, 266–272

Verschuuren, J. J. G. M. (1989). Experimental Autoimmune Myasthenia Gravis. Antibodies, Idiotypes and Anti-idiotypes. PhD Thesis, University of Limburg at Maastricht, The Netherlands

Wada, K., Ballivet, M., Boulter, J., Connolly, J., Wada, E., Deneris, E. S., Swanson, L. W., Heinemann, S. and Patrick, J. (1988). Functional expression of a new pharmacological subtype of brain nicotinic acetylcholine receptor. *Science, N.Y.*, **240**, 330–334

Wan, K. and Lindstrom, J. (1985). Effects of monoclonal antibodies on the function of purified acetylcholine receptor from *Torpedo californica* reconstituted into liposomes. *Biochemistry*, **24**, 1212–1221

Ward, E. S., Gussow, D., Griffiths, A. D., Jones, P. T. and Winter, G. (1989). Binding activities of a repertoire of single immunoglobulin variable domains secreted from *Escherichia coli*. *Nature*, **341**, 544–546

Watters, D. and Maelicke, A. (1983). Organization of ligand binding sites at the acetylcholine receptor: A study with monoclonal antibodies. *Biochemistry*, **22**, 1811–1819

Whiting, P. and Lindstrom, J. (1986). Purification and characterization of a nicotinic acetylcholine receptor from chick brain. *Biochemistry*, **25**, 2082–2093

Whiting, P. J. and Lindstrom, J. M. (1988). Characterization of bovine and human neuronal nicotinic acetylcholine receptors using monoclonal antibodies. *J. Neurosci.*, **8**, 3395–3404

Whiting, P. J., Schoepfer, R., Swanson, L. W., Simmons, D. M. and Lindstrom, J. M. (1987). Functional acetylcholine receptor in PC12 cells reacts with a mab to brain nicotinic receptors. *Nature*, **327**, 515–518

Whiting, P. J., Vincent, A. and Newsom-Davis, J. (1986). Myasthenia gravis: Monoclonal antihuman acetylcholine receptor antibodies used to analyse antibody specificities and responses to treatment. *Neurology*, **36**, 612–617

Wilson, P. T. and Lentz, T. L. (1988). Binding of α-bungarotoxin to synthetic peptides corresponding to residues 173–204 of the α subunit of *Torpedo*, calf, and human acetylcholine receptor and restoration of high-affinity binding by sodium dodecyl sulfate. *Biochemistry*, **27**, 6667–6674

Wood, H., Beeson, D., Vincent, A. and Newsom-Davis, J. (1989). Epitopes on human acetylcholine receptor α-subunit: binding of monoclonal antibodies to recombinant and synthetic peptides. *Biochem. Soc. Trans.*, **17**, 220–221

Xu, Q., DuPont, B. L., Fairclough, R. H. and Richman, D. P. (1988). An anti-acetylcholine receptor monoclonal antibody that blocks agonist binding also modifies antibody binding to the main immunogenic region of the receptor. *Neurology*, **38**, Suppl. 1, 135

Zhang, Y., Barkas, T., Juillerat, M., Schwendimann, B. and Wekerle, H. (1988a). T cell epitopes in EAmyasthenia gravis of the rat: strain-specific epitopes and cross-reaction between two distinct segments of the α chain of the nicotinic acetylcholine receptor (*Torpedo californica*). *Eur. J. Immunol.*, **18**, 551–557

Zhang, Y., Tzartos, S. J. and Wekerle, H. (1988b). B–T lymphocyte interactions in experimental autoimmune myasthenia gravis: antigen presentation by rat/mouse hybridoma lines secreting monoclonal antibodies against the nicotinic acetylcholine receptor. *Eur. J. Immunol.*, **18**, 211–218

7

Studies on [3H]Glutamate Binding in Nervous Tissues. What are the Pitfalls?

YUKIO YONEDA and KIYOKAZU OGITA

Department of Pharmacology, Faculty of Pharmaceutical Sciences, Setsunan University, Hirakata, Osaka 573–01, Japan

Contents

Current Aspects of the Neurosciences, Vol. 3. Edited by N. N. Osborne. © The Macmillan Press Ltd 1991

1. *Introduction*

Some free acidic amino acids enriched in the brain, such as L-glutamic acid
(Glu) and L-aspartic acid (Asp), are believed to play a role as excitatory
amino acid neurotransmitters in the mammalian central nervous system
(Curtis and Johnston, 1974; Fonnum, 1984). For instance, Glu is synthesized
in presynaptic nerve terminals from which it is released during the neuronal
excitation in a Ca^{2+}-dependent fashion. A high-affinity and Na^+-dependent
uptake system is responsible for the termination of neurotransmission mediated by these acidic amino acids. Recently it has been demonstrated that Glu
is released from an exocytotic pool in cerebral cortical synaptosomes on
depolarization of the plasma membranes (Nicholls and Sihra, 1986; Sanchez-
Prieto *et al.*, 1987). These findings are consistent with the successful isolation
of synaptic vesicles with a Na^+-independent and ATP-dependent accumulation system for the acidic amino acid, which is distinctly different from the
abovementioned Na^+-dependent uptake system (Naito and Ueda, 1983,
1985). An immunohistochemical study has revealed the localization of
vesicular structures accumulating Glu in nerve terminals (Storm-Mathisen *et
al.*, 1983). In addition, human fibroblasts are shown to contain an acidic
amino acid exchange system between cystine and Glu across plasma membranes (Bannai, 1986).

On the other hand, synaptic receptors for these putative excitatory amino
acid neurotransmitters are classified into at least three subtypes according to
difference in the sensitivity to exogenous acidic compounds, such as *N*-
methyl-D-aspartic acid (NMDA), quisqualic acid (QA) and kainic acid (KA)
(Watkins and Evans, 1981; Foster and Fagg, 1984). Biochemical labelling of
these receptor sites has been carried out using [³H]Glu as a radioligand. In
addition to radiolabelling of the receptor sites, however, [³H]Glu is useful in
detecting the association with substrate-recognition sites of some membrane-
bound enzymes with a substantially high affinity for the neurotransmitter
candidate. The radioligand is also able to associate with various transport
sites described above. Therefore, it is conceivable that specific binding of
[³H]Glu may not only reflect the association of the ligand with synaptic
receptor sites, but also represent the association with membranous proteins
other than receptors under some particular experimental conditions. In fact,
radioligand labelling of the NMDA-sensitive receptors often encounters
numerous methodological difficulties (Ferkany and Coyle, 1983; Foster and
Fagg, 1987; Murphy *et al.*, 1987). Biochemical binding studies using [³H]Glu
as a radioligand are sometimes inconsistent with the findings obtained in

experiments by physiological techniques. Furthermore, a displaceable adsorption of [³H]Glu occurs with microfuge tubes made of polypropylene as well as glass fibre and nitrocellulose filters, which depends on the incubation buffer employed (Ito *et al.*, 1986). These methodological problems are undoubtedly obstructive to the progress of biochemical and physiological studies on the excitatory amino acid receptors. In this chapter, therefore, we have attempted to settle various arguments about the receptors by overcoming the methodological pitfalls in radioligand binding assays of [³H]Glu.

2. Pitfalls in Radioactive Ligand

Displaceable Adsorption

Commercially obtained [³H]Glu was incubated at 30 °C for 60 min in 50 mM Tris-acetate buffer (pH 7.4) in the absence of brain synaptic membranes. After adding chilled buffer, the incubation mixture was filtered through a Whatman GF/B glass fibre filter under constant vacuum (Yoneda and Ogita, 1987a). A considerable amount of radioactivity was still retained on the filter rinsed four times with the buffer. This type of adsorption was greatly increased by the use of a filter previously soaked in polyethyleneimine (PEI) solution (Bruns *et al.*, 1983). The adsorption was markedly reduced by incubation in the presence of 1 mM unlabelled Glu, independently of the PEI treatment of filters. Therefore, it is evident that a displaceable adsorption indeed occurs with glass fibre filters, as demonstrated previously (Ito *et al.*, 1986). Similar marked adsorption was seen with nitrocellulose filters, but not with centrifuge tubes made of polypropylene or polyethylene. The displaceable adsorption was observed irrespective of commercial sources of [³H]Glu. To characterize the radioactive adsorbate, an attempt was made to determine whether or not the adsorption is affected by the use of a filter previously soaked in excess Glu. However, the use of Glu-treated filters did not alter the total binding or non-specific binding found in the presence of 1 mM Glu. These results suggest that the radioactive adsorbate is not [³H]Glu itself.

Contaminant

To investigate the purity of [³H]Glu, commercially obtained [³H]Glu solutions were applied to a plastic column packed with a slurry of cation exchange resin (Dowex 50W × 8, 200–400 mesh). The column was first eluted with distilled, deionized and sterilized water, and then with 0.5 M HCl. One-millilitre fractions were successively collected and the radioactivity of each fraction was measured. As shown in Figure 1, two radioactive materials were eluted from the column. Fraction I was eluted with water and Fraction II was

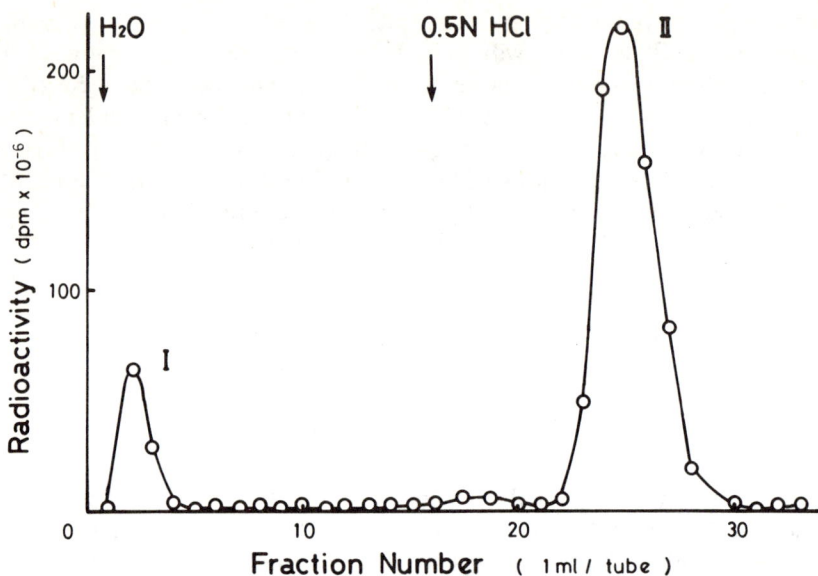

Figure 1 Elution profile of commercially obtained [³H]Glu on cation exchange column. Commercial [³H]Glu solution was applied to a plastic column packed with a slurry of Dowex 50W × 8 resin (200–400 mesh, 5 × 50 mm). The column was eluted with water and then with 0.5 M HCl. One-ml fractions were successively collected and the radioactivity was measured. Data shown are from a representative experiment which was repeated three times with similar results

eluted with HCl. Fraction I accounted for less than 5% of fraction II. Accordingly, commercially obtained [³H]Glu preparations seem to contain a radioactive contaminant with the chemical property of not being adsorbed to cation exchange resin.

'Binding' or 'Adsorption'

To examine the properties of these two radioactive materials, each fraction was individually incubated in 50 mM Tris-acetate buffer (pH 7.4) at 30°C for 60 min in either the presence or the absence of synaptic membrane preparations obtained from the rat brain (Ogita and Yoneda, 1986). Radioactivity found in the presence of synaptic membranes was referred to as 'binding', and 'adsorption' was derived from radioactivity found in the absence of membranes. After terminating the incubation with [³H]Glu before cation exchange chromatography (crude [³H]Glu) in the absence of synaptic membranes by the addition of cold buffer, the incubation mixture was subsequently filtered through a Whatman GF/B glass fibre filter under constant vacuum. Unidentified radioactive material was adsorbed to the filter extensively rinsed with the buffer in a manner displaceable by unlabelled Glu, as described

Table 1 Effect of purification of [³H]Glu on binding and adsorption

	Binding (dpm/*assay*)		*Adsorption* (dpm/*assay*)	
	None	*1 mM Glu*	*None*	*1 mM Glu*
Crude [³H]Glu	4 000 ± 340	1 200 ± 160	3 100 ± 300	1 150 ± 50
Fraction I	12 200 ± 730	12 500 ± 800	10 500 ± 650	12 900 ± 600
Fraction II	5 500 ± 120	560 ± 39	4 600 ± 340	260 ± 50

Commercially obtained [³H]Glu was applied to the Dowex column, and the column was first eluted with water and then HCl as shown in Figure 1. Each radioactive fraction (500 000 dpm) eluted from the column was individually incubated at 30 °C for 60 min in either the presence (binding) or the absence (adsorption) of brain synaptic membranes. Unlabelled Glu at 1 mM was also included in the incubation mixture to determine the non-specific binding or displaceable adsorption as needed. Values are from four separate experiments done in triplicate.

above. Incubation of crude [³H]Glu with synaptic membranes resulted in a slight increase in radioactivity retained on the filter after an extensive rinsing (Table 1). Addition of excess unlabelled Glu also decreased the radioactivity found in the presence of synaptic membranes. Specific binding, which was estimated by subtracting the radioactivity found in the presence of unlabelled Glu from the total amount of bound radioactivity, was slightly higher in the presence of synaptic membranes than in the absence of membranes.

Subsequently, incubation was carried out in either the presence or the absence of synaptic membranes, using two radioactive fractions obtained from the cation exchange chromatography. Incubation of fraction I resulted in an extremely high radioactivity retained on the filter after an extensive rinsing, irrespective of the presence of synaptic membranes (Table 1). The radioactivity was not reduced by incubation in the presence of 1 mM unlabelled Glu. These results, with the elution profile on the Dowex column, clearly indicate that fraction I is not [³H]Glu but a radioactive contaminant which is adsorbed to glass fibre filters in a manner not displaced by Glu. In contrast, fraction II caused a displaceable adsorption in the absence of synaptic membranes. Incubation of fraction II with brain synaptic membranes almost doubled the specific binding obtained in the experiments using crude [³H]Glu. However, the adsorption found in the absence of added Glu was more than eight times higher than the non-specific binding found in the presence of 1 mM Glu.

The latter value should be somewhat higher than the former value if non-specific binding to membranous proteins occurs to a significant extent. These problems have to be solved to enable an accurate and reproducible assay system for [³H]Glu binding to be run. Since a direct filtration of fraction II did not induce any displaceable adsorption, it seems possible that unidentified radioactive adsorbate is formed during the incubation of fraction II in the buffer at 30 °C. Judging from the elution profile and the data described above, [³H]Glu is responsible for the radioactive material in fraction II. Since the formation of radioactive adsorbate was drastically reduced by incubation in the presence of 1 mM unlabelled Glu, the radioactive adsorbate seems to be derived from [³H]Glu.

Settlement

The amount of radioactive contaminant increased in proportion to the duration of storage of the ligand. More than 20% of a radioactive material other than [³H]Glu was evolved in commercially obtained [³H]Glu solution under storage conditions of 2 °C for 1 month in 0.01 M HCl. To minimize the contribution of this artefactual contamination to the binding, the commercial [³H]Glu should be purified by cation exchange chromatography, and the purified [³H]Glu has to be frozen at −80 °C until use after being divided into small quantities. On the day of experiments, the necessary quantity of frozen [³H]Glu has to be thawed and diluted with 0.01 M HCl made by addition of glass-distilled, deionized and sterilized water to an appropriate concentration. The dilute ratioactive endogenous ligand should be used up in a day and should not be stocked.

3. *Formation of Adsorbates*

To confirm the formation of a radioactive adsorbate from [³H]Glu during incubation, chromatographic profiles of the incubation mixtures were compared on the Dowex column before and after incubation of fraction II (purified [³H]Glu) in the buffer at 30 °C for 60 min in the absence of synaptic membranes. The column was first eluted with water and then with HCl. When an incubation medium was applied to the column before incubation, a single peak of radioactivity was detected in the HCl eluate but not in the water eluate. In contrast, a peak of radioactivity was found in the water eluate in addition to that in the HCl eluate following the application of a medium after incubation at 30 °C (Yoneda and Ogita, 1989a).

This radioactive fraction eluted with water was collected and directly poured on a glass fibre filter in order to see whether or not the fraction is indeed adsorbed to the filters. An extremely high level of radioactivity was detected on the filter without rinsing, which gradually decreased in proportion to increasing times of rinsing. A substantial quantity of radioactivity was still retained on the filter after rinsing with the buffer twelve times under vacuum. This adsorption was not diminished by rinsing with buffers containing various acids at a concentration of 0.1 mM. These included pyroglutamic, citric, oxalic, malic, succinic, glutaric, adipic and α-ketoglutaric acids (Yoneda and Ogita, 1989a). Accordingly, there is no doubt that unidentified radioactive adsorbate is really formed from [³H]Glu during the incubation of purified [³H]Glu in the buffer at 30 °C for 60 min in the absence of brain synaptic membrane preparations.

4. Properties of Adsorbates

Reversibility

To begin with evaluation of the radioactive adsorbate, the effects of incubation time and temperature on the formation of adsorbate were examined in the absence of synaptic membranes. Incubation was performed at 2 °C or 30 °C for varying periods, and was terminated by filtration through a glass fibre filter. The radioactivity retained on the filter after rinsing increased linearly with incubation time up to 40 min at 30 °C, and reached a plateau 60 min after the initiation of incubation. A significant amount of this adsorbate was already formed even 1 min after incubation at 30 °C. The adsorption was not rapidly reduced by the addition of excess unlabelled Glu 60 min after the initiation of incubation at 30 °C, about 30% of the radioactivity being eliminated within 10 min. Reduction of the incubation temperature from 30 °C to 2 °C resulted in complete abolition of the formation of radioactive adsorbate. The data cited here indicate that the formation of radioactive adsorbate from [³H]Glu is entirely dependent on the incubation temperature and is an irreversible process.

Saturability

Formation of the adsorbate increased in proportion to increasing ligand concentrations in a range of 10–200 nM, and reached a steady state level at concentrations above 200 nM. Scatchard analysis of these data revealed that the displaceable adsorption consisted of a single component with an apparent dissociation constant of 73 ± 20 nM. Therefore, the formation of radioactive adsorbate is saturable with increasing concentrations of [³H]Glu.

Pharmacology

Subsequently, the effects of incubation in the presence of numerous acidic compounds analogous to Glu on the formation of radioactive adsorbate were examined (Table 2). Addition of L-Glu as well as L-Asp at a concentration of 0.1 mM completely abolished the formation of adsorbate, whereas their respective D isomers caused a relatively weak inhibition. Both L-cysteinesulphinic (CSA) and L-cysteic acids more potently inhibited the formation of adsorbate than did D-Glu. Among the other sulphur-containing amino acids tested, reduced glutathione was most effective in inhibiting the formation of adsorbate, with a potency similar to that of CSA, followed by L-homocysteic acid, cysthathionine, L-methionine, DL-homocysteine, taurine, L-cysteine and homotaurine in that order of potency. These results make it

Table 2 Effects of Glu analogues on the formation of radioactive adsorbate from
[³H]Glu

Addition (0.1 mM)	Adsorption (% control)	Addition (0.1 mM)	Adsorption (% control)
Control	100 ± 5.6		
Amino acids		Agonists and antagonists	
L-Glu	0	NMDA	96.3 ± 9.2
L-Asp	0.4 ± 0.2[a]	CPP	100.5 ± 5.2
D-Glu	18.7 ± 4.9[a]	MK-801	92.1 ± 10.6
D-Asp	47.0 ± 4.7[a]	PCP	53.2 ± 4.6[a]
L-CA	5.7 ± 0.6[a]		
L-CSA	9.2 ± 2.1[a]	QA	5.4 ± 1.5[a]
L-CysH	78.5 ± 3.2[a]	AMPA	58.4 ± 1.3[a]
L-HCA	19.6 ± 7.6[a]	KA	72.2 ± 5.8[a]
DL-HCysH	44.9 ± 12.7[a]		
L-Met	40.3 ± 6.2[a]	KYNA	95.0 ± 15.1
Tau	62.1 ± 10.3[a]	α-AAA	73.2 ± 12.3[a]
HTau	149.6 ± 37.9	GDEE	32.1 ± 10.1[a]
Aminophos-phonates			
DL-AP3	66.6 ± 4.1[a]	DL-AP4	28.2 ± 5.8[a]
DL-AP5	34.9 ± 4.7[a]	DL-AP6	24.5 ± 5.4[a]
DL-AP7	39.2 ± 5.9[a]		

[a] $P < 0.01$, compared with the control value obtained in the absence of any drug (6600 ± 370 dpm/assay).
Abbreviations: α-AAA, α-amino-adipic acid; L-CA, L-cysteic acid; L-CSA, L-cysteinesulphinic acid; L-CysH, L-cysteine; GDEE, L-glutamic acid diethylester; L-HCA, L-homocysteic acid; DL-HCysH, DL-homocysteine; HTau, hypotaurine; KYNA, kynurenic acid.
Purified [³H]Glu (fraction II) was incubated in the buffer containing various analogues indicated at a concentration of 0.1 mM at 30 °C for 60 min in the absence of brain synaptic membrane preparations. Each value was obtained in three different experiments performed in triplicate.

clear that the formation of adsorbate is a stereospecific and structure selective phenomenon.

Of three different agonists used for subclassification of the central excitatory amino acid receptors, QA most potently inhibited the formation of adsorbate, to an extent similar to that produced by L-cysteic acid. The agonist more specific to the QA-sensitive receptors than QA itself, DL-α-amino-3-hydroxy-5-methylisoxazole-4-propionic acid (AMPA), also induced a moderate inhibition at 0.1 mM. The other agonist, KA, induced a slightly less potent inhibition than did AMPA. In contrast, NMDA did not significantly affect the formation of adsorbate at 0.1 mM. Similarly, a competetitive antagonist, (±)-3-(2-carboxypiperazin-4-yl)propyl-1-phosphonic acid (CPP), as well as a non-competitive antagonist (+)-5-methyl-10,11-dihydro-5H-dibenzo[a,d]cyclohepten-5,10-imine (MK-

801), for the NMDA-sensitive receptors did not inhibit the formation of radioactive adsorbate from [³H]Glu at 0.1 mM. However, the other non-competitive NMDA antagonist, phencyclidine (PCP), induced a moderate inhibition similar to that induced by AMPA. A non-selective antagonist, L-glutamic acid diethylester (GDEE), rather potently inhibited the adsorption, while kynurenic acid did not significantly affect the formation of adsorbate.

Both DL-2-amino-4-phosphonobutyric (AP4) and DL-2-amino-6-phosphonohexanoic (AP6) acids potently inhibited the formation of adsorbate from [³H]Glu, among various aminophosphonic acids examined. Progressively lower potencies were found for DL-2-amino-5-phosphonovaleric (AP5), DL-2-amino-7-phosphonoheptanoic (AP7) and DL-2-amino-3-phosphonopropionic (AP3) acids. Consequently, most of the putative agonists and antagonists for the brain excitatory amino acid receptors, except NMDA and CPP, were effective as inhibitors of the formation of radioactive adsorbate from [³H]Glu, in addition to being active at the receptor sites. In other words, these positive compounds are obviously not specific to the excitatory amino acid receptors in the brain, in terms of having a relatively high affinity for the adsorbate formation system. Therefore, identification and characterization of the receptor subtype using these compounds ought to be carefully carried out as much as possible.

Biochemical Characteristics

The formation of adsorbate was markedly reduced by incubation with some chemical modifiers, such as N-bromosuccinimide, N-ethylmaleimide and p-chloromercuribenzoic acid, at 0.1 mM. Neither 5,5'-dithio-bis(2-nitrobenzoic acid) nor dithiothreitol inhibited the formation of adsorbate at a similar concentration. No significant alteration of the adsorption occurred following incubation in the presence of some inorganic ions known to potentiate [³H]Glu binding in brain synaptic membranes, including Cl^-, Cl^-/Ca^{2+} and Na^+ ions (Yoneda and Ogita, 1989a).

Enzymatic Treatment

The abovementioned findings all show that the displaceable adsorption is a structure-selective, stereospecific, temperature-dependent, non-reversible and saturable process which is sensitive to some SH-reactive agents. Therefore, an attempt was next made to determine whether protein constituents are responsible for the formation of adsorbate. Incubation was carried out in the presence of varying concentrations of several proteases, such as trypsin, chymotrypsin, papain and pronase E (Table 3). Neither trypsin nor chymo-

Table 3 Effects of proteases and phospholipases on the formation of radioactive adsorbate from [^{3}H]Glu

Addition	Adsorption (% control)	Addition	Adsorption (% control)
Control	100 ± 12		
Proteases (µg/ml)		Phospholipases (units/ml)	
Trypsin		Phospholipase A$_2$	
1	90 ± 2	0.01	103 ± 12
10	116 ± 39	0.1	127 ± 23
100	128 ± 16	1.0	119 ± 11
1000	118 ± 26	10	109 ± 27
Chymotrypsin		Phospholipase C	
1	126 ± 16	0.01	129 ± 20
10	132 ± 21	0.1	105 ± 10
100	120 ± 35	1.0	95 ± 30
1000	84 ± 18	10	12 ± 7^a
Papain		Phospholipase D	
1	128 ± 22	0.01	117 ± 10
10	117 ± 20	0.1	128 ± 35
100	62 ± 15^a	1.0	106 ± 17
1000	40 ± 14^a	10	101 ± 32
Pronase E			
1	122 ± 14	BSA	
10	82 ± 12	1 mg/ml	97 ± 8
100	53 ± 27		
1000	0		

[a] $P<0.05$, compared with the control value obtained in the absence of any added protein (6300 ± 870 dpm/assay).
Purified [^{3}H]Glu (fraction II) was incubated in the buffer containing varying concentrations of proteins indicated at 30 °C for 60 min in the absence of brain synaptic membranes. Values were obtained in four independent determinations performed in triplicate.
BSA, bovine serum albumin.

trypsin exerted a marked effect on the formation of adsorbate at a concentration range of 1–1000 µg/ml. However, both papain and pronase E significantly inhibited the formation in a concentration-dependent manner at a similar concentration range. Pronase E at a concentration of 1 mg/ml completely abolished the formation at radioactive adsorbate from [^{3}H]Glu. Similarly, phospholipase C at a concentration of 10 units/ml inhibited the formation by more than 80%, while the other phospholipases, including phospholipases A$_2$ and D, were ineffective in inhibiting the formation at the concentrations employed. These results imply that the displaceable adsorption may be attributed to the formation of radioactive adsorbate from [^{3}H]Glu by protein constituents with a relatively high affinity for Glu under lipophilic environments sensitive to phospholipase C during incubation.

5. Pitfalls in Incubation Buffer

Micro-organisms

Throughout these binding studies, 50 mM Tris-acetate buffer (pH 7.4) was freshly prepared each time before use by diluting 500 mM Tris-acetate buffer (pH 7.4) stored at 2 °C for various periods with glass-distilled, deionized and sterilized water. We noticed that the adsorption seemed to increase in proportion to the duration of storage of the original concentrated buffer. No significant displaceable adsorption occurred when the original buffer was freshly made, whereas the use of original concentrated buffer stored at 2 °C for 3 days resulted in a marked formation of radioactive adsorbate during the incubation. These findings strongly suggest that the original buffer may be contaminated with some micro-organisms present in the air during storage at 2 °C.

Settlement

To study such a possibility, an attempt was made to determine whether sterilization of the buffer completely abolishes the formation of radioactive adsorbate from [³H]Glu. The original buffer was stored at 2 °C for various periods, and diluted with glass-distilled, deionized and sterilized water immediately before each use on the day of experiments. Then the diluted buffer was used directly, or after sterilization by boiling at 100 °C for 30 min or by filtration through a nitrocellulose membrane filter with a pore size of 450 nm. The use of buffer before sterilization induced a marked displaceable adsorption in proportion to the duration of storage of the original buffer, in spite of diluting the original buffer with sterilized water. A displaceable adsorption of more than 5000 dpm/assay was detected on the filter after an extensive rinsing with the original buffer stored at 2 °C for 14 days. Consequently, this radioactivity would be calculated as a pseudospecific binding of [³H]Glu.

In contrast, boiling of the diluted buffer entirely eliminated the formation of adsorbate from [³H]Glu, even when the original buffer stored at 2 °C for 84 days was used. Similarly, no significant displaceable adsorption was detected so long as the diluted buffer was sterilized before each use by filtration through a nitrocellulose filter with a pore size of 450 nm. The use of incubation buffer diluted from the original concentrated buffer stored at 2 °C for 84 days after filtration did not cause any detectable adsorption. These results provide strong support for the proposal that the displaceable adsorption may be due to the formation of a radioactive adsorbate from [³H]Glu by micro-organisms evolved in the incubation buffer, such as bacteria and moulds, which have an ability to deaminate Glu. It thus appears that [³H]Glu binding may not only represent the specific binding of the neurotransmitter to its receptor sites, but also reflect the association of [³H]Glu with substrate-recognition sites of some microbial enzymes having a relatively high affinity for Glu, in addition to the artefactual adsorption of the radioactive product of [³H]Glu according to the experimental conditions employed. At any rate, the incubation buffer should be sterilized immediately before each use in order to run accurate and reproducible assays for [³H]Glu binding. These microbial artefacts may be operative in a temperature-dependent area of the apparent specific binding of miscellaneous neurotransmitters, hormones and autacoids.

6. Pitfalls in Membrane Preparations

Brain

In addition to the artefactual problems mentioned above, another methodo-logical pitfall is found with [³H]Glu binding assays using brain synaptic membrane preparations. As described in the introductory statements, the mammalian brain contains several neuronal constituents with an ability to associate with [³H]Glu. For example, [³H]Glu could associate with substrate-recognition sites of Glu transport systems in the brain, such as Na^+-dependent uptake, ATP-dependent vesicular accumulation and acidic amino acid exchange, in addition to binding to receptor sites. An association with substrate-recognition sites of membrane-bound enzymes with a relatively high affinity would also be responsible for the apparent binding of [³H]Glu in brain synaptic membranes. In fact, Cl^--dependent binding of [³H]Glu is shown to be associated with a temperature-dependent transport of Glu into resealed vesicular structures (Pin et al., 1984). Cystine is used to differentiate the specific binding of [³H]Glu from the sequestration in brain synaptic membrane preparations (Kessler et al., 1987).

As shown in Figure 2, [³H]Glu binding would be contaminated with the association with substrate-recognition sites of a membrane-bound enzyme with a considerable affinity for Glu. Brain synaptic membranes were incu-bated with [³H]Glu at 30 °C for 60 min in the presence of some inorganic ions known to potentiate the binding (Foster and Fagg, 1984). After terminating the incubation by centrifugation at $50\,000\,g$ for 30 min, the supernatant fractions were applied to a Dowex column. The column was first eluted with water and then with 0.5 M HCl. No significant radioactivity was eluted from the column with water following the application of an incubation mixture after the incubation in the absence of membrane preparations. As shown in Table 4, however, incubation in the presence of brain synaptic membranes resulted in a drastic increase in the radioactivity eluted with water from the column. Addition of 20 mM ammonium chloride markedly potentiated the binding at 30 °C without significantly affecting the radioactivity in the water eluate. Chloride ions at a similar concentration failed to enhance [³H]Glu binding at 2 °C. Further addition of 2.5 mM calcium acetate caused an

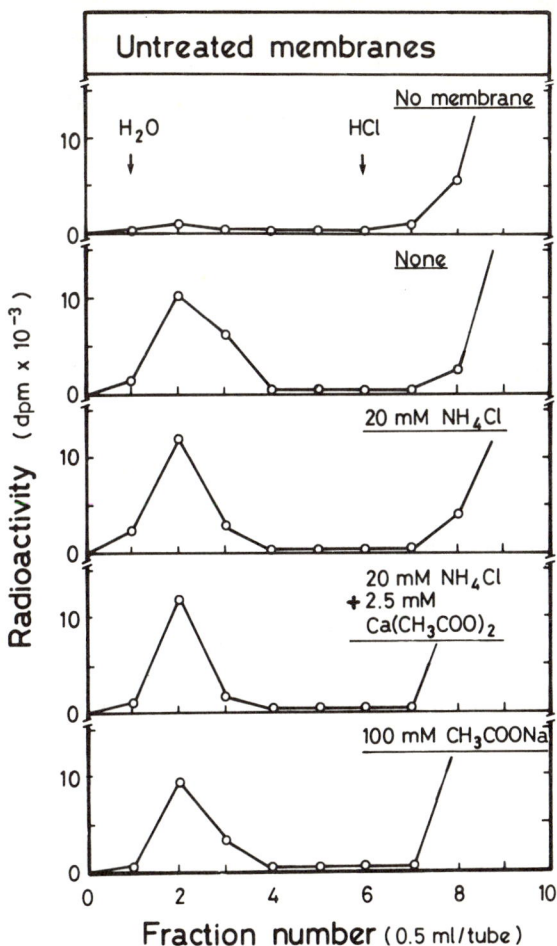

Figure 2 Elution profiles of incubation mixtures after incubation under different conditions. Untreated synaptic membrane preparations were incubated with 10 nM purified [³H]Glu in the sterilized buffer at 30 °C for 60 min in either the presence or absence of several inorganic ions indicated. After terminating the incubation by centrifuging at 50 000 g for 20 min, resultant pellets were superficially rinsed with the buffer twice and the radioactivity was measured. The supernatant fractions were individually applied to plastic columns packed with slurries of Dowex 50W × 8 resin (5 × 20 mm). The columns were eluted with water and then with 0.5 M HCl, and 0.5 ml fractions were successively collected to determine the radioactivity. Data shown are from a representative experiment which was repeated four times with similar results

additional potentiation of the binding in the presence of 20 mM ammonium chloride at 30 °C, the radioactive water eluate being unaltered. Addition of 100 mM sodium acetate did not alter the amount of radioactive water eluate, the binding being potentiated irrespective of the incubation temperature.

Table 4   Radioactivities in water eluate of Dowex column

Addition	Radioactivity in water eluate (dpm × 10⁻³/mg *protein*)	Binding (fmol/mg *protein*)
None	97 ± 7	74 ± 4
20 mM NH₄Cl	98 ± 6	184 ± 16
20 mM NH₄Cl + 2.5 mM Ca(CH₃COOH)₂	101 ± 4	269 ± 24
100 mM CH₃COONa	74 ± 2	260 ± 7

Brain synaptic membranes were incubated with purified [³H]Glu (fraction II) in the buffer containing several inorganic ions indicated at 30 °C for 60 min. This incubation was terminated by centrifugation at 50 000 g for 20 min, and resultant supernatants were applied to the Dowex column. The column was first eluted with water and then with HCl. The water eluate was collected and the radioactivity was measured by a liquid scintillation spectrometer. The resultant pellets were subjected to the determination of bound radioactivity after rinsing twice. Values were from four separate experiments performed in triplicate.

Similarly, a significant amount of the radioactive water eluate was formed during the incubation of [³H]Glu with brain synaptic membranes at 2 °C for 60 min in the absence of added ions (Ogita and Yoneda, 1988). From the data cited here, there is no doubt that [³H]Glu is metabolized into a radioactive water eluate of the Dowex column during incubation with brain synaptic membranes, irrespective of the incubation temperature. It is also suggested that the stimulatory ions may not potentiate the binding of [³H]Glu in brain synaptic membranes through enhancing the association with substrate-recognition sites of some membrane-bound enzymes.

Central Distribution

Table 5 shows regional variation of [³H]Glu bindings determined under different experimental conditions in the rat central nervous system. Homogenates of each central structure were treated or not treated with Triton X-100. In homogenate particulate preparations not treated with Triton X-100, [³H]Glu binding was enhanced by the addition of several inorganic ions, such as Cl^-, Cl^-/Ca^{2+} and Na^+ ions. The striatum exhibited the highest basal binding at 2 °C, with progressively lower bindings in the cerebral cortex, hypothalamus, midbrain, hippocampus, cerebellum, medulla pons and spinal cord, while the highest basal binding at 30 °C was found in the midbrain, followed by the hypothalamus, medulla pons, cerebellum, striatum, spinal cord, cerebral cortex and hippocampus. Sodium-dependent binding was highest in the cerebral cortex at 2 °C, accompanied by striatum, hippocampus, midbrain, hypothalamus, spinal cord, medulla pons and cerebellum in a decreasing order of binding. Elevation of incubation temperature from 2 °C to 30 °C resulted in a more than threefold reduction of the Na^+-dependent

Table 5 Regional variation of [³H]Glu bindings determined under different conditions in rat brain

	[³H]*Glu binding (fmol/mg protein)*						
	Basal		Na⁺-*dependent*		Cl⁻-*dependent*	Ca²⁺-*stimulated*	NMDA-*sensitive*
Region	2 °C (10)	30 °C (10)	2 °C (10)	30 °C (10)	(10)	30 °C (10)	2 °C (6)
CC	49.6 ± 6.9	49.8 ± 8.3	1400 ± 124	397 ± 20	144 ± 12	88 ± 9	372 ± 18
HPC	38.2 ± 9.6	47.0 ± 6.0	1082 ± 87	266 ± 16	129 ± 10	97 ± 14	392 ± 29
ST	61.3 ± 9.9	70.3 ± 9.6	1089 ± 132	343 ± 31	127 ± 11	97 ± 20	242 ± 30
HT	47.7 ± 9.2	86.6 ± 9.3	351 ± 68	281 ± 36	349 ± 34	192 ± 29	90 ± 11
MB	40.6 ± 5.4	98.6 ± 9.4	527 ± 50	166 ± 17	255 ± 19	181 ± 40	63 ± 16
MP	27.1 ± 4.5	85.6 ± 9.1	87 ± 14	121 ± 11	223 ± 18	126 ± 23	26 ± 5
CB	35.6 ± 5.8	81.2 ± 9.2	75 ± 13	39 ± 11	80 ± 7	33 ± 10	36 ± 7
SC	7.0 ± 2.6	58.9 ± 7.6	176 ± 29	181 ± 17	277 ± 29	66 ± 16	9 ± 4

Each brain region was dissected according to the procedures described by Glowinski and Iversen (1966), and homogenized in 40 vol. glass-distilled, deionized and sterilized water. The homogenates were centrifuged at 50 000 *g* for 20 min and resultant pellets were washed three times by the suspension and subsequent centrifugation. The final pellets were suspended in 0.32 M sucrose and the suspensions were frozen at −80 °C until use. On the day of experiments, the frozen suspensions were thawed at room temperature and the thawed suspensions were washed twice to determine the basal, Na⁺-dependent, Cl⁻-dependent and Ca²⁺-stimulated bindings. An aliquot of these membranes was incubated with 10 nM purified [³H]Glu at 2 °C or 30 °C for 60 min in either the presence or the absence of several inorganic ions. Sodium-dependent binding was calculated from the difference in radioactivity found in the absence and in the presence of 100 mM sodium acetate. Chloride-dependent binding was estimated by subtracting the basal binding from the binding found in the presence of 20 mM ammonium chloride. Calcium-stimulated binding was obtained from the difference between radioactivity found in the presence of 20 mM ammonium chloride alone and that found in the presence of 20 mM ammonium chloride plus 2.5 mM calcium acetate. NMDA-sensitive [³H]Glu binding was determined by incubating 10 nM purified [³H]Glu for 10 min at 2 °C with membranous preparations after treatment with a low concentration of Triton X-100, as described previously (Yoneda *et al.*, 1989). Values were obtained in various numbers of separate experiments indicated in the parentheses.
Abbreviations: CB, cerebellum; CC, cerebral cortex; HPC, hippocampus; HT, hypothalamus; MB, midbrain; MP, medulla pons; SC, spinal cord; ST, striatum.

binding in the cerebral cortex, with a concomitant slight enhancement of that in the medulla pons and spinal cord. The hypothalamus had the highest Cl⁻-dependent as well as Ca²⁺-stimulated binding among various central structures. Progressively lower Cl⁻-dependent bindings were found for the spinal cord, midbrain, medulla pons, cerebral cortex, hippocampus, striatum and cerebellum in order of decreasing activity, whereas the spinal cord possessed a relatively low Ca²⁺-stimulated binding. These results obviously indicate that no clear correlation was observed among distribution profiles of [³H]Glu bindings enhanced by inorganic ions in membranous preparations of the central structures.

In contrast to those preparations not treated with a detergent, the latter stimulatory ions did not enhance [³H]Glu binding in membranous preparations treated with Triton X-100, irrespective of the incubation temperature. In these Triton-treated membranes, both NMDA and CPP markedly displaced [³H]Glu binding in a concentration-dependent manner, AMPA and KA being inactive (Yoneda *et al.*, 1989). The hippocampus contained the highest NMDA-sensitive binding among various central structures examined.

Progressively lower NMDA-sensitive bindings were found for the cerebral
cortex, striatum, hypothalamus, midbrain, cerebellum, medulla pons and
spinal cord, when membranous preparations of each structure were treated
with a low concentration of Triton X-100 (Table 5). These findings make it
possible to propose that some of the abovementioned bindings in membranous preparations not treated with a detergent may be derived from an
artefactual association of the radioactive endogenous ligand with substrate-
recognition sites of membrane-bound constituents, such as enzymes, Na^+-
dependent uptake, ATP-dependent vesicular accumulation or acidic amino
acid exchange, rather than with agonist-recognition sites of central excitatory
amino acid receptors.

Retina

Glu has been also proposed to play a neurotransmitter role in the vertebrate
retina. Glu is released from photoreceptor cells (Dowling and Ripps, 1973;
Cervetto and Piccolino, 1974; Brandon and Lam, 1983; Slaughter and Miller,
1985), and retinal bipolar cells have synapses activated by excitatory amino
acids such as L-Glu and L-Asp (Slaughter and Miller, 1983; Bolz et al., 1984).
In accord with these physiological studies, several mammalian retinal membrane preparations exhibited a [^{3}H]Glu binding with a relatively high affinity
similar to that found in brain synaptic membranes. These included retinas of
the chick (Lopez-Colome, 1981; Lopez-Colome and Somohano, 1984, 1987),
calf (Hockel and Muller, 1982; Mitchell and Redburn, 1982) and rat (Yoneda
et al., 1987). These previous findings are all suggestive of the validity of
[^{3}H]Glu binding as a biochemical measure for synaptic receptors of the
excitatory amino acids in the retina.

However, our recent results raised the possibility that retinal [^{3}H]Glu
binding may be at least in part attributable to the association of [^{3}H]Glu with
substrate-recognition sites of some unidentified membrane-bound enzyme
with a considerable affinity for the putative neurotransmitter. The retinal
binding was temperature-dependent, and sensitive to displacement by QA
but not to that by NMDA and KA (Yoneda et al., 1987). Treatment of retinal
membrane preparations with Nonidet P-40 resulted in a significant solubilization of [^{3}H]Glu binding, which was a protein-dependent, temperature-
dependent, stereospecific, structure-selective, reversible and saturable process with a relatively high affinity for Glu (K_d: 0.17 ± 0.04 μM at 2 °C;
0.25 ± 0.03 μM at 30 °C). One agonist for the excitatory amino acid receptor
QA was effective as an inhibitor of the solubilized binding in a concentration-
dependent manner at concentrations above 1 μM, the other two different
agonists such as NMDA and KA being inactive as inhibitors. The solubilized
binding was not sensitive to an agonist more specific to the QA-sensitive
receptors than QA itself, AMPA (Table 6). However, cation exchange
chromatography of the incubation media revealed that unidentified radioac-

tive water eluate was indeed formed from [³H]Glu in a temperature-dependent manner during incubation (Yoneda and Ogita, 1989b). This radioactive metabolite was also formed during the incubation of solubilized preparations, even at 2 °C. Therefore, the solubilized binding seems to be at least in part derived from the association of [³H]Glu with substrate-recognition sites of some unidentified membrane-bound enzyme with a relatively high sensitivity to QA. It thus appears that QA sensitivity is not supporting evidence for the possible involvement of the QA-sensitive subclass of the central excitatory amino acid receptors in any central events.

Pituitary

In addition to the central structures described above, several peripheral excitable tissues are shown to contain a significant binding of [³H]Glu. In rat pituitary, neurohypophysis had a binding of [³H]Glu higher than that found in adenohypophysis by a factor of more than 2 (Yoneda and Ogita, 1986a). The binding was sensitive to displacement by QA but not to displacement by NMDA and KA, as seen with the retinal binding. The pituitary binding was solubilized by treating the membranous preparations with Nonidet P-40

Table 6 Effects of numerous putative agonists and antagonists on [³H]Glu binding solubilized from retina, pituitary and adrenal

Addition (0.1 mM)	[³H]Glu binding (% of control)		
	Retina	Pituitary	Adrenal
Control	100.0 ± 8.5	100.0 ± 12.7	100.0 ± 10.3
QA (Sigma)	33.7 ± 9.7[a]	33.1 ± 1.2[a]	6.1 ± 0.5[a]
QA (CRB)	35.4 ± 1.1[a]	25.1 ± 7.2[a]	34.2 ± 4.6[a]
AMPA	109.8 ± 11.5	86.6 ± 12.9	93.7 ± 5.6
Willardiine	107.4 ± 5.3	81.2 ± 3.6	98.8 ± 5.1
NMDA	101.3 ± 8.9	105.6 ± 9.3	102.1 ± 3.1
CPP	100.7 ± 6.7	92.8 ± 17.9	98.1 ± 2.9
PCP	104.9 ± 8.7	90.8 ± 12.1	96.5 ± 1.7
MK-801	114.6 ± 8.1	102.3 ± 5.9	107.0 ± 3.6
KA	102.6 ± 7.8	101.1 ± 9.0	103.0 ± 5.1
α-AAA	94.6 ± 6.6	105.0 ± 7.0	100.6 ± 7.8
γ-DGG	108.8 ± 8.6	94.8 ± 2.9	93.4 ± 3.5

[a] $P < 0.01$, compared with each control value.
Suspensions of each neuronal tissue were treated with 1% Nonidet P-40 in the buffer containing 0.1 mM phenylmethylsulphonyl fluoride, 0.02% bacitracin and 0.1 mM EDTA after repeating the washing procedures four times, and then centrifuged at 100 000 g for 60 min. The resultant supernatants were dialysed against the buffer for 14 h and these dialysis procedures were repeated three times. An aliquot of the individual supernatants was incubated with purified [³H]Glu at 30 °C for 60 min in either the presence or the absence of numerous compounds indicated. Values were from four independent determinations.

(Yoneda and Ogita, 1989c). The solubilized binding exhibited a protein-dependency, temperature-dependency, stereospecificity, reversibility, saturability and relatively high affinity (K_d: 0.31 ± 0.07 μM at 2 °C; 0.34 ± 0.07 μM at 30 °C). The solubilized binding was also sensitive to QA but insensitive to NMDA, KA and AMPA (Table 6). Among various putative agonists and antagonists, QA was the only compound which inhibited the solubilized binding. Cation exchange chromatography of the incubation media again revealed that some unidentified radioactive metabolite was in fact formed from [³H]Glu during the incubation of pituitary solubilized preparations, even at 2 °C for 60 min. The possibility that the pituitary binding may originate in a QA-sensitive and membrane-bound enzyme with a considerable affinity for Glu, rather than the QA-sensitive synaptic receptors for Glu, is strongly suggested. Sensitivity to QA is evidently not a useful criterion for the possible involvement of QA-sensitive receptors in the central incidents examined.

Adrenal

QA-sensitive [³H]Glu binding was also detected in the rat adrenal, and the binding was more than four times greater in the medullary part than in the cortical part (Yoneda and Ogita, 1986b). The binding was inhibited by sodium ions in a temperature-dependent manner (Yoneda and Ogita, 1987b). Treatment of adrenal membranous preparations with Nonidet P-40 resulted in a significant solubilization of temperature-dependent, stereospecific, structure-selective, reversible and saturable binding of [³H]Glu (Yoneda and Ogita, 1987c). Both QA and GDEE were active in inhibiting the solubilized binding, the other agonists, NMDA and KA, being ineffective. Recrystallized QA also inhibited the solubilized binding, while the more specific agonist AMPA had no significant effect (Table 6). The solubilized binding was sensitive to pronases, phospholipase C and β-galactosidase (Yoneda and Ogita, 1989d). As seen with the other QA-sensitive bindings described above, some unidentified radioactive metabolite was formed from [³H]Glu during the incubation of the adrenal solubilized preparations, even at 2 °C (Yoneda and Ogita, 1989d). Accordingly, the sensitivity to QA does not mean a possible QA contribution of the QA-sensitive subclass of excitatory amino acid receptors to the [³H]Glu binding observed. Several independent lines of evidence have demonstrated that this compound is not a specific agonist for the QA-sensitive subclass of the brain excitatory amino acid receptors (Honore et al., 1982; Robinson et al., 1986, 1987).

Triton X-100 Treatment

To avoid possible contribution of the association of the radioactive endogenous ligand with substrate-recognition sites of some membrane-bound enzymes, membranous preparations should be treated with a low concentration of a detergent prior to the determination of specific binding. For example, synaptic membranes were obtained from the rat brain and extensively washed with buffer by suspension and subsequent centrifugation. Then membranes were treated with 0.08% Triton X-100 at an approximate protein concentration of 0.32 mg/ml at 2 °C for 10 min with gentle stirring (Ogita and Yoneda, 1988). This treatment was terminated by centrifuging at 50 000 g for 20 min, and the pellets thus obtained were washed again to remove excess detergent. Under these conditions, no radioactive metabolite was formed from [³H]Glu during the incubation so long as a low incubation temperature was employed. Elevation of the incubation temperature resulted in a marked formation of radioactive metabolite of [³H]Glu during the incubation with synaptic membranes treated with Triton X-100 (Ogita and Yoneda, 1988). Consequently, [³H]Glu binding assay ought to be carried out in the sterilized buffer at a low temperature for a short period, using an incubation of purified [³H]Glu with brain synaptic membranes treated with a low concentration of Triton X-100, in order to predominantly detect the receptor sites. Otherwise, several independent methodological artefacts described above could obscure the biochemical studies on radioligand labelling of excitatory amino acid receptors in the brain.

7. Pitfalls in Separation Assay

Filtration?

Current thinking on the separation method of binding assays is that a centrifugation method but not a filtration method is useful for accurate and reproducible detection of a simple binding process of a radioligand with a relatively low affinity ($K_d > 100$ nM) to the specific binding sites. However, the centrifugation method is quite time-consuming and troublesome when a large number of samples have to be handled, as compared with the filtration method. In addition, the fact that termination of assay by centrifugation often takes much more time than termination of assay by filtration makes it difficult to accurately analyse kinetics of the binding, such as initial association and dissociation. Therefore, it is evidently beneficial to determine [³H]Glu binding to the specific receptor sites by a filtration method, in addition to a centrifugation method, for the development and introduction of novel neuroactive drugs acting at the latter sites.

Rinsing Times

In order to evaluate the possible rapid dissociation of a ligand with a relatively

Table 7   Effect of rinsing of filters on [³H]Glu binding in brain synaptic membranes

Rinsing times	Total	Non-specific	Specific	
		(dpm/mg *protein*)		Specific/Total
Untreated membranes				
0	66 104 ± 3 639	63 160 ± 1 762	2 944 ± 1 903	4.0 ± 2.6
1	21 789 ± 1 254	17 384 ± 867	4 405 ± 389	20.1 ± 0.6
2	9 589 ± 392	6 600 ± 220	2 989 ± 484	30.8 ± 3.9
3	7 679 ± 172	5 689 ± 221	1 989 ± 124	26.0 ± 1.7
4	7 200 ± 312	4 040 ± 200	3 160 ± 131	43.9 ± 0.8
5	6 875 ± 829	4 154 ± 174	2 721 ± 996	35.9 ± 10.5
7	5 704 ± 158	3 400 ± 189	2 304 ± 342	40.0 ± 4.8
10	5 019 ± 74	2975 ± 66	2 044 ± 130	40.6 ± 2.1
Triton-treated membranes				
0	120 175 ± 2 645	97 116 ± 4 666	23 059 ± 7 053	18.8 ± 5.6
1	50 740 ± 3 205	26 412 ± 1 422	24 328 ± 4 288	47.0 ± 5.2
2	31 398 ± 178	6 879 ± 283	24 520 ± 300	78.1 ± 0.9
3	28 932 ± 1 102	5 667 ± 421	23 266 ± 826	80.5 ± 1.0
4	26 689 ± 566	4 003 ± 230	22 686 ± 717	85.0 ± 1.1
5	25 328 ± 419	3 689 ± 290	21 638 ± 522	85.4 ± 1.2
7	23 997 ± 590	2 831 ± 28	21 167 ± 611	88.2 ± 0.4
10	22 757 ± 192	2 480 ± 130	20 277 ± 323	89.1 ± 0.7

Thawed synaptic membrane suspensions were washed twice by repeating the centrifugation and suspension to obtain 'untreated membranes'. An aliquot of thawed membranes was treated with 0.08% Triton X-100 at an approximate protein concentration of 0.32 mg/ml at 2 °C for 10 min with gentle stirring. This treatment was terminated by the centrifugation at 50 000 *g* for 20 min and resultant pellets were resuspended in the buffer. The suspensions were washed once more to obtain 'Triton-membranes' (Ogita and Yoneda, 1988). These membrane preparations were incubated with 10 nM purified [³H]Glu in the sterilized buffer at 2 °C for 10 min. Incubation was terminated by the addition of 3 ml ice-cold buffer (2 °C) and subsequent filtration, as described previously (Ogita and Yoneda, 1988). After rinsing the filter with chilled buffer (2 °C), various times indicated, radioactivity retained on the filter was measured by a liquid scintillation spectrometer using Triton–toluene scintillant. Values were obtained in three different experiments.

low affinity during the separation of bound ligand from free ligand by a filtration method, an attempt was made to determine whether extensive rinsing of filters with cold buffer (2 °C) affects the specific binding.

When brain synaptic membranes not treated with a detergent (untreated membranes) were used as membranous preparations, no significant difference was detected between the total and the non-specific bindings obtained in filters without any rinsing (Table 7). Increasing number of times of rinsing decreased both the total and the non-specific bindings in untreated membranes up to 10 times, while the ratio between specific binding and total binding increased in proportion to increasing number of times of rinsing up to four times. However, further rinsing of filters did not markedly affect the ratio obtained in filters rinsed with cold buffer four times.

In contrast, the use of Triton-treated membranes resulted in a drastic potentiation of total binding of [³H]Glu without significantly altering the non-specific binding. Abolition of the rinsing led to a slight difference between the total and the non-specific bindings. Both the total and the non-specific binding decreased with increasing times of rinsing up to 10 times as seen with untreated membranes, whereas the use of Triton-treated membranes doubled the ratio between specific and total binding obtained in untreated membranes. The ratio was fairly constant in filters rinsed with cold buffer more than four times, in contrast to the sudden elevation of the ratio in filters rinsed less than four times. Therefore, it is evident that the radioactive ligand is not dissociated to a significant extent from its specific binding sites during the rinsing of filters in spite of a relatively low affinity, even when determined by a filtration method. Similar retention of the bound ligand is seen with strychnine-insensitive [³H]glycine (Gly) binding, which has a K_d of 202 ± 53 nM (Ogita *et al.*, 1989; Yoneda *et al.*, 1990).

Temperature of Rinsing Buffer

To demonstrate the accuracy of a filtration method for the termination of binding assay, the effect of temperature of rinsing buffer was examined. The routine incubation was carried out at 2 °C, using brain synaptic membranes treated or not treated with Triton X-100. After terminating the incubation by the addition of buffers at different temperatures and subsequent filtration, the filters were rinsed four times with buffers at various temperatures. As shown in Table 8, both total and non-specific bindings decreased in proportion to

Table 8   Effect of temperature of rinsing buffer on [³H]Glu binding

Temperature (°C)	Total	Non-specific	Specific	Specific/Total
		(dpm/mg *protein*)		
Untreated membranes				
2	6751 ± 119	4088 ± 325	2663 ± 440	39.2 ± 5.7
5	6467 ± 265	4675 ± 97	1791 ± 283	27.3 ± 3.5
10	5837 ± 107	4265 ± 314	1572 ± 396	26.7 ± 6.5
15	5346 ± 272	5047 ± 11	298 ± 266	4.9 ± 4.4
20	4132 ± 152	3612 ± 51	519 ± 125	12.3 ± 2.7
30	3416 ± 212	3302 ± 251	114 ± 167	3.2 ± 5.1
Triton-treated membranes				
2	25989 ± 377	4650 ± 199	21339 ± 267	82.1 ± 0.6
5	22393 ± 770	4263 ± 83	18130 ± 794	80.9 ± 0.8
10	22975 ± 608	3825 ± 160	19150 ± 767	83.3 ± 1.1
15	18955 ± 585	4500 ± 396	14455 ± 954	76.0 ± 2.7
20	17099 ± 559	4333 ± 327	12766 ± 644	74.6 ± 2.1
30	11856 ± 232	3910 ± 326	7946 ± 556	66.8 ± 3.4

An aliquot of untreated or Triton-treated membranes was incubated with 10 nM purified [³H]Glu in the sterilized buffer at 2 °C for 10 min. Incubation was terminated by the addition of buffer at different temperatures indicated and subsequent filtration through a Whatman GF/B glass fibre filter as described in the legend to Table 7. The filter was rinsed four times with the buffer at various temperatures indicated, and radioactivity retained on the filter after rinsing was measured. Values were from three independent experiments.

increasing temperatures of rinsing buffer, independently of membrane preparations used, which resulted in a proportional decrease in the specific binding. The ratio between specific and total binding also decreased with the elevation of temperature of rinsing buffer up to 15 °C, while further elevation almost eliminated the specific binding in untreated membranes. In contrast, the specific binding was fairly stable in Triton-treated membranes at a rinsing temperature below 10 °C. Rinsing of filters with buffer at 30 °C still retained on the filters more than 60% of the ligand bound to its specific binding sites in Triton-treated membranes. Accordingly, Triton-treated membranes are undoubtedly superior to untreated membranes in terms of the strong retention of the bound ligand when determined by a filtration method. In other words, dissociation of the bound ligand occurs during the rinsing of filters in untreated membranes to a more significant extent than in Triton-treated membranes. The Triton treatment would be crucial to the establishment of a rapid, accurate and reproducible filtration assay method for studying the specific binding of excitatory amino acids to the receptor sites.

8.   *Future Trends*

Agonist Binding

The abovementioned correction of the experimental conditions provides us with accurate and reproducible assay methods for detecting the specific binding of an agonist to the receptor sites. Most radioligand binding studies on the NMDA-sensitive receptors have been carried out using radiolabelled antagonists, such as [³H]AP5 (Olverman *et al.*, 1984), [³H]AP7 (Ferkany and Coyle, 1983), [³H]CPP (Olverman *et al.*, 1986; Murphy *et al.*, 1987; Ogita and Yoneda, 1990) and [³H]*cis*-4-phosphonomethyl-2-piperidine carboxylic acid (CGS 19755) (Murphy *et al.*, 1988), with a few exceptions (Fagg and Matus, 1984; Monahan and Michel, 1987; Ogita and Yoneda, 1988). Overcoming these methodological pitfalls makes it easy to compare the properties of recognition sites for agonists and antagonists within the NMDA receptor complex in the brain.

The NMDA-sensitive subclass is proposed to form a receptor ion channel complex consisting of at least three distinctly different domains: (1) NMDA recognition site, (2) ion channel site and (3) strychnine-insensitive Gly recognition site (Gly_B site) (Ogita *et al.*, 1989) (for reviews, see Robinson and Coyle, 1987; Yoneda *et al.*, 1988). Moreover, recent biochemical binding studies have raised the possibility that several endogenous polyamines may participate in physiological and/or pathophysiological responses mediated by the NMDA-sensitive subclass through a novel fourth site within the complex in rodent brain (Ransom and Stec, 1988; Yoneda and Ogita, 1990). On the other hand, L-Glu surprisingly has a higher affinity for the NMDA-sensitive subclass than for the other two subclasses, judging from the data cited in literatures (Hampson *et al.*, 1987; Olsen *et al.*, 1987; Errami and Nieoullon, 1988; Henley and Barnard, 1989). Accordingly, accurate and reproducible detection of [³H]Glu binding provides a useful tool for evaluating biochemical and pharmacological profiles of the NMDA-recognition site on the complex. For instance, [³H]Glu binding is valuable in biochemical elucidation of the proposal that the NMDA-sensitive subclass is anatomically classified into two different subpopulations such as agonist-preferring and antagonist-preferring forms (Monaghan *et al.*, 1988). Indeed, NMDA agonists exhibit a higher affinity for [³H]Glu binding than for [³H]CPP binding under the correct experimental conditions, and vice versa (Ogita and Yoneda, 1990). Furthermore, possible conversion between these two subpopulations could be analysed by the rapid filtration method for [³H]CPP as well as [³H]Glu binding. Evaluation of the functional role of GTP-binding proteins in the NMDA-mediated responses will not be possible until binding assays using agonists are established independently of the termination method. Purification of the NMDA receptor complex should be accomplished using [³H]Glu binding as one of several biochemical measures, in order to see whether the NMDA recognition site is a membranous constituent distinctly different from the other molecules, including ion channel and Gly_B site, within the complex.

In this way, liquidation of numerous methodological pitfalls in [³H]Glu binding assays is beneficial not only for the development and introduction of novel drugs acting at the excitatory amino acid receptors, but also for the progress of physiological as well as biochemical studies on the receptors.

Re-evaluation of 'Temperature-dependent Binding'

Since substantial numbers of radioreceptor bindings using endogenous ligands occur in a temperature-dependent manner, it is conceivable that some of these temperature-dependent bindings may give rise to methodological pitfalls in their binding assays, as shown here. Microbial contamination would be responsible for the temperature-dependent association of a radiolabelled endogenous ligand in the absence of added receptor preparations. The temperature-dependent portion of the apparent specific binding of an endogenous ligand could be at least in part derived from the association with substrate-recognition sites of some membrane-bound components, such as enzymes and transport carriers, in brain synaptic membrane preparations. Putative agonists and antagonists may have a relatively high affinity for the substrate-recognition sites of these membranous constituents other than receptors. Elucidation of a temperature-dependent binding of a radiolabelled endogenous ligand might need to be started all over again, taking into consideration numerous methodological pitfalls described in this chapter. A receptor binding assay is easily performed in any laboratory, and it should be carefully carried out as often as possible.

9. Summary

[³H]Glutamate has been widely used as a radioligand to label sites responsible for mediating the excitatory amino acid neurotransmission in the brain. Indeed, Na^+-dependent and Na^+-independent bindings of [³H]Glu were detected in brain synaptic membrane preparations. However, binding assays of [³H]Glu often involve several methodological pitfalls which result in a serious misunderstanding of the findings. For example, commercially obtained [³H]Glu contained less than 2% of some radioactive contaminant which was adsorbed to glass fibre filters routinely used for the binding assays, independently of a commercial source. This adsorption was not displaced by Glu and was greatly increased by the pretreatment of filters with polyethyleneimine used for the purpose of reducing the non-specific binding. Furthermore, some unidentified micro-organisms were evolved in the incubation buffer during storage, even at 2 °C. The radioactive endogenous ligand associated with substrate-recognition sites of these microbial membrane-bound enzymes with a relatively high affinity for Glu and was metabolized into some unidentified radioactive adsorbate to glass fibre filters during incubation in a temperature-dependent manner. This enzymatic formation of radioactive adsorbate from [³H]Glu was significantly inhibited by most putative agonists and antagonists for the brain excitatory amino acid receptors, except N-methyl-D-aspartate (NMDA) and (±)-3-(2-carboxypiperazin-4-yl)propyl-1-phosphonate (CPP). Therefore, temperature-dependent bindings of [³H]Glu may be at least in part attributable to the association with substrate-recognition sites of microbial enzymes contaminated in the incubation buffer. In addition, some radioactive metabolite was indeed formed during the incubation of purified [³H]Glu, even at 2 °C with brain synaptic membrane preparations not treated with a detergent. Treatment of brain synaptic membranes with a low concentration of Triton X-100 resulted in a drastic disclosure of [³H]Glu binding sensitive to displacement by both NMDA and CPP, with a concomitant abolition of the formation of radioactive metabolite of [³H]Glu. Triton-treated membranes are also superior to untreated membranes in terms of freedom from a rapid dissociation of the bound ligand during an extensive rinsing of filters when determined by a filtration method. There is no doubt, from the data cited in this chapter, that the filtration method is also quite useful for predominantly detecting the binding of [³H]Glu to its specific receptor sites, so long as the experimental conditions are carefully controlled in details.

References

Bannai, S. (1986). Exchange of cystine and glutamate across plasma membrane of human fibroblasts. *J. Biol. Chem.*, **261**, 2256–2263

Bolz, J., Wassle, H. and Thier, P. (1984). Pharmacological modulation of ON and OFF ganglion cells in the cat retina. *Neuroscience*, **12**, 875–885

Brandon, C. and Lam, D. M. K. (1983). L-Glutamic acid: a neurotransmitter candidate for cone photoreceptors in human and rat retinas. *Proc. Natl Acad. Sci. USA*, **80**, 5117–5121

Bruns, R. F., Lawson-Wendling, K. and Pugsley, T. A. (1983). A rapid filtration assay for soluble receptors using polyethyleneimine-treated filters. *Anal. Biochem.*, **132**, 74–81

Cervetto, L. and Piccolino, M. (1974). Synaptic transmission between photoreceptors and horizontal cells in the turtle retina. *Science, N.Y.*, **183**, 417–419

Curtis, D. R. and Johnston, G. A. R. (1974). Amino acid transmitters in the mammalian central nervous system. *Ergeb. Physiol.*, **69**, 94–188

Dowling, J. E. and Ripps, H. (1973). Effect of magnesium on horizontal cell activity in the skate retina. *Nature*, **242**, 101–103

Errami, M. and Nieoullon, A. (1988). α-[³H]Hydroxy-5-methyl-4-isoxazolepropionic acid binding to rat striatal membranes: Effects of selective brain lesions. *J. Neurochem.*, **51**, 579–586

Fagg, G. E. and Matus, A. (1984). Selective association of N-methyl aspartate and quisqualate types of L-glutamate receptor with brain postsynaptic densities. *Proc. Natl Acad. Sci. USA*, **81**, 6876–6880

Ferkany, J. M. and Coyle, J. T. (1983). Specific binding of [³H](±)-2-amino-7-phosphonoheptanoic acid to rat brain membranes *in vitro*. *Life Sci.*, **33**, 1295–1305

Fonnum, F. (1984). Glutamate: a neurotransmitter in mammalian brain. *J. Neurochem.*, **42**, 1–11

Foster, A. C. and Fagg, G. E. (1984). Acidic amino acid binding sites in mammalian neuronal membranes: their characteristics and relationships to synaptic receptors. *Brain Res. Rev.*, **7**, 103–164

Foster, A. C. and Fagg, G. E. (1987). Comparison of L-[³H]glutamate, D-[³H]aspartate, DL-[³H]AP5 and [³H]NMDA as ligands for NMDA receptors in crude postsynaptic densities from rat brain. *Eur. J. Pharmacol.*, **133**, 291–300

Glowinski, J. and Iversen, L. L. (1966). Regional studies of catecholamines in the rat brain. I. The disposition of [³H]norepinephrine, [³H]dopamine and [³H]DOPA in various regions of the brain. *J. Neurochem.*, **13**, 655–669

Hampson, D. R., Huie, D. and Wenthold, R. J. (1987). Solubilization of kainic acid binding sites from rat brain. *J. Neurochem.*, **49**, 1209–1215

Henley, J. M. and Barnard, E. A. (1989). Kainate receptors in *Xenopus* central nervous system: Solubilisation with n-octyl-β-D-glucopyranoside. *J. Neurochem.*, **52**, 31–37

Hockel, S. H. J. and Muller, W. E. (1982). L-Glutamate receptor binding in bovine retina. *Exp. Eye Res.*, **35**, 55–60

Honore, T., Lauridsen, J. and Krogsgaard-Larsen, P. (1982). The binding of [³H]AMPA, a structural analogue of glutamic acid, to rat brain membranes. *J. Neurochem.*, **38**, 173–178

Ito, M., Periyasamy, S. and Chiu, T. H. (1986). Displaceable binding of [³H]L-glutamic acid to non-receptor materials. *Life Sci.*, **38**, 1089–1096

Kessler, M., Baudry, M. and Lynch, G. (1987). Use of cystine to distinguish glutamate binding from glutamate sequestration. *Neurosci. Lett.*, **81**, 221–226

Lopez-Colome, A. M. (1981). High-affinity binding of L-glutamate to chick retinal membranes. *Neurochem. Res.*, **6**, 1019–1033

Lopez-Colome, A. M. and Somohano, F. (1984). Localization of L-glutamate and L-aspartate synaptic receptors in chick retinal neurons. *Brain Res.*, **298**, 159–162

Lopez-Colome, A. M. and Somohano, F. (1987). Characterization of quisqualate-type L-glutamate receptors in the retina. *Brain Res.*, **414**, 99–108

Mitchell, C. K. and Redburn, D. A. (1982). 2-Amino-4-phosphonobutyric acid and N-methyl-D-aspartate differentiate between ³H-glutamate and ³H-aspartate binding sites in bovine retina. *Neurosci. Lett.*, **28**, 241–246

Monaghan, D. T., Olverman, H. J., Nguyen, L., Watkins, J. C. and Cotman, C. W. (1988). Two classes of N-methyl-D-aspartate recognition sites: Differential distribution and differential regulation by glycine. *Proc. Natl Acad. Sci. USA*, **85**, 9836–9840

Monahan, J. B. and Michel, J. (1987). Identification and characterization of an N-methyl-D-aspartate-specific L-[³H]glutamate recognition site in synaptic plasma membranes. *J. Neurochem.*, **48**, 1699–1708

Murphy, D. E., Hutchinson, A. J., Hurt, S. D., Williams, M. and Sills, M. A. (1988). Characterization of the binding of [³H]-CGS 19755: a novel N-methyl-D-aspartate antagonist with nanomolar affinity in rat brain. *Br. J. Pharmacol.*, **95**, 932–938

Murphy, D. E., Schneider, J., Boehm, C., Lehmann, J. and Williams, M. (1987). Binding of [³H]3-(2-carboxypiperazin-4-yl)propyl-1-phosphonic acid to rat brain membranes: a selective, high-affinity ligand for N-methyl-D-aspartate receptors. *J. Pharmacol. Exp. Ther.*, **240**, 778–784

Naito, S. and Ueda, T. (1983). ATP-dependent uptake of glutamate into protein I-associated synaptic vesicles. *J. Biol. Chem.*, **258**, 696–699

Naito, S. and Ueda, T. (1985). Characterization of glutamate uptake into synaptic vesicles. *J. Neurochem.*, **44**, 99–109

Nicholls, D. G. and Sihra, T. S. (1986). Synaptosomes possess an exocytotic pool of glutamate. *Nature*, **321**, 772–773

Ogita, K., Suzuki, T. and Yoneda, Y. (1989). Strychnine-insensitive binding of [³H]glycine to synaptic membranes in rat brain, treated with Triton X-100. *Neuropharmacology*, **28**, 1263–1270

Ogita, K. and Yoneda, Y. (1986). Characterization of Na⁺-dependent binding sites of [³H]glutamate in synaptic membranes from rat brain. *Brain Res.*, **397**, 137–144

Ogita, K. and Yoneda, Y. (1988). Disclosure by Triton X-100 of NMDA-sensitive [³H]glutamate binding sites in rat brain synaptic membranes. *Biochem. Biophys. Res. Commun.*, **153**, 510–517

Ogita, K. and Yoneda, Y. (1990). Temperature-independent binding of [³H](±)-3-(2-carboxypiperazin-4-yl)propyl-1-phosphonic acid in brain synaptic membranes treated by Triton X-100. *Brain Res.*, **515**, 51–56

Olsen, R. W., Szamraj, O. and Houser, C. R. (1987). [³H]AMPA binding to glutamate receptor subpopulations in rat brain. *Brain Res.*, **402**, 243–254

Olverman, H. J., Jones, A. W. and Watkins, J. C. (1984). L-Glutamate has higher affinity than other amino acids for [³H]-D-AP5 binding sites in rat brain membranes. *Nature*, **307**, 460–462

Olverman, H. J., Monaghan, D. T., Cotman, C. W. and Watkins, J. C. (1986). [³H]CPP, a new competitive ligand for NMDA receptors. *Eur. J. Pharmacol.*, **131**, 161–162

Pin, J.-P., Bockaert, J. and Recasens, M. (1984). The Ca²⁺/Cl⁻ dependent L-[³H]glutamate binding: a new receptor or a particular transport process? *FEBS Lett.*, **175**, 31–36

Ransom, R. W. and Stec, N. L. (1988). Cooperative modulation of [³H]MK-801 binding to the N-methyl-D-aspartate receptor-ion channel complex by L-glutamate, glycine and polyamines. *J. Neurochem.*, **51**, 830–836

Robinson, M. B., Blakely, R. D., Couto, R. and Coyle, J. T. (1987). Hydrolysis of the brain dipeptide-N-acetyl-L-aspartyl-L-glutamate. Identification and characterization of a novel N-acetylated α-linked acidic dipeptidase activity from rat brain. *J. Biol. Chem.*, **262**, 14498–14506

Robinson, M. B., Blakely, R. D. and Coyle, J. T. (1986). Quisqualate selectively inhibits a brain peptidase which cleaves N-acetyl-aspartyl-glutamate *in vitro*. *Eur. J. Pharmacol.*, **130**, 345–347

Robinson, M. B. and Coyle, J. T. (1987). Glutamate and related acidic excitatory neurotransmitters: from basic to clinical application. *FASEB Jl*, **1**, 446–455

Sanchez-Prieto, J., Sihra, T. S. and Nicholls, D. G. (1987). Characterization of the exocytotic release of glutamate from guinea-pig cerebral cortical synaptosomes. *J. Neurochem.*, **49**, 58–64

Slaughter, M. M. and Miller, R. F. (1983). Bipolar cells in the mudpuppy retina use an excitatory amino acid neurotransmitter. *Nature*, **303**, 537–538

Slaughter, M. M. and Miller, R. F. (1985). Identification of a distinct synaptic glutamate receptor on horizontal cells in mudpuppy retina. *Nature*, **314**, 96–97

Storm-Mathisen, J., Leknes, A. K., Bore, A. T., Vaaland, J. L., Edminson, P., Haug, F.-M. S. and Ottersen, O. P. (1983). First visualization of glutamate and GABA in neurones by immunocytochemistry. *Nature*, **301**, 517–519

Watkins, J. C. and Evans, R. H. (1981). Excitatory amino acid transmitters. *Ann. Rev. Pharmacol. Toxicol.*, **21**, 165–204

Yoneda, Y. and Ogita, K. (1986a). [³H]Glutamate binding sites in the rat pituitary. *Neurosci. Res.*, **3**, 430–435

Yoneda, Y. and Ogita, K. (1986b). Localization of [³H]glutamate binding sites in rat adrenal medulla. *Brain Res.*, **383**, 387–391

Yoneda, Y. and Ogita, K. (1987a). Are Ca²⁺-dependent proteases really responsible for Cl⁻-dependent and Ca²⁺-stimulated binding of [³H]glutamate in rat brain? *Brain Res.*, **400**, 70–79

Yoneda, Y. and Ogita, K. (1987b). Enhancement of [³H]glutamate binding by N-methyl-D-aspartic acid in rat adrenal. *Brain Res.*, **406**, 24–31

Yoneda, Y. and Ogita, K. (1987c). Solubilization of novel binding sites for [³H]glutamate in rat adrenal. *Biochem. Biophys. Res. Commun.*, **142**, 609–616

Yoneda, Y. and Ogita, K. (1989a). Microbial methodological artifacts in [³H]glutamate receptor binding assays. *Anal. Biochem.*, **177**, 250–255

Yoneda, Y. and Ogita, K. (1989b). Solubilization of quisqualate-sensitive [³H]glutamate binding activity from rat retina. *J. Neurochem.*, **52**, 1501–1507

Yoneda, Y. and Ogita, K. (1989c). Solubilization of stereospecific and quisqualate-sensitive activity of [³H]glutamate binding in the pituitary of the rat. *Neuropharmacology*, **28**, 611–616

Yoneda, Y. and Ogita, K. (1989d). Characterization of quisqualate-sensitive [³H]glutamate binding activity solubilized from rat adrenal. *Neurochem. Int.*, **15**, 137–143

Yoneda, Y. and Ogita, K. (1990). Neurochemical aspects of the *N*-methyl-D-aspartate receptor complex. *Neurosci. Res.*, **8**, in press

Yoneda, Y., Ogita, K., Nakamuta, H., Fukuda, Y., Koida, M. and Ogawa, Y. (1987). Comparative study of [³H]glutamate binding sites in rat retina and cerebral cortex. *Biochem. Pharmacol.*, **36**, 772–774

Yoneda, Y., Ogita, K., Ohgaki, T., Uchida, S. and Meguri, H. (1989). *N*-Methyl-D-aspartate-sensitive [³H]glutamate binding sites in brain synaptic membranes treated with Triton X-100. *Biochem. Biophys. Acta*, **1012**, 74–80

Yoneda, Y., Ogita, K. and Suzuki, T. (1988). Multiple binding sites on the NMDA receptor/ion channel complex in brain synaptic membranes. In *Neurotransmitters: Focus on Excitatory Amino Acids* (ed. I. Kanazawa). Excerpta Medica, Tokyo, pp. 47–65

Yoneda, Y., Ogita, K. and Suzuki, T. (1990). Interaction of strychnine-insensitive glycine binding with MK-801 binding in brain synaptic membranes. *J. Neurochem.*, **55**, 237–244

8

Neuropeptide Gene Families that Control Reproductive Behaviour and Growth in Molluscs

[1]W. P. M. GERAERTS, [1]A. B. SMIT, [1]K. W. LI,
[2]E. VREUGDENHIL and [2]H. VAN HEERIKHUIZEN

[1]Biological Laboratory, and [2]Biochemical Laboratory, Vrije Universiteit,
PO Box 7161, 1007 MC Amsterdam, The Netherlands

Contents

Current Aspects of the Neurosciences, Vol. 3. Edited by N. N. Osborne. © The Macmillan Press Ltd 1991

1. *Introduction*

Peptidergic neuroendocrine cells play an important role in the control of complex and interrelated life processes, such as growth, reproduction and behaviour. These neurons function as transducer cells; they integrate (neural) signals carrying information on the internal and external environment and convert these signals into peptide messages, which, in a co-ordinated fashion, activate the appropriate target systems of the body to produce a specific response. For a complete understanding of the basic mechanisms underlying the functioning of peptidergic cells, information on many aspects of the cell is needed. To study these different processes (input, integrative capacities, branching patterns, ultrastructural characteristics, biosynthesis and release activities, etc.), a multidisciplinary approach is needed. Unfortunately, the peptidergic systems of most animal groups are not optimally suited for this approach. The identification of the cells *in vivo* is often impossible; the cells are often too small for specific techniques, such as the intracellular recording of membrane potentials; and furthermore, the physiological and behavioural systems of many animals, especially vertebrates, are very complicated, which seriously hampers studies on the role of peptidergic neurons in the control of physiological processes and behaviour.

Invertebrates provide simple physiological and behavioural systems that may be very useful here. The gastropod molluscs, *Lymnaea stagnalis* and *Aplysia californica* (Figure 1), are particularly advantageous models for neurobiological studies, because the central nervous systems (CNS) of these animals consist of only about 15 000 neurons clustered into a small number of major ganglia. Many of these neurons are of a giant size and can be easily identified. In addition, the peptidergic systems controlling specific behaviours and physiological processes have been intensively studied (e.g. Kandel, 1979; Geraerts *et al.*, 1988a,b; Joosse, 1988). Egg-laying in *Lymnaea* and *Aplysia* is a clear example of a stereotyped behaviour consisting of a limited number of behavioural acts that are controlled by specific sets of neuropeptides. Similarly, body growth and energy metabolism in *Lymnaea* is an example of a complex vital life process that is controlled by a set of unique insulin-related peptides. Studies concerning these peptides have been extended in recent years to include the genes encoding them. In this review we shall discuss several aspects of the peptidergic systems and the genes involved in the regulation of egg-laying and growth in *Lymnaea* and *Aplysia*. We shall first consider the egg-laying peptide genes, and the anatomy, morphology and role in reproduction of the peptidergic systems that express these genes. In the section that follows, we shall review the genes encoding the insulin-related peptides of *Lymnaea*.

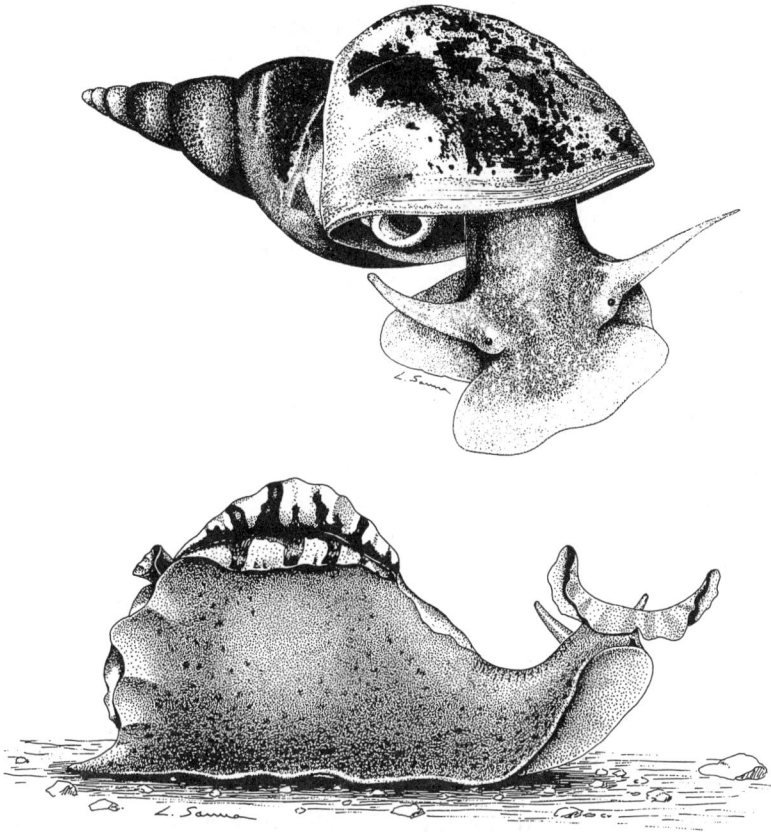

Figure 1 The freshwater gastropod *L. stagnalis* (top) and the marine gastropod *A. californica* (bottom). *Lymnaea*, the pond snail, is a basommatophoran pulmonate. The head possesses one pair of tentacles, which have simple eyes at their base. *Lymnaea* is common in fresh water, where it can be found crawling on leaves of plants, on which the egg masses are preferentially deposited. The animal has a sac-like lung cavity, the opening of which is located near the rim of the shell. *L. stagnalis* can reach a shell height of 35–60 mm. In laboratory breeding conditions, it begins egg-laying at a shell height of about 23 mm. *Aplysia*, the sea hare, is an opisthobranchean gastropod. The head possesses two pairs of tentacles, the anteriors being large and earlike (hence the animal's name), while those of the second pair are small and have each an eye at their base. The animal dwells in the tidal and subtidal zones, where it feeds on seaweeds. The egg string is deposited on non-movable objects, such as rocks and stones. Respiration occurs by a kind of gill, which is covered up in the figure by upwardly directed flaps, the parapodia, which can be used for swimming. *A. californica* can become very large; animals weighing over 1 kg are no exception

2.   *Genes Controlling Egg-laying Behaviour in* Lymnaea *and* Aplysia

Anatomy and Cytology of the Peptidergic Systems Controlling Egg-laying

The anatomy and cytology of the peptidergic cells that control egg-laying and associated behaviours in *Lymnaea* and *Aplysia* will be briefly reviewed here. The reader is referred to Roubos (1984) and Geraerts *et al.* (1988a) for more detailed descriptions of these peptidergic systems.

Anatomy and Topology

In *Lymnaea* the somata of the egg-laying controlling caudodorsal cells (CDCs) are located in the caudodorsal part of each cerebral ganglion (Figure 2) (Joosse, 1964; Wendelaar Bonga, 1970). Each cluster contains about 50 cells and the individual CDC somata can reach a maximal size of 90 µm. The axons emerge excentrically from the somata and first run to the anterior part of the cerebral ganglia, then form a loop in the 'loop area', where they run close together and contact each other eletrotonically (Figure 3). After leaving the loop area the axons run toward the ipsilateral part of the intercerebral commissure (COM) and form many thin branches that contain the neurosecretory granules and that end blindly in the neurohaemal area. The ventral CDCs form an additional axon branch, which runs straight to and through the COM, passes through the contralateral loop area, and then returns to the contralateral half of the neurohaemal area. In this way the ventral CDCs connect electrotonically both CDC clusters via the crossing axons and the loops. The proximal, unbifurcated part of the axon is studded with side-branches, which are involved in the reception of synaptic input (e.g., cholinergic input). Thus, the function of the subset of specialized ventral CDCs is to receive the sensory egg-laying inducing stimuli and to relay these to the other CDCs. Furthermore, the crossing axons give rise to collaterals, which ramify and form an extensive diffuse network, the collateral system, throughout the inner compartment (Figure 4) (Schmidt and Roubos, 1987). It seems likely that the collaterals enable the CDCs to communicate with targets within the CNS in a nonsynaptic ('paracrine', 'hormone-like') fashion (see page 280).

The somata of the bag cells (BCs) that control egg-laying in *Aplysia* are localized in two homogeneous clusters of 250–400 cells, each at the ventral surface of the pleurovisceral connective at the rostral margin of the abdominal ganglion (Figure 5; Coggeshall, 1967). The BCs (diameter 60 µm) are heteropolar and the major processes travel out of the BC clusters into different directions. The connective tissue sheath surrounding the abdominal ganglion and the pleurovisceral connectives constitutes the neurohaemal area of the BCs. The BCs within a cluster are electrotonically coupled and there is also electrotonic coupling between the BCs of the two clusters via BC branches that run to the contralateral clusters.

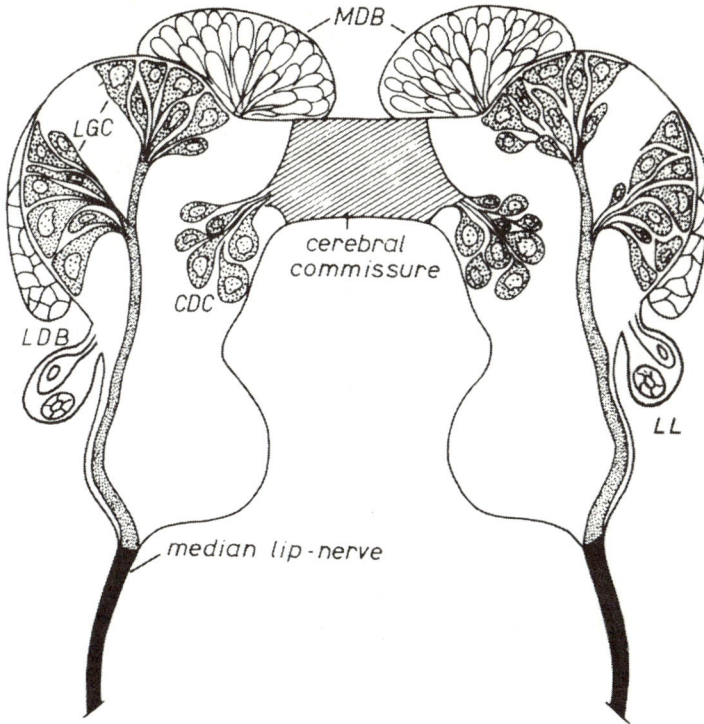

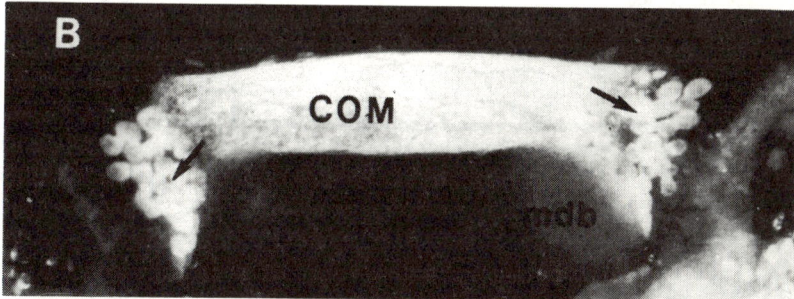

Figure 2 Location of the CDCs in the cerebral ganglia of *L. stagnalis*. A: Diagrammatic transverse section through the cerebral ganglia showing the location of the various neuroendocrine and endocrine centres. CDC, caudodorsal cells; LGC, light green cells; LL, lateral lobes; MDB and LDB, mediodorsal and laterodorsal bodies. The periphery of the cerebral commissure is the neurohaemal area of the CDCs. The peripheries of the median lip nerves are the neurohaemal areas of the LGCs. B: Ventral view of both cerebral ganglia of *L. stagnalis in situ*. The cluster of whitish CDCs (arrows) in each ganglion are clearly visible. The neurohaemal area of the CDCs, the periphery of the intercerebral commissure (COM), also has a whitish appearance, due to stored neurosecretory products of the CDCs. Note the mediodorsal bodies (mdb) that are located dorsal on the cerebral ganglia

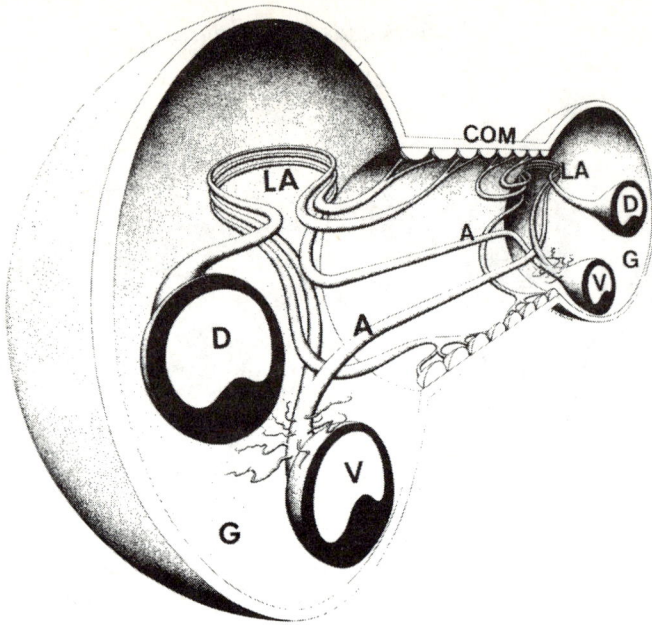

Figure 3 Schematic representation of the cerebral ganglia (G) of *Lymnaea* with dorsal (D) and ventral (V) CDCs. Each CDC has an axon branch that runs through the ipsilateral loop area (LA). Ventral CDCs have an additional branch (crossing axon, A) running via the COM through the contralateral loop area. All axon branches form neurohaemal terminals in the periphery of the COM

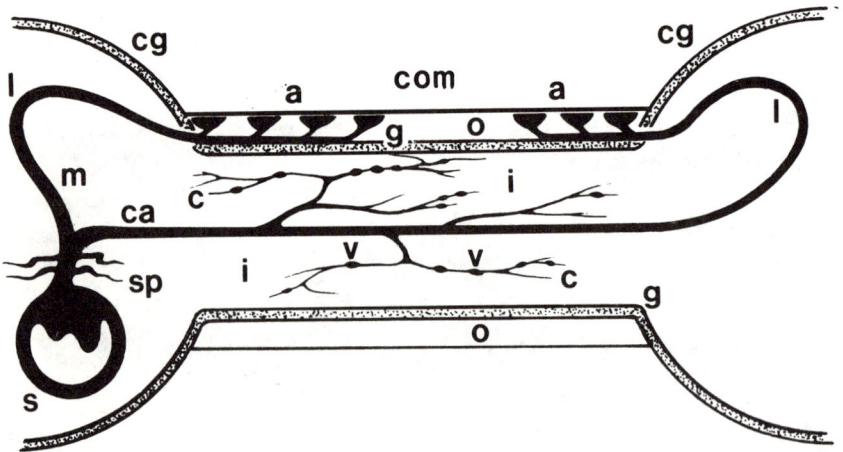

Figure 4 Outer and inner compartments of the COM of *L. stagnalis*. The compartments are separated by a glial sheath (g). Shown is the anatomy of one ventral CDC. The main axon (m) of the ventral CDC runs through the loop area (l) to the neurohaemal area in the outer compartment (o), where the axon terminals (a) end blindly. A branch of the main axon, the crossing axon (ca), runs through the inner compartment (i) of the COM, passes through the contralateral loop area, and then runs to the outer compartment. In the inner compartment the crossing axon gives rise to the collaterals (c). cg, cerebral ganglion; s, soma; sp, spines; v, varicosity. From Schmidt and Roubos (1987)

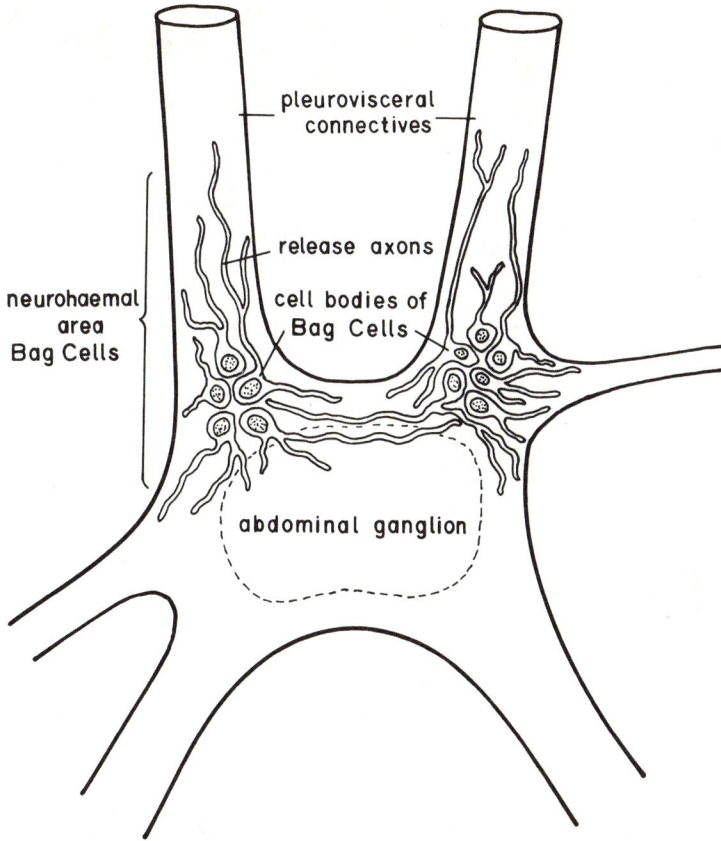

Figure 5 Dorsal view of the abdominal ganglion of *A. californica* with the bag cells. Only a small number of the numerous bag cells with their release axons in the neurohaemal area are indicated. From each cluster of bag cells, some axons cross over and make electrotonic contacts with cells in the contralateral cluster

Cytology

CDCs and BCs are polyploid (Coggeshall *et al.*, 1970; Boer *et al.*, 1977). The neurons exhibit the typical characteristics of protein-synthesizing cells, with elaborate stacks of granular endoplasmic reticulum, a well-developed Golgi apparatus and numerous neurosecreteory granules (Figure 6). In the Golgi apparatus proteinergic secretory material is condensed, possibly modified, and finally budded off as neurosecretory granules that contain the egg-laying-inducing peptides (Figure 6A). The internal axon structure is characterized by the occurrence of microtubules and neurosecretory granules (Figure 6B). Numerous gap junctions occur between processes of the CDCs or BCs (Kaczmarek *et al.*, 1979; Roubos *et al.*, 1985). In the CDCs these occur frequently in the loop areas. The contents of the neurosecretory granules are

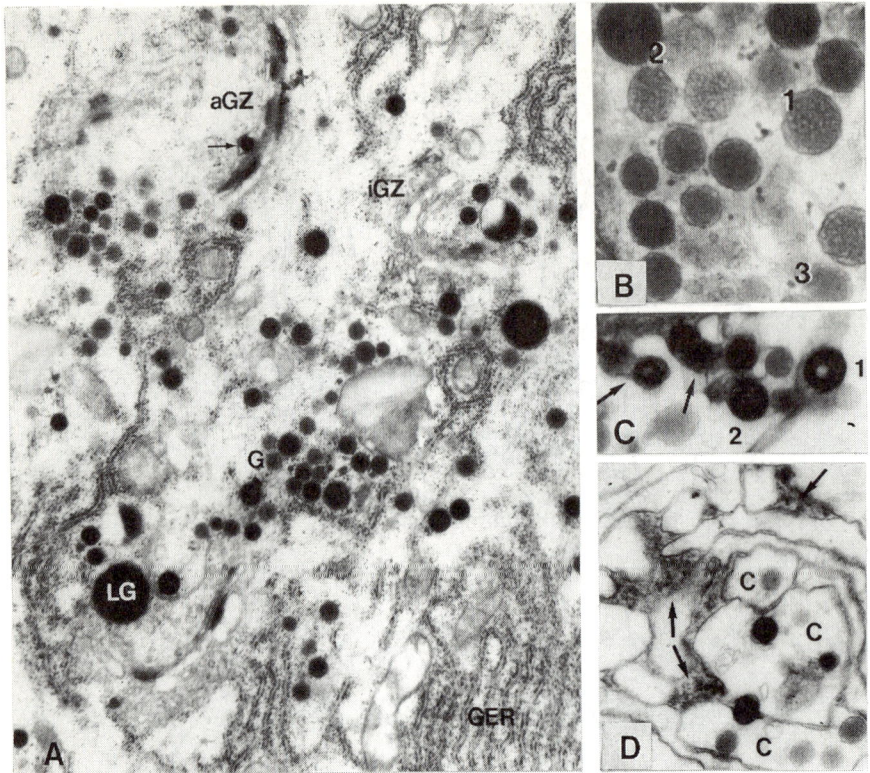

Figure 6 CDC soma and axons of *Lymnaea*. A: Soma showing granular endoplasmic reticulum (GER), Golgi zones (active, aGZ; inactive, iGZ), neurosecretory granules (G) and large electron-dense granules (LG). Arrow indicates formation of immature neurosecretory granules. ×25 000. B: Axon terminal in the neurohaemal area. Three types (1–3) of neurosecretory granule are indicated. Uranyl and lead stains. ×90 000. C: Two types (1 and 2) of multiple exocytosis (arrows) in CDC terminal in the neurohaemal area. TARI method. ×110 000. D: Non-synaptic release from CDC collaterals in the inner compartment of the COM. Large intercellular spaces filled with flocculent electron-dense material (arrows) near highly active non-synaptic release sites of CDC collaterals (C). TARI method. ×35 000. From Roubos (1984); Schmidt and Roubos (1987)

released extracellularly by exocytosis (Figure 6C). The exocytosis frequency in CDC terminals located in the neurohaemal area is low in CDC systems that are not electrically active but increases dramatically during discharges of the CDCs, when large amounts of ovulation hormone and other peptides are released into the haemolymph. Calcium ions play an important role in exocytosis, and mitochondria and several vesicular structures in addition to calcium channels are involved in the control of the axoplasmic calcium concentration (Buma *et al.*, 1983). In the collateral system exocytosis occurs into various directions from the release sites that lack any morphological synaptic specialization (Figure 6D), suggesting nonsynaptic release (Schmidt and Roubos, 1987).

The Role of the CDCs and the BCs in Reproduction

L. stagnalis and *A. californica* are functional simultaneous hermaphrodites (Figure 7). In the ovotestis, male and female gametes are produced. There is one (small) hermaphroditic duct arising from the gonad. In the next part of the system, male and female gametes are transported via separate paths. These may be either two separate ducts, as in *Lymnaea*, or functionally separate channels within a common duct, as in *Aplysia*. At ovulation numerous oocytes are transported to the female duct and after fertilization the egg cells are surrounded one by one by perivitellin fluid of the albumen gland (this fluid serves as nutrition during embryonic development). The eggs are packaged into a compact egg mass (*Lymnaea*) or a long egg string (*Aplysia*). This process may take up to several hours and is accompanied by a series of stereotyped overt behaviours.

In the hermaphrodite gastropods, complex (neuro)endocrine systems have evolved to control reproductive activities, and peptidergic neurons controlling egg-mass production and associated overt behaviours are present, in addition to the centres regulating hermaphroditism (Kupfermann, 1967; Geraerts and Bohlken, 1976). It is only in certain habitats in the environment that conditions favourable for the development of embryos and hatchlings prevail. Some conditions in the preferred habitats act as microenvironmental stimuli for the release activities of the CDCs and BCs and, hence, for egg-laying. During oviposition, the egg masses or egg strings must be firmly attached to non-moving objects, such as rocks and leaves of plants. The main purpose of the overt behaviours that accompany egg-laying is to ensure that the eggs are deposited in the preferred habitats.

From the CDCs and BCs several peptides involved in the regulation of egg-laying have been structurally identified. These peptides include the egg-release-inducing peptides, caudodorsal cell hormone (CDCH) of *L. stagnalis* (Ebberink *et al.*, 1985) and egg-laying hormone (ELH) of *A. californica* (Chiu *et al.*, 1979). Other peptides, such as α-bag cell peptide (α-BCP; Rothman *et al.*, 1983) and calfluxin (Dictus *et al.*, 1987) were subsequently purified and their regulatory roles in the egg-laying process were studied. Peptides capable of inducing egg-laying also appeared to be present in accessory sex glands—i.e. the atrial gland of *A. californica* and the male and female glands of *L. stagnalis*. Biologically active peptides, as a rule, are synthesized as part of a high-molecular-weight prohormone. In the next subsections we shall review our knowledge concerning the egg-laying prohormones and the genes encoding them.

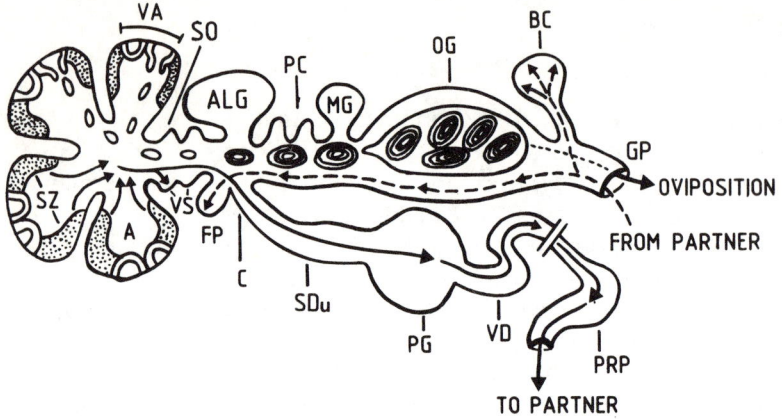

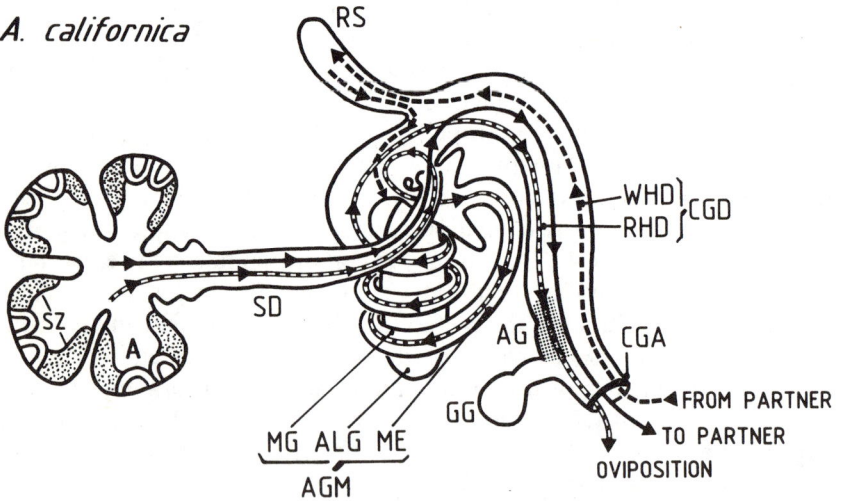

Figure 7 Diagrammatic representation of the functional anatomy of the reproductive systems of *L. stagnalis* and *A. californica*. In the *Lymnaea* system are indicated ovulation, egg formation and egg mass formation. Dotted line and broken/enclosed line: passage of eggs and egg mass or egg string. Continuous line: passage of autosperm. Sperm is transported to the functionally female copulation partner. Heavy dashed line: passage of foreign sperm. Foreign sperm is transported to the fertilization pocket or receptaculum seminis, where it is stored until ovulated oocytes appear for fertilization. The atrial gland (AG) of the *Aplysia* system is shaded. A, acinus of the ovotestis; AG, atrial gland; AGM, accessory genital mass; ALG, albumen gland; BC, bursa copulatrix; C, carrefour; CGA, common genital aperture; CGD, common genital duct; FP, fertilization pocket; GG, gametolytic gland; GP, genital pore; ME, membrane gland; MG, muciparous gland; OG, oothecal gland; PC, pars contorta; PG, prostate gland; PRP, praeputium; RHD, red hemiduct; RS, receptaculum seminis; SD, small hermaphroditic duct; SDu, sperm duct; SO, sperm oviduct; SZ, spermatogenic zone; VA, vitellogenic area; VD, vas deferens; VS, vesiculae seminalis; WHD, white hemiduct

The Organization of the Egg-laying Peptide Genes

The recombinant DNA technology has been the method of choice to demonstrate that the biologically active peptides in the CDCs and BCs are initially synthesized as part of a large common prohormone. Using these methods, the structure of the gene encoding ELH, which is expressed in the BCs of *A. californica*, was first established (Scheller *et al.*, 1982; Mahon *et al.*, 1985) and subsequently the cDNA encoding the precursor of CDCH, which is produced in the CDCs of *L. stagnalis*, was determined (Vreugdenhil *et al.*, 1988). The *ELH* gene, which is schematically diagrammed in Figure 8, spans 10 kilobasepairs (kbp) and contains one large intron and three exons. The large exon III contains an open reading frame that encodes the ELH preprohormone, including part of the 5' and the entire 3' untranslated regions of the mRNAs. Remaining sequences coding for 5' untranslated regions of

ELH-GENE FAMILY OF *APLYSIA CALIFORNICA*

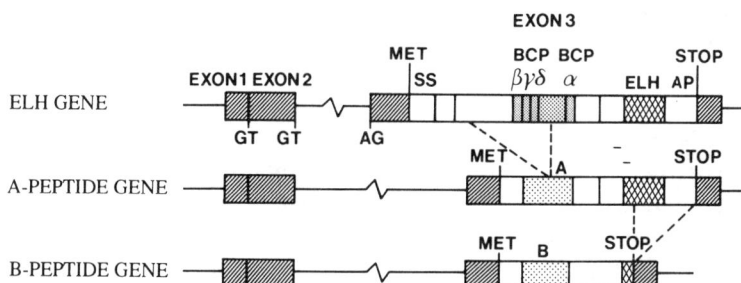

CDCH-GENE FAMILY OF *LYMNAEA STAGNALIS*

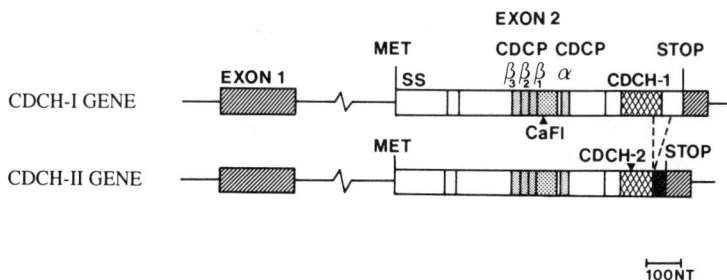

Figure 8 Organization of the *ELH* and *CDCH* gene families. Indicated are exons, introns, splice junction donor (GT) and acceptor (AG) sites, the translation initiating codon methionine (MET), the stop codon (STOP) and the various possible proteolytic cleavage sites (vertical bars). SS, signal sequence; BCP, bag cell peptide; ELH, egg-laying hormone; AP, acidic peptide; A, peptide A; B, peptide B; CDCP, caudodorsal cell peptide; CDCH, caudodorsal cell hormone; CaFl, calfluxin; NT, nucleotides

the ELH mRNA are found further upstream (at least 6 kbp) on two smaller linked exons (exons I and II). 'TATA' and 'CAAT' boxes, which serve as transcriptional signals in eukaryotic genes, are present upstream from exon I, and sequences for polyadenylation were identified in the 3' untranslated region. The *CDCH* gene is similarly organized and contains two exons, of which exon I contains the 5' non-coding part and exon II the complete coding region (Figure 8).

Both the *ELH* gene and the *CDCH* gene are members of multigene families consisting of a small number of highly homologous genes that are expressed in a tissue-specific fashion (Figure 8) (Scheller *et al.*, 1982; Mahon *et al.*, 1985; Nambu and Scheller, 1986; Shyamala *et al.*, 1986; van Minnen *et al.*, 1988, 1989). In *A. californica* the *ELH* gene family consists of approximately five genes per haploid genome, and many or even all members of the gene family probably are linked. Three members of the family have been studied in detail. These include the *ELH* gene and the *peptide A* and *B* genes. These genes are more than 90% homologous at the DNA level. The major structural difference between the *ELH* gene and the *peptide A* and *B* genes is a 240-nucleotide insert in the A/B peptide coding region. In addition, small differences in the DNA sequence, such as point mutations, have occurred, many of which have led to significant changes of the residues constituting the proteolytic processing sites. Thus, different sets of peptides are generated from the precursors. The homology between genes dramatically declines upstream from the sequence directing transcription initiation, and it has been suggested that changes in the DNA sequences upstream to transcription initiation may be important in the evolution of the tissue-specific expression of the gene family (Mahon *et al.*, 1985). Recent peptide sequencing data suggest that in the atrial gland two more genes, called *peptide A'* and *B'* genes, are expressed, which are closely related to the *peptide A* and *B* genes (Nagle *et al.*, 1988, 1989). The *CDCH* gene of *L. stagnalis* belongs to a small gene family, which consists of at least two types: the *CDCH I* and *II* genes. The most striking difference is a 17 bp deletion near the C-terminal region of CDCH, including its proteolytic processing site. This gives rise to a truncated form of CDCH, which is flanked C-terminally by a completely different peptide. In addition, several amino acid substitutions occur in other peptide domains. As a result, each type of *CDCH* gene encodes a different though overlapping set of peptides.

Expression of the Egg-laying Peptide Genes

The *ELH* gene family is differentially expressed in both neural and non-neural tissues in *A. californica*. The *ELH* gene is preferentially expressed in the BCs, while the *peptide A/A'* and *B/B'* genes are expressed in the atrial gland (cf. Figure 7) of the reproductive tract of *Aplysia* (Mahon *et al.*, 1985; see also the reviews of Geraerts *et al.*, 1988a; Nagle *et al.*, 1989). It has further

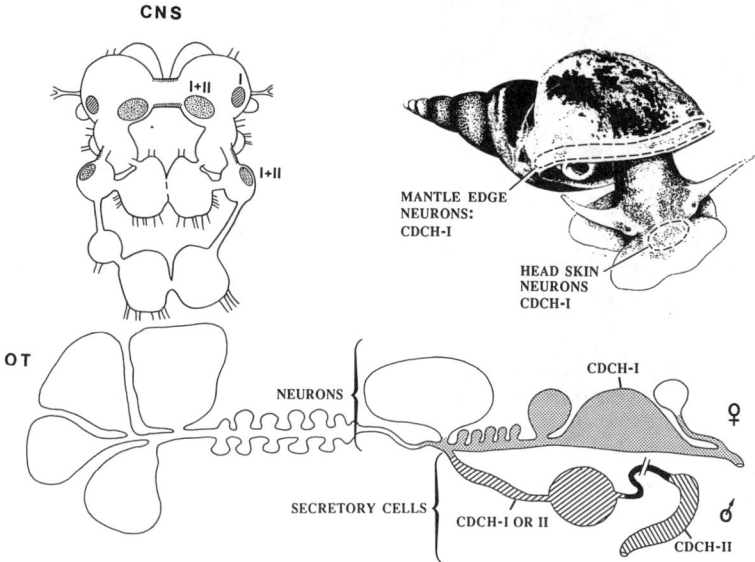

Figure 9 Summary of the central and peripheral expression of the *CDCH I* and *II* genes (indicated as I and II) in *L. stagnalis*. The *CDCH* genes are expressed in neurons of the CNS, the skin of the head region, the mantle edge and the female part of the reproductive duct, except for the albumen gland. In the male glands (cross-hatched), the genes are expressed in exocrine cells. OT, ovotestis. Courtesy of Dr Joosse

been shown that the *ELH* gene is expressed in other neurons of the CNS, in addition to the BCs. The *peptide A'* gene is also expressed in a number of neurons of the CNS. The atrial gland is an exocrine gland and its products are secreted into the oviduct. It has been suggested that the peptides encoded by the *peptide A/A'* and *B/B'* genes may be secreted on to the egg cordon as it is transported through the oviduct and that these peptides may subsequently act as pheromones to induce or facilitate mating behaviour (Nagle *et al.*, 1989).

In *Lymnaea* the members of the *CDCH* gene family are also expressed, in a tissue-specific way, both in the CNS in cell clusters or dispersed throughout the ganglia, and in neurons or secretory cells in the skin, the mantle edge, and the male and female accessory sex organs (Figures 9–11; van Minnen *et al.*, 1988, 1989). In the female glands the *CDCH I* gene is expressed in neurons that control the activities of muscles and glandular cells involved in egg mass production. In the male glands, the *CDCH I* and *II* genes are expressed in glandular cells. The materials of these cells are secreted and passed on to the partner during copulation. They possibly regulate reproductive behaviour of the partner acting as the female copulant. It is furthermore suggested that sensory and other types of neuron that express the *CDCH* genes in the skin, female tract and CNS are involved in transmitting egg-laying-inducing stimuli to the CDC clusters in the cerebral ganglia.

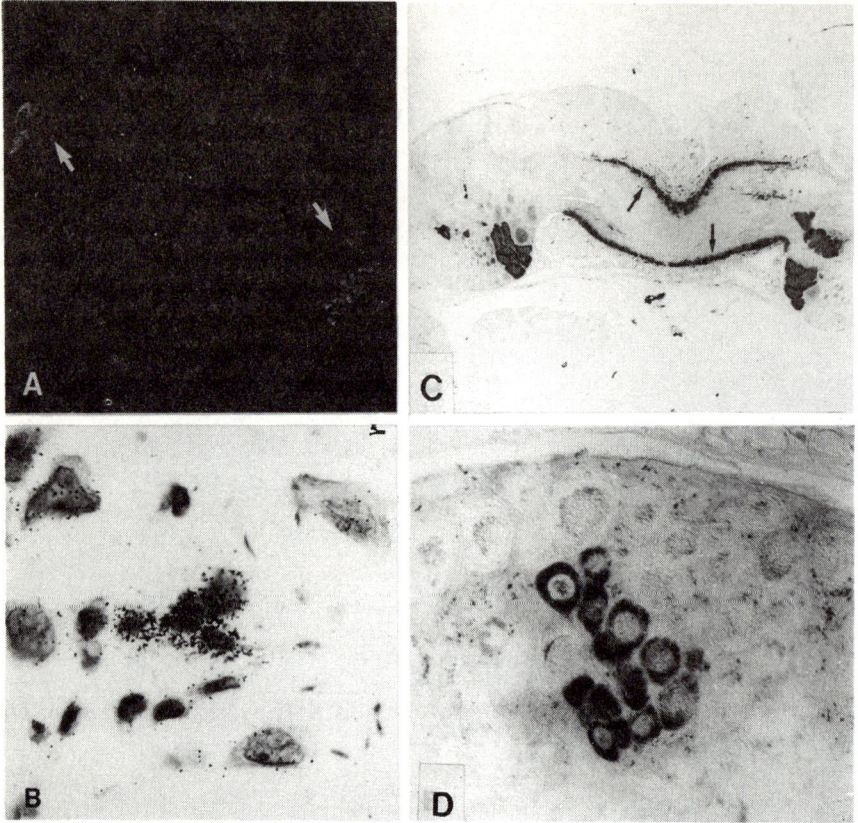

Figure 10 *In situ* hybridization and immunocytochemical localization of CDCH and CDCH-like peptide expressing neurons in the CNS of *L. stagnalis*. A, B: *In situ* hybridization. Bouin-fixed and frozen sections of the CNS were exposed to a CDCH-specific cDNA probe labelled with ^{35}S. The probe hybridized with CDCH mRNA, whose location was revealed by autoradiography. A: Dark-field autoradiograph. Arrows show hybridization in the clusters of CDCs in the cerebral ganglia. ×40. B: The black dots show hybridization in cells other than the CDCs in the cerebral ganglia. ×400. C, D: Immunocytochemistry using a polyclonal antibody to synthetic CDCH. C: AntiCDCH-positive perikarya of the CDCs in the cerebral ganglia and their axon terminals in the COM (arrows). ×40. D: AntiCDCH-positive perikarya of a group of cells other than the CDCs in the left cerebral ganglion. These cells express only the *CDCH I* gene (cf. Figure 9). ×500. Courtesy Dr van Minnen

Figure 11 (*opposite*)   CDCH-immunoreactive cells and processes in the accessory sex organs of *L. stagnalis*. A: Oothecal gland. Arrows show antiCDCH-positive perikarya of neurons as well as positive varicosities of axons apparently contacting secretory cells. ×200. B: AntiCDCH-positive perikaryon and a ramifying process (arrows) of a neuron in the oothecal gland. ×500. C: Cross-section of the spermduct (SD) and the oothecal gland (OG). The secretory cells of the spermduct are filled with antiCDCH-positive material. In the oothecal gland, antiCDCH-positive neurons and varicosities of axons are present (arrows). ×40. C: Cross-section of the prostate gland with secretory cells containing antiCDCH-positive secretory granules (SG). ×500. Courtesy Dr van Minnen

Structure of the Egg-laying Peptide Precursor Proteins

The ELH and CDCH precursors of *A. californica* and *L. stagnalis*, respectively, together with the ELH precursor of a second *Aplysia* species, *A. parvula* (Nambu and Scheller, 1986), are shown in Figure 12. Comparison of the precursors and peptides is of interest with regard to the evolutionary

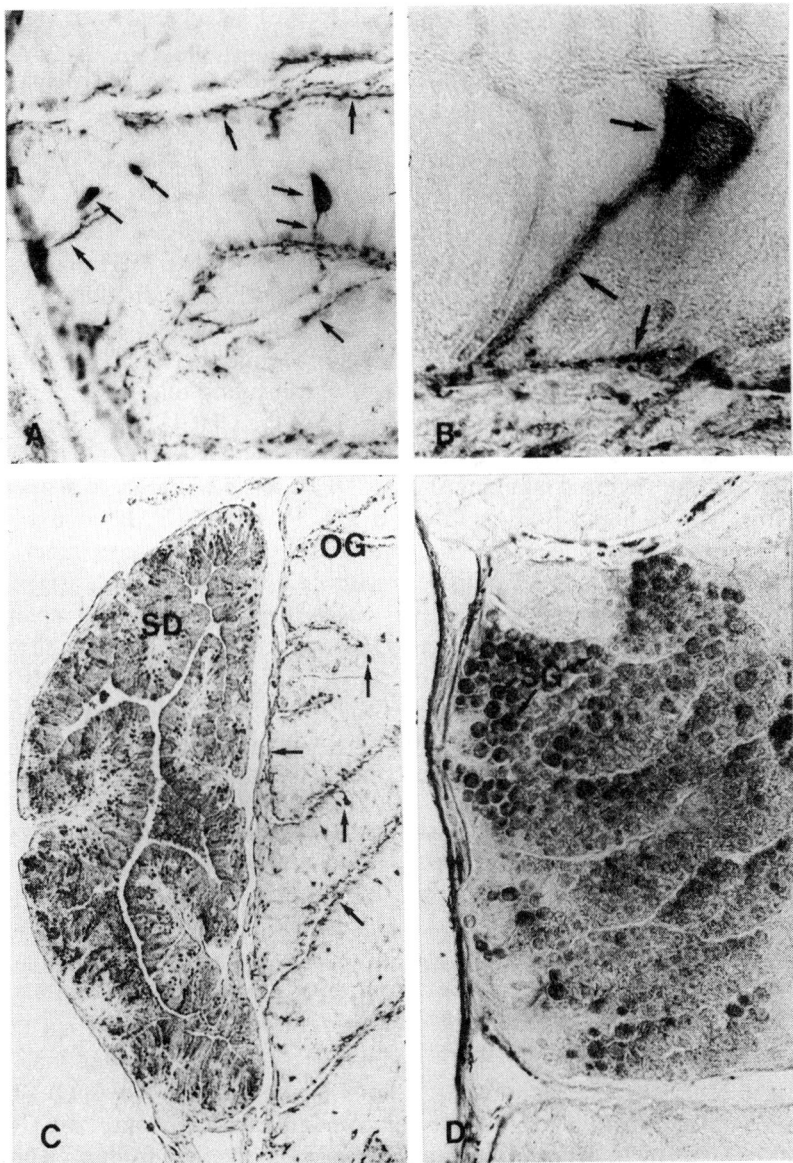

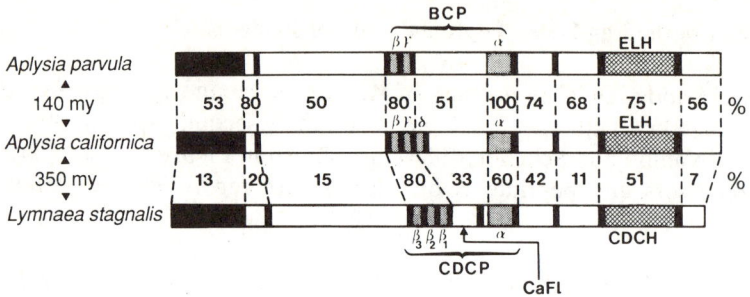

Figure 12 Comparison of the CDCH and ELH precursors from the CDCs of *L. stagnalis* and the BCs of *A. californica* and *A. parvula*. Percentage homologies between regions are indicated. Further indicated are the positions of the identified peptides, including CDCH and ELH, α-BCP and α-CDCP, β-, γ-BCP and β1-3-CDCP, and calfluxin (CaFl). Cleavage sites are shown as vertical black bars. Signal peptides are shown as black areas

history of these species. The structural organizations of the ELH precursors of both *Aplysia* species are quite similar, with conservation of all but one of the potential proteolytical cleavage sites. The overall amino acid homology between the ELH precurors is 66%. The regions containing ELH, α-BCP and the β-BCPs are even more highly conserved, indicating that these peptides are of importance in egg-laying. Three regions of the CDCH precursor are of interest: CDCH has a high degree of homology with ELH; α-CDCP with α-BCP; and the region containing the β-CDCPs has a remarkable sequence homology with β- and γ-BCP, and with α-CDCP and α-BCP. In comparison with ELH precursors, one extra pentapeptide (β2-CDCP) has been generated in the CDCH precursor. Compared with *A. parvula* and *L. stagnalis* precursors, the δ-BCP region in the *A. californica* precursor is completely different. The region between the β-CDCPs and α-CDCP is much shorter than the counterpart on the ELH precursor. This difference suggests the occurrence of one or more deletions in the *Lymnaea* gene during the course of evolution. Another difference between the CDCH and ELH precursors is that, apart from the homologies described above, the CDCH and ELH precursors are not homologous.

CDCH and the ELHs each consists of 36 amino acids (Figure 13). They have a basic character. The ELHs of both *Aplysia* species exhibit 78% homology, with nearly all of the amino acid alterations in the middle third of the molecule. CDCH shows 44% homology with ELH of *A. californica*, with amino acid alterations predominantly in the middle part of the peptide. α-BCPs share 100% homology, and α-CDCP has five uninterrupted amino acids in common with the α-BCPs (Figure 14), suggesting that α-CDCP exhibits similar functions to α-BCP, including the autotransmitter function (see page 278). β1-CDCP is completely homologous with the *Aplysia* β-BCPs (Figure 14), and further exhibits strong homology with β2- and β3-CDCP, and with the γ-BCPs. *A. californica* and *A. parvula* diverged from each other

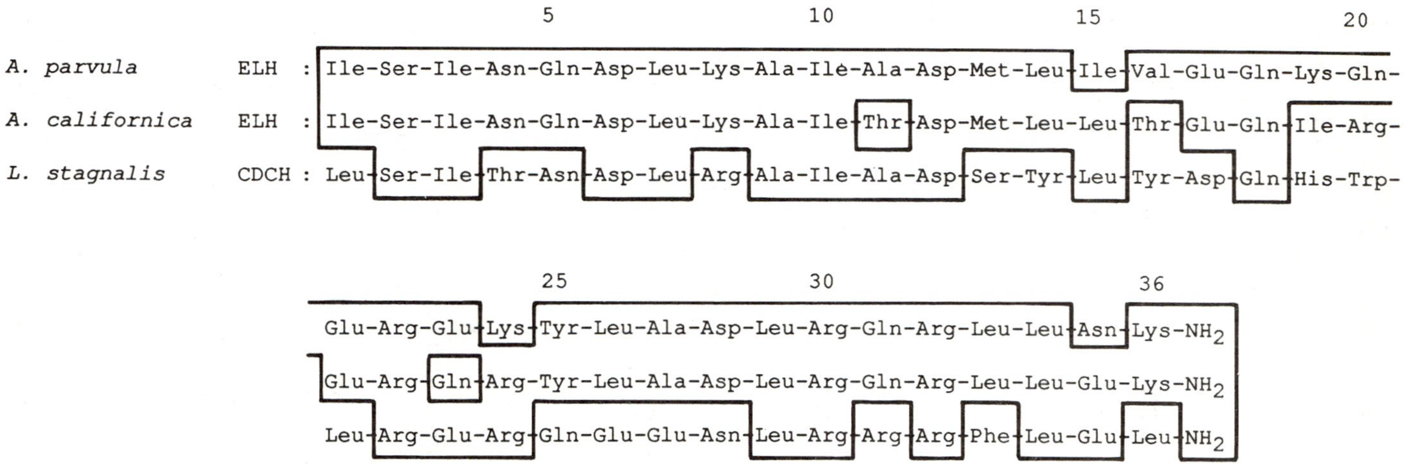

```
                    5              10             15            20

A. parvula      ELH  : Ile-Ser-Ile-Asn-Gln-Asp-Leu-Lys-Ala-Ile-Ala-Asp-Met-Leu-Ile-Val-Glu-Gln-Lys-Gln-

A. californica  ELH  : Ile-Ser-Ile-Asn-Gln-Asp-Leu-Lys-Ala-Ile-Thr-Asp-Met-Leu-Leu-Thr-Glu-Gln-Ile-Arg-

L. stagnalis    CDCH : Leu-Ser-Ile-Thr-Asn-Asp-Leu-Arg-Ala-Ile-Ala-Asp-Ser-Tyr-Leu-Tyr-Asp-Gln-His-Trp-


                    25             30             36

                     Glu-Arg-Glu-Lys-Tyr-Leu-Ala-Asp-Leu-Arg-Gln-Arg-Leu-Leu-Asn-Lys-NH₂

                     Glu-Arg-Gln-Arg-Tyr-Leu-Ala-Asp-Leu-Arg-Gln-Arg-Leu-Leu-Glu-Lys-NH₂

                     Leu-Arg-Glu-Arg-Gln-Glu-Glu-Asn-Leu-Arg-Arg-Arg-Phe-Leu-Glu-Leu-NH₂
```

Figure 13 Amino acid sequence homologies among CDCH and the ELHs. Identical amino acids are enclosed within boxes

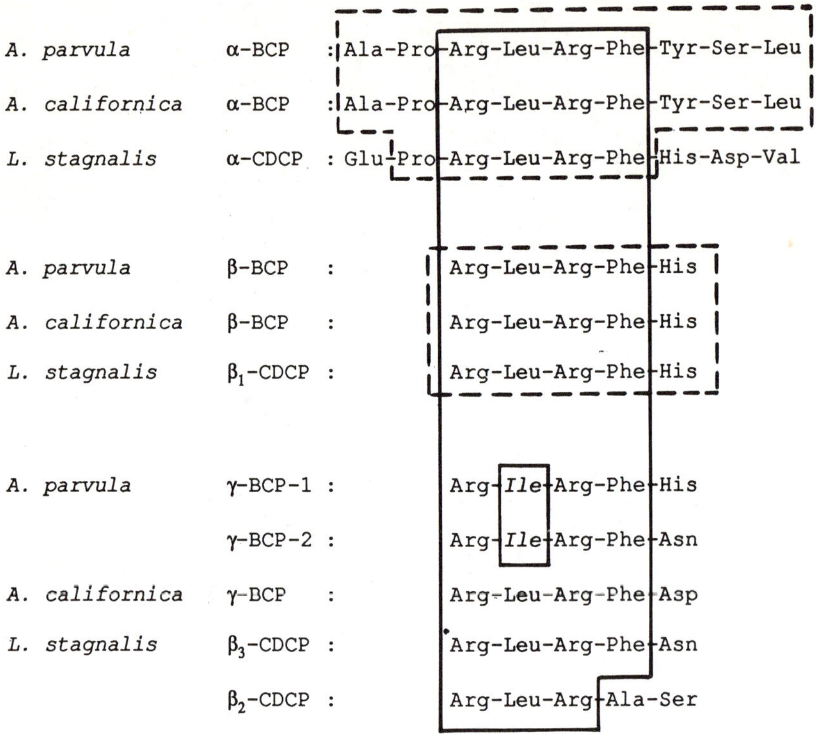

```
A. parvula        α-BCP    :|Ala-Pro-Arg-Leu-Arg-Phe-Tyr-Ser-Leu|

A. californica    α-BCP    :|Ala-Pro-Arg-Leu-Arg-Phe-Tyr-Ser-Leu|

L. stagnalis      α-CDCP   : Glu-Pro-Arg-Leu-Arg-Phe-His-Asp-Val


A. parvula        β-BCP    :       Arg-Leu-Arg-Phe-His

A. californica    β-BCP    :       Arg-Leu-Arg-Phe-His

L. stagnalis      β₁-CDCP  :       Arg-Leu-Arg-Phe-His


A. parvula        γ-BCP-1  :       Arg-Ile-Arg-Phe-His

                  γ-BCP-2  :       Arg-Ile-Arg-Phe-Asn

A. californica    γ-BCP    :       Arg-Leu-Arg-Phe-Asp

L. stagnalis      β₃-CDCP  :       Arg-Leu-Arg-Phe-Asn

                  β₂-CDCP  :       Arg-Leu-Arg-Ala-Ser
```

Figure 14 Amino acid sequence homologies among α-CDCP, α-BCPs and the pentapeptides. Identical amino acids are enclosed within boxes

some 140 million years ago, while pulmonate and opisthobranch gastropod subclasses diverged from each other about 350 million years ago. Also, the Lymnaeidae are evolved from marine-based molluscs through land-based intermediates, and are only distantly related to the Aplysiids. Regions on the precursors that exhibit strong homology are peptides that control egg-laying. Apparently these peptides have been under intense selective pressure. It is tempting to speculate that the diverged peptides regulate aspects of egg-laying that are species-specific.

It has long been thought that the egg-laying peptides were restricted to the gastropod molluscs. However, a cDNA encoding a novel prohormone in the rat, the melanin-concentrating hormone precursor (Nahon *et al.*, 1989), has been shown to be evolutionary related to the peptide A prohormone of *Aplysia*. The amino acid similarities are low, though statistically significant. The gene encoding the melanin-concentrating hormone precursor is expressed in the rat hypothalamus and, in addition, might possibly be transcribed in tissues other than the brain.

Processing of the Egg-laying Peptide Precursors

The precursors of neuropeptides undergo a variety of post-translational modifications resulting in biologically active peptides that are released by exocytosis. The hydrophobic signal sequence is removed as the nascent precursor enters the lumen of the endoplasmic reticulum. The prohormone is then transported to the Golgi apparatus, where glycosylation, sulphation and packaging into secretory granules takes place. The bioactive domains on prohormones most frequently are flanked by basic amino acid residues, which serve as proteolytic processing sites. Processing of the prohormones involves a number of enzymes, such as endopeptidases, exopeptidases and non-proteolytic enzymes which modify the N- or C-terminus of the peptide. The processing of the ELH precursor in the BCs and of the peptide A/A' and B/B' precursors in the atrial gland of *Aplysia* are studied in detail.

The processing of the ELH prohormone in the BCs shows some unique features. The ELH prohormone is cleaved at eight sites, which results in nine peptide products, some of which are further modified by amidation or proteolytic trimming of the N- or C-terminal ends (Figure 15) (Newcomb and

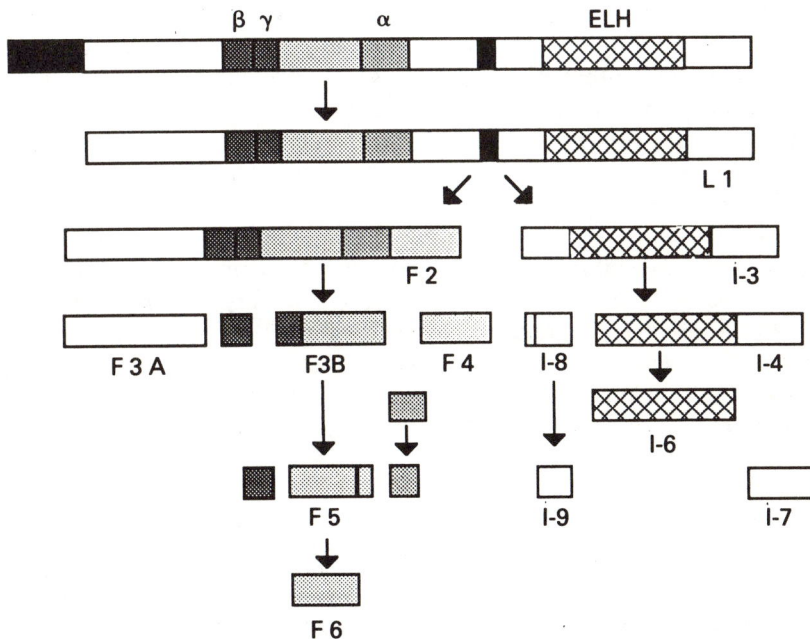

Figure 15 Proteolytic processing of the ELH prohormone in the BCs of *A. californica*. The N-terminally located large black area represents the signal sequence. Small vertical bars represent the endoproteolytical cleavage sites. The first cleavage occurs at the tetrabasic sequence ArgArgLysArg, separating the precursor into N- and C-terminal fragments (F-2 and I-3), which are further processed as shown. Modified after Fisher *et al.* (1988)

Scheller, 1987; Newcomb *et al.*, 1988). The first endoproteolytic cleavage occurs at a site consisting of four consecutive basic residues. The C-terminal region of the precursor is then rapidly further processed to yield three peptides including ELH. The N-terminal intermediate is processed more slowly, yielding three physiologically active peptides, the α-, β- and γ-BCPs, together with a number of other peptides. The peptides C-terminal to the first cleavage, including ELH, are present at much higher levels, 3–8-fold greater than the N-terminal cleavage products, including the BCPs. The reason for this phenomenon is not well understood. There is some evidence suggesting that the first cleavage of the ELH prohormone occurs in the Golgi apparatus (Fisher *et al.*, 1988). Next, via an unknown mechanism, sorting takes place and vesicles bud off the trans Golgi, containing either the C-terminal intermediate, the N-terminal intermediate, or both. Vesicles containing the C-terminal peptides are transported to the BC axon terminals in the neurohaemal area in much larger quantities than vesicles containing the N-terminal peptides. Also, in the BC soma large, BCP-containing vesicles are present, the biogenesis of which is still a mystery. These vesicles are not seen in the axon terminals. The differential vesiculation and transport is significant in the context of the physiological functions of the peptides. ELH functions largely as a circulatory hormone, whereas the BCPs are thought to have autocrine actions on the BCs and in addition have local actions on abdominal ganglion neurons (Rothman *et al.*, 1983; Kauer *et al.*, 1987) and thus are not released into the circulatory system in large quantities. The CDCH precursors of *Lymnaea* are also processed via intermediates, and quantification of peptide amounts, together with immunocytochemistry, suggests that in the CDCs also differential packaging and transport occurs.

The processing of the egg-laying peptide precursors in the atrial gland of *A. californica* has been investigated in considerable detail (Nagle *et al.*, 1988; review of Nagle *et al.*, 1989). In Figure 16 a summary of the processing of three prohormones, the peptide A/A' and B' precursors, is presented. No products of a peptide B precursor have as yet been detected. Processing occurs via intermediates, and end-products include peptides A/A' and B and various complexes of ELH-related and acidic peptide-related peptides.

Figure 16 (*opposite*)   Proteolytic processing of the egg-laying peptide precursors in the atrial gland of *A. californica*. Several intermediates are formed, which are further processed as shown. End products include the nominal peptides and various complexes of ELH-related and acidic peptide-related peptides, which are produced by formation of disulphide bonds (S—S) and various degrees of processing of the C- and N-terminals of the ELH-related peptide. Peptide purification and sequencing has as yet not demonstrated processing of the peptide B prohormone. Peptides derived from the peptide A' prohormone are very similar to those derived from the peptide A prohormone. Homologous peptide domains are represented by similar shading. Vertical black bars represent the endoproteolytic cleavage sites. SS, signal sequence; NTP, N-terminal peptide; PEP, peptide; ELH, egg-laying hormone-related peptide;

A PRECURSOR

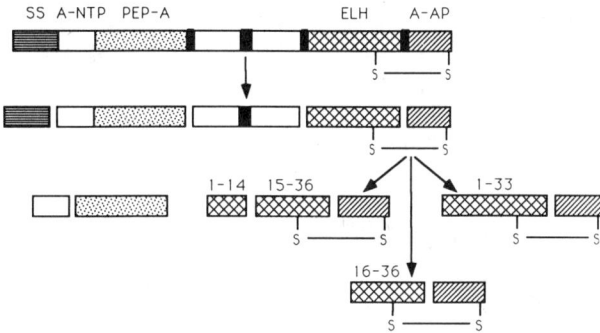

A' PRECURSOR

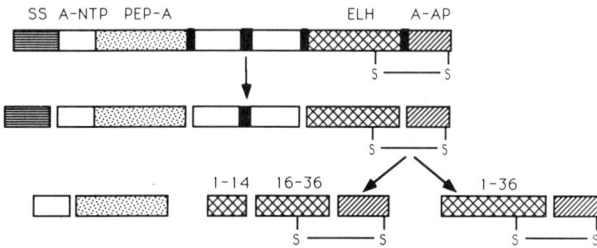

B PRECURSOR

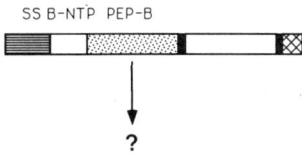

B' PRECURSOR

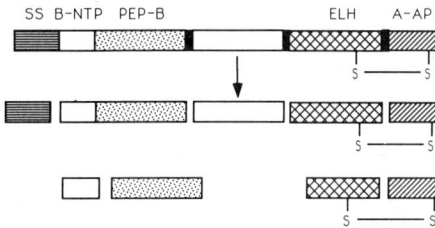

AP, acidic peptide-related peptide; numbers above bars relate to amino acid positions in the peptides. Modified after Nagle *et al.* (1989)

Discharges, Exocytosis and Peptide Release

Electrophysiologically the CDCs and BCs are characterized by three different states of excitability—the active, inhibited and resting state (Kits, 1980). Their occurrence is closely related to the egg-laying cycle (Figure 17). The central event in egg-laying is a long-lasting period of electrical activity (discharge) of the cells (Figure 18). *In vivo* recordings using chronically

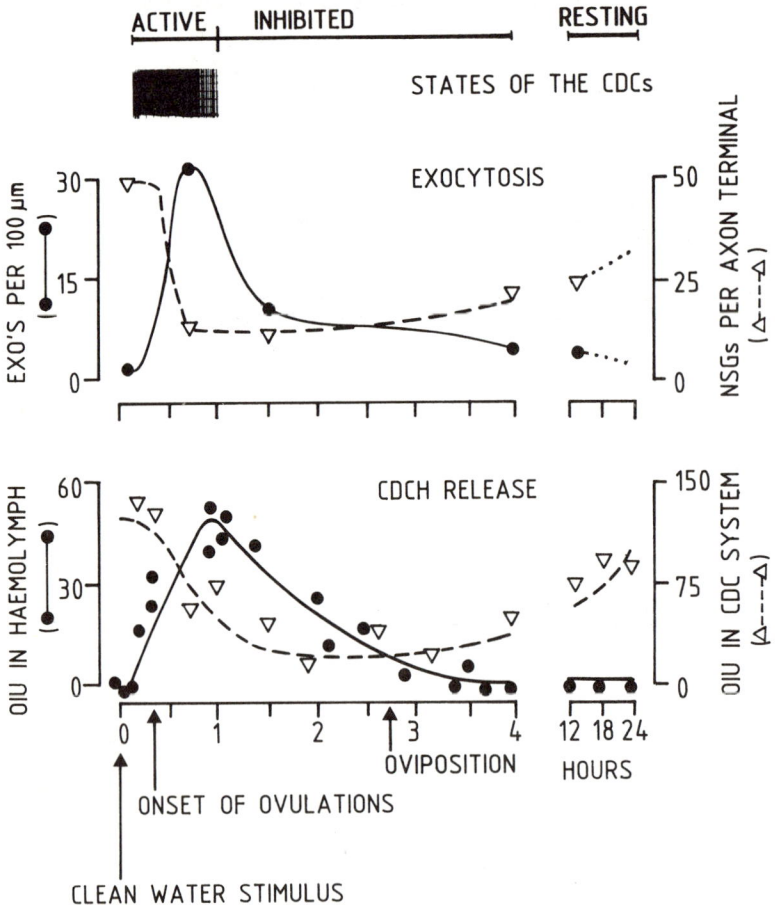

Figure 17 Discharge, exocytosis, CDCH release and egg laying in *L. stagnalis.* Animals were induced to lay egg masses by application of the clean water stimulus. Top, the physiological cycle of the CDCs (active, inhibited and resting state). Middle part, morphometry of CDC axon terminals. Storage of neurosecretory granules, expressed as numbers of granules (NSG) per axon terminal profile; release of granule contents expressed as numbers of exocytoses (EXO's) per outline of the COM (100 μM). Bottom, CDCH titres in the blood and CDCH contents of the CDC system, expressed in ovulation inducing units (OIU). (1 OIU is the threshold dose for the induction of ovulation)

implanted cuff- and fine wire electrodes on CDCs and BCs have revealed that discharges always precede spontaneous egg-laying (e.g. Ter Maat *et al.*, 1986). The CDC discharges last about 60 min, whereas BC discharges last considerably shorter (about 20 min). During the discharge all cells of the network are simultaneously active. Synchrony between the cells of a network

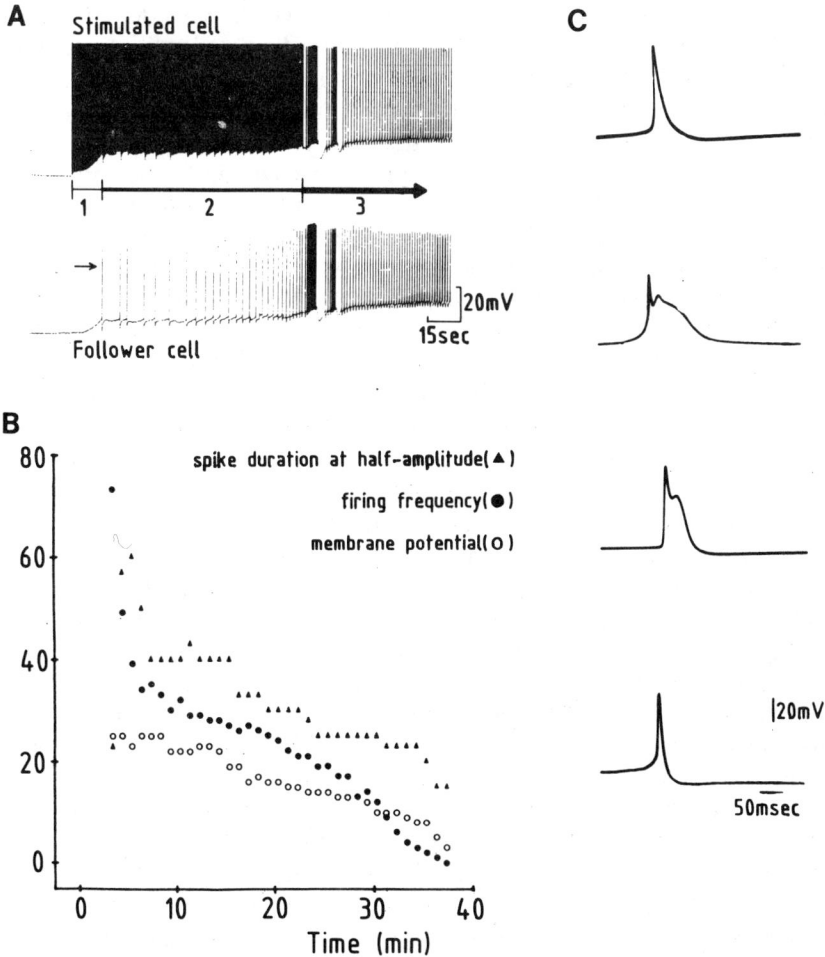

Figure 18 Characteristics of the CDC discharge in *L. stagnalis*. A: Activation of all CDCs by stimulation of one cell of the system. After an initial depolarization (1), other CDCs are recruited (note the spikes in the follower cell), and additional spikes are fired with increasing frequency (2) until stimulation can be stopped and the afterdischarge develops (3). B: Time courses of spike width, firing frequency and membrane potential. C: Shapes of spikes in resting and active states. From top to bottom: action potentials in resting state, after 1 and after 5 min following the onset of the afterdischarge and near the end of the afterdischarge. Note the considerable broadening during the active state, which is due to an additional slow Ca/Na-component. Courtesy Dr Kits

is achieved through electrotonic connections (Kaczmarek *et al.*, 1979; de Vlieger *et al.*, 1980). In the laboratory, discharges can be triggered by environmental conditions that are favourable for survival of offspring, such as clean water, optimal temperature and high oxygen content (Ter Maat *et al.*, 1983a,b). First and second messengers, as well as autotransmission, play a role in generating discharges. First-messenger regulation of the CDCs involves a biphasic response to acetylcholine, which is mediated through nicotinic and muscarinic acetylcholine receptors. *In vitro* studies have shown that there is an initial transient depolarization and a late hyperpolarization (Ter Maat *et al.*, 1983a). The initial response may play a role in the initiation of the CDC discharge. The hyperpolarizing response considerably decreases the excitability of the CDCs and thus prevents CDC discharge activity and egg-laying. It probably plays a role in interrupting egg-mass production during escape behaviour of the animal—e.g. when it is attacked by predators. The effects of the molluscan tetrapeptide, FMRFamide, on the CDCs have been studied in detail (Brussaard *et al.*, 1988). This peptide has a powerful dual inhibitory action consisting of a transient hyperpolarizing response and a suppression of the excitability of the cells. Anti-FMRFamide positive varicosities and axons close to the CDC somata, axons and axon terminals in the neurohaemal area were demonstrated immunocytochemically.

The way in which a discharge is triggered can be viewed as a two-stage process. An external stimulus is relayed to the system and excites (a subset of) the peptidergic network sufficiently to trigger spikes and hence the release of autotransmitters. The next stage is one of amplification. As a result of excitatory action of the autotransmitters, all cells constituting the network are depolarized until maximum excitation is achieved (Brussaard *et al.*, 1990). In this respect, it is interesting to note that the hormonal output of the CDC system during the discharge is as high as 50 times the threshold dose of CDCH for the triggering of egg-laying in *Lymnaea* (Figure 17) (Geraerts *et al.*, 1984). Thus, this positive feedback mechanism ensures the maximum output of the system once triggered.

Autotransmitters are released by the CDCs upon depolarization of the cells (Ter Maat *et al.*, 1987; Brussaard *et al.*, 1990). It has been demonstrated that a specific combination of four peptides is necessary and sufficient to elicit the CDC discharge (Brussaard *et al.*, 1990). These peptides—CDCH, α-CDCP and two peptides derived from α-CDCP—are encoded by the *CDCH I* gene and partly by the *CDCH II* gene. The CDCs offer the first example of an excitatory feedback mechanism employing peptides to build up their characteristic firing pattern. Similar mechanisms might apply to functionally related systems, such as the BCs in *Aplysia* and the oxytocin and vasopresin cells in vertebrates. The biochemical mechanisms underlying CDC and BC discharges involve the phosphorylation of proteins, both enzymes and ionic channels. Several second messengers, such as cAMP, calcium, phorbol esters and pH, appear to be involved and the reader is referred to the review of Geraerts *et al.* (1988a) for a more detailed discussion of this topic.

There is a close relationship between electrical activity, exocytosis, and release of peptides by CDCs or BCs (Ter Maat *et al.*, 1983a; Geraerts *et al.*, 1984; Roubos, 1984). This is particularly clear from experiments with *L. stagnalis*, in which the animals were induced to lay eggs with the help of the clean water stimulus. The onset of the CDC discharge precedes the appearance of CDCH in the blood and, furthermore, ovulations do not begin until the hormone has appeared in the blood (Figure 17). Release of CDCH takes place almost exclusively during the CDC discharge and is accompanied by a decrease in the CDCH contents of the CDC system. These phenomena are closely paralleled by an enormous increase of exocytosis profiles in CDC terminals of the neurohaemal area in the COM during the CDC discharge. *In vitro* experiments have shown that during a discharge of an isolated CDC system (Geraerts and Hogenes, 1985) or an isolated BC cluster (Stuart *et al.*, 1980), prelabelled with radioactive amino acids, various different peptides are released that are encoded by the egg-laying peptide genes.

Role of the CDC and BC Peptides in the Control of Egg-laying

The onset of the discharge marks the start of egg-laying behaviour. The egg-laying behaviour comprises both internal (covert) and externally observable (overt) behaviours. The covert behaviours relate to egg-mass formation and the overt behaviours consist of a number of action patterns that serve to prepare the substrate for egg-mass deposition. The covert and overt behaviours are similar (though not identical) in *Lymnaea* and *Aplysia*, and will be briefly described for *Lymnaea*. The reader is referred to Geraerts *et al.* (1988a) for a summary of the *Aplysia* egg-laying behaviours.

In *Lymnaea*, 100–200 oocytes are released within 5–10 min after the start of the CDC discharge and the subsequent appearance of the ovulation hormone in the blood. The oocytes are fertilized and packaged one by one into eggs and subsequently into an egg mass (cf. Figure 7), which appears on the substrate about 2 h following the onset of the discharge. The overt egg-laying behaviour is illustrated in Figure 19. Its onset is characterized by a cessation of locomotion and a period during which the animal retains a fixed posture with the shell drawn over the anterior head-foot and tentacles drooping (the 'resting' phase). After about 60 min the animal starts crawling about, very slowly, along a tortuous path such that it virtually remains in the same place. At this point the animal cleans the surface of the substrate with rasping movements of the buccal mass, exactly where the egg mass is to be deposited. This 'turning' phase is followed by the actual deposition of the egg mass and by 'inspection' of the egg mass. Thus, overt egg-laying behaviour in *Lymnaea* is a rather complex sequence of behavioural acts that involve a variety of command and motor systems. The effects of CDC peptides on these systems and on the reproductive tract have been studied in quite some detail,

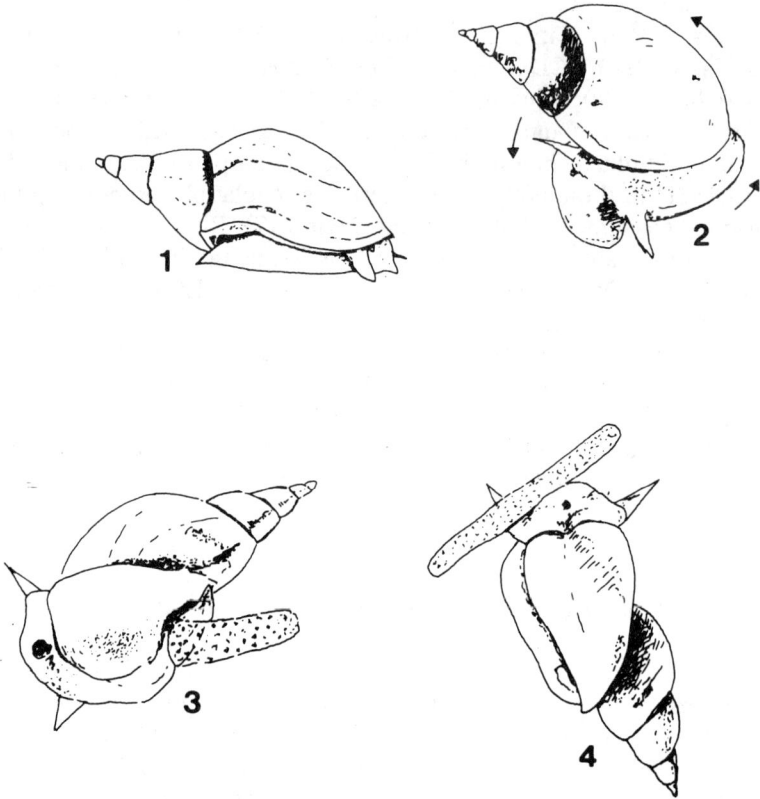

.**Figure 19**   Overt egg-laying behaviour of *L. stagnalis*. Postures during the four phases of egg-laying behaviour: 1, resting; 2, turning; 3, deposition of the egg mass; 4, inspection

and our present knowledge of the organization of egg-laying in *Lymnaea* is summarized in Figure 20.

The unpaired Ring Neuron of the right cerebral ganglion of *Lymnaea* deserves special attention, because it plays a crucial role in egg-laying behaviour. The Ring Neuron provides a direct pathway from the CDCs to the musculature involved in the early phase of egg-laying. This neuron projects towards the pedal ganglia where it shows extensive branching and traverses the pedal commissure, thus completing a ring (Figure 21; Jansen and Bos, 1984). Some of the motor neurons that innervate the columellar muscle, which causes the movements of the shell, receive excitatory input and others inhibitory input from the Ring Neuron (Jansen and Ter Maat, 1985). The CDC discharge increases the firing rate of the Ring Neuron. This effect has a latency of seconds, and it may last as long as the CDC discharge (Jansen and Bos, 1984). It seems very likely that these responses are the result of local actions of CDC peptides, probably mediated via nonsynaptic (paracrine)

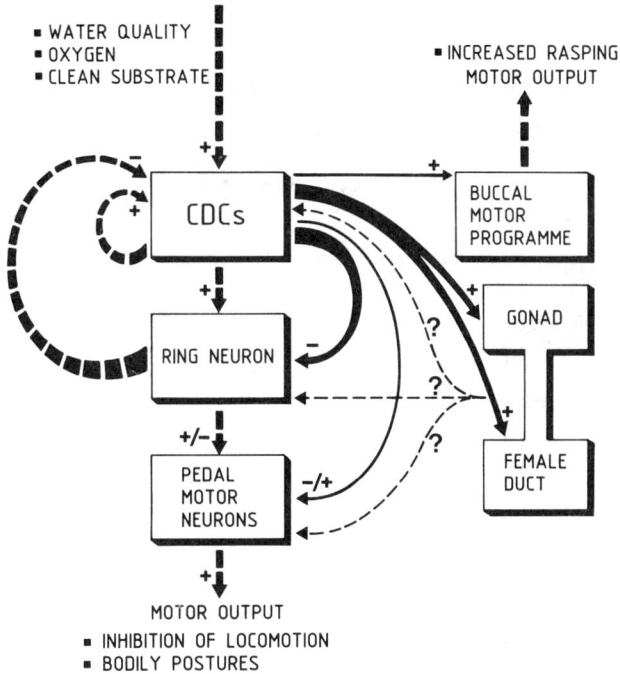

Figure 20 Scheme summarizing the organization of egg-laying in *Lymnaea*. External known stimuli trigger the CDC discharge. Autoexcitation leads to maximal output of the CDC system and hence to ovulation. There is an immediate excitation of the Ring Neuron, which in turn affects the firing of pedal motor neurons. In addition, there are hormonal effects on the Ring Neuron and on motor neurons in both pedal and buccal ganglia. The activities of the motor neurons can explain the elevated rate of rasping and the shell forward position, which are characteristic of egg-laying. Heavily dashed arrow, neuronal pathway within the brain; solid arrow, blood-borne; lightly dashed arrow, presumed neuronal or hormonal pathway

release of material from the collateral system in the inner compartment of the COM (see p. 263). As the excitation of the Ring Neuron lasts as long as the CDC discharge, it is sufficient to explain the first part of the egg-laying behaviour (the 'resting' phase). Thus, *Lymnaea* provides a neural analogue for parts of the egg-laying behaviour, in that within the brain a pathway is present that relays the activity of the CDCs through the Ring Neuron to motor neurons innervating the columellar muscle and probably also the muscle systems involved in locomotion. BC afterdischarges also affect the activities of a variety of neurons in the CNS of *Aplysia*—in particular, in the abdominal ganglion (Mayeri *et al.*, 1979a,b; Brownell, 1983; Rothman *et al.*, 1983), and it is thought that the effects will be reflected in behaviour. Notably, the inhibition of the inking motor neurons predicts that the inking reflex is altered during egg-laying. Likewise, since the firing patterns of neuron R15 are affected, it is thought that osmoregulation and circulatory

EGG-LAYING

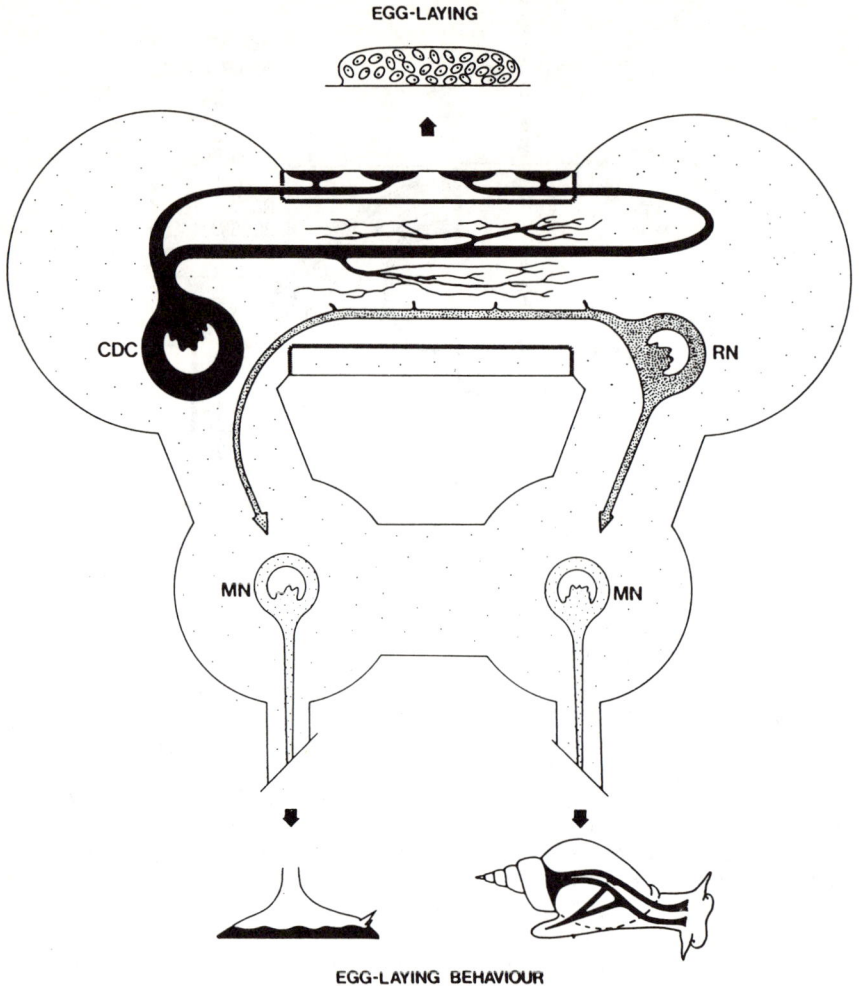

EGG-LAYING BEHAVIOUR

Figure 21 Tentative scheme of the role of neurohormonal and nonsynaptic release of peptides from the CDC neurohaemal and collateral systems in the control of egg-laying behaviour in *L. stagnalis*. The peptides are released in the circulatory system to act on peripheral and central targets. In addition, the peptides are released in intercellular spaces in the inner compartment of the COM and influence the activities of the Ring Neuron (RN). The Ring Neuron in turn modulates the activities of motor neurons (MN) in the pedal ganglia controlling muscle systems involved in the control of movement and of shell position

regulation are altered, and because the L10 neuronal activities are changed, it is hypothesized that the heart rate is influenced. Furthermore, visceromotor behaviours such as gill and siphon contractions are affected by BC discharges. ELH and α-BCP seem to account for most of the observed effects. These peptides exert their effects by nonsynaptic transmission (Mayeri *et al.*, 1979a,b).

3. Genes Encoding Insulin-related Peptides Involved in the Control of Growth and Associated Processes in Lymnaea

Animal growth is characterized by an increase in dry weight of the organic material (mainly protein) of the body. Body growth and body structure are highly interrelated and the organs—in particular, the skeleton—grow in proportion to the body as a whole. In vertebrates this is achieved by an intricate interaction of many hormones—e.g. growth hormone, prolactin, thyroid hormones, androgens, insulin and insulin-like growth factors (IGFs I and II). In the next subsection we shall review our knowledge of the neuroendocrine regulation of growth by the light-green cells (LGCs) in *Lymnaea*. Next we focus on the genes that code for the insulin-related peptides that are released by the LGCs.

LGCs and the Control of Body Growth

In molluscs neuroendocrine centres are involved in the regulation of body growth (see reviews of Joosse, 1988; Geraerts *et al.*, 1988b). This has been studied in detail in *L. stagnalis*, where the LGCs regulate the growth of the soft body parts and the shell. The LGCs are giant neurons (diameter 90 μm), which are located in the cerebral ganglia in two paired groups with together about 200 cells (Figure 22). They use the periphery of the long median lip nerves as their neurohaemal area (Joosse, 1964; Wendelaar Bonga, 1970). The LGCs show all the characteristics of protein-synthesizing cells, with elaborate stacks of endoplasmic reticulum, many active Golgi apparatus, numerous neurosecretory granules and exocytosis profiles, typical of peptidergic (neuroendocrine) cells.

The experimental proof that the LGCs are involved in the control of growth of *Lymnaea* comes from classical endocrinological extirpation and implantation experiments. Cauterization of the LGCs of rapidly growing juvenile snails results in a markedly retarded body growth, which can be restored by implantation of cerebral ganglia containing the LGCs (Figure 23; Geraerts, 1976a). The LGCs affect also various aspects of the metabolism related to growth (Geraerts *et al.*, 1988b; reviewed in Joosse, 1988). Thus, factors of the LGCs control the breakdown of glycogen stores, and stimulate the activity of ornithine decarboxylase, an enzyme which shows high levels of activity in growing animal tissues. Moreover, the LGCs produce a peptide stimulating the uptake of sodium through the integument. The LGCs further stimulate various processes of shell growth: formation of the periostracum, the proteinaceous component of the shell; calcium and bicarbonate incorporation into the shell edge; and the maintenance of high concentrations of a calcium-binding protein, important for cellular calcium transport in the mantle edge.

In *Lymnaea* a second centre involved in growth control is located in the

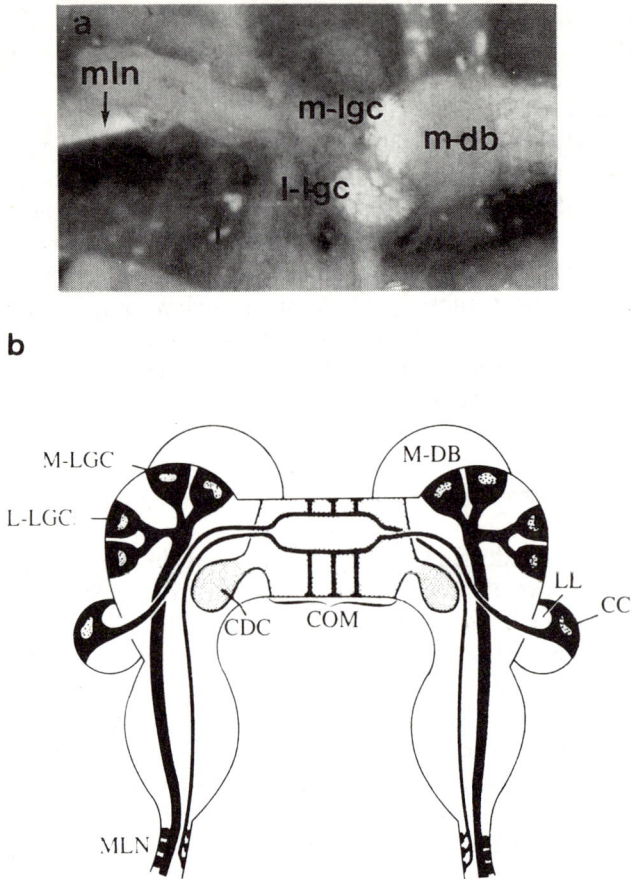

Figure 22 Location and anatomical organization of the LGC system in the cerebral ganglia of *L. stagnalis*. a: Dorsal view of the left cerebral ganglion *in situ*. The mediodorsal cluster of the LGCs (m-lgc) and the laterodorsal cluster (l-lgc) are clearly visible. Each cluster consists of about 50 large LGC cell bodies. A part of the left median lip nerve (mln) can also be seen. The periphery of the mln serves as the neurohaemal area of the LGCs. m-db, the female gonadotropin-producing mediodorsal bodies. b: Schematic representation of the anatomical organization of the LGC system, based on Lucifer Yellow fillings (Benjamin *et al.* (1976) and light and electron microscopy (Wendelaar Bonga, 1970; van Minnen *et al.*, 1980). Notice the intricate axonal topology of the canopy cells (CC) in the lateral lobes (LL), which strongly suggests that the CC control the activities of the other LGCs

lateral lobes (Figure 22). Cauterization of the lobes results in giant growth, whereas reimplantation of cerebral ganglia with lateral lobes restores normal growth (Figure 23; Geraerts, 1976b). These effects of the lateral lobes are mediated via changes of the synthetic activities of the LGCs (Geraerts, 1976b). The lobes exert also strong hormonal effects on glycogen metabolism, probably via the LGCs. This is based on the observation that removal of the

A

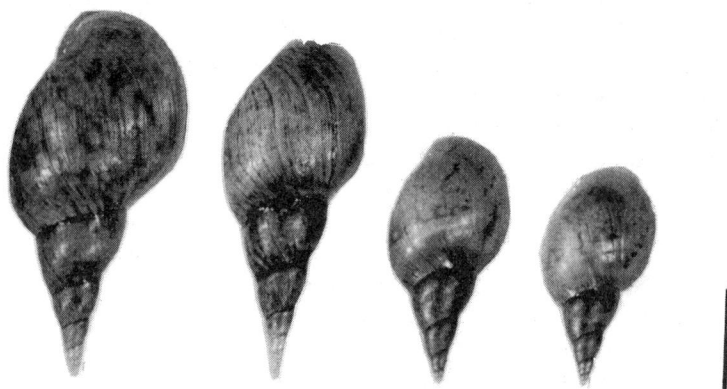

B

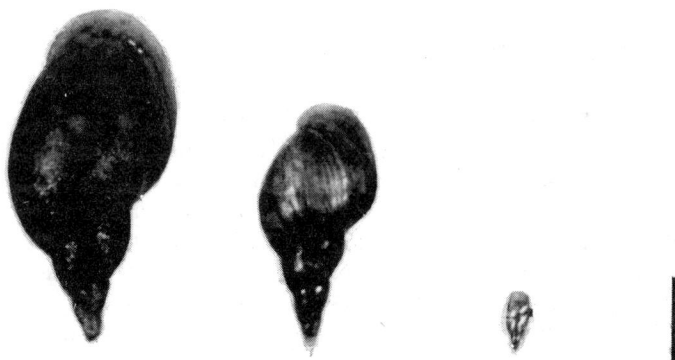

Figure 23   The effects of the LGCs and lateral lobes on body growth of *L. stagnalis*. A: The effects of the LGCs. From right to left: size of the snails at the onset of the cauterization and reimplantation experiments; snails deprived of the LGCs at the end of the experiment, 42 days after cauterization; cauterized snails implanted with cerebral ganglia containing the LGCs; sham-operated control snails. B: The effects of the lateral lobes. From right to left: size of the snails at the beginning of the experiment; sham-operated controls (and cauterized snails reimplanted with lateral lobes); giant snails without lateral lobes. Vertical bars represent 1 cm

lobes results in a low glycogen content of almost all tissues, which could be restored by implantation of the lobes (Geraerts *et al.*, 1988b; Joosse, 1988). An interesting observation is that in each lobe an ectopic LGC, the canopy cell, is located. The axons of the canopy cells show an intricate branching pattern and run very close to axons coming from the clusters of LGCs in the cerebral ganglia (Figure 22) (Benjamin *et al.*, 1976; van Minnen *et al.*, 1980). This suggests that the canopy cells are specialized LGCs that transmit regulatory stimuli to the LGC clusters in the cerebral ganglia.

The peptide messengers produced by the LGCs have been identified using the methodologies of molecular biology and peptide chemistry. The LGCs produce at least four insulin-related peptides, called molluscan insulin-related peptides (MIPs), each of which is thought to control a different aspect of growth and associated processes in *Lymnaea* (Smit *et al.*, 1988; A. B. Smit, unpublished results). The MIPs possess the basic three-dimensional configuration, with disulphide bridges, a hydrophobic core, α-helices and sharp turns of the peptide chains, typical of other members of the insulin superfamily—i.e. the insulins, IGFs and relaxins of the vertebrates (Blundell and Wood, 1975; Blundell and Humbel, 1980; Froesch *et al.*, 1985; Steiner *et al.*, 1985), the bombyxins of the insects (Kawakami *et al.*, 1989) and the insulin-related peptide of the sponges (Robitzki *et al.*, 1989). The organization, expression and evolutionary aspects of the MIPs and the gene family encoding them are reviewed in the subsections that follow.

The Organization of the *MIP* Gene Family

Using a plus/minus screening strategy, four LGC-specific cDNA clones encoding the precursors of MIPs I, II, III and V were identified. The corresponding *MIP I, II, III* and *V* genes were isolated with the help of radioactive probes made from the MIP cDNAs and from synthetic gene-specific oligonucleotide sequences derived from the cDNAs. Two more genes, the *MIP IV* and *VI* genes, were identified in the course of the genomic analysis (Smit *et al.*, 1988; A. B. Smit, unpublished results). Highly interesting features of the organization of the *MIP* genes were revealed when the *MIP* genes were compared with the vertebrate insulin genes—e.g. the human insulin gene (Figure 24). All *MIP* genes show the overall structure typical of the insulin genes, with three exons interspaced by two introns. The exons code for similar domains of the precursors in both the *MIP* genes and *insulin* genes. The positions of the introns are also conserved, one within the sequence coding for the mRNA leader region and the other interrupting the C peptide coding region. The six *MIP* genes are present in the genome as three couples of closely linked genes, which are transcribed in the same direction. They represent all homologous members of the *MIP* gene family in the *Lymnaea* genome, as indicated by genomic Southern blotting and restriction analysis of separate genomic clones. The family may, however,

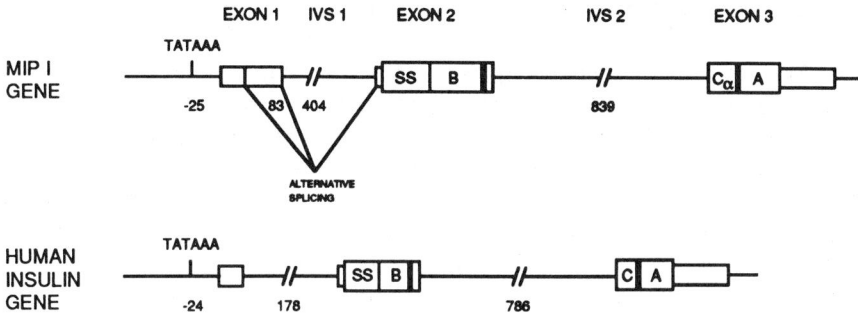

Figure 24 Schematic representation of the *MIP I* gene and the human insulin gene. The *MIP* genes *II–VI* have a similar organization. Indicated are the exons and the intervening sequences (IVSs). SS, signal sequence; B, B chain; A, A chain; Cα, Cα peptide; C, C peptide. Goldberg–Hogness box, TATAAA. Numbers refer to nucleotide length. The alternative splicing in exon 1 of the *MIP I* gene is also indicated

include additional members with undetectably low homology to the identified *MIP* genes. The genomic organization of the *MIP* gene family differs markedly from that of the *bombyxin* gene family (Kawakami *et al.*, 1989). *Bombyxin* genes do not contain introns and are arranged as transcription units of paired genes with opposite orientation.

A TATA box is present at the expected position (approx. −25) in the 5′-region of the *MIP I, II, III* and *V* genes. By contrast, in both the *MIP IV* and *VI* genes, a putative TATA box is located further upstream (at position −178). Two transcripts, which differ in their leader sequence by 83 nucleotides, can be generated from the *MIP I* gene by alternative splicing. The stretches of the 5′-flanking regions near the transcription initiation sites of the *MIP I* and *II* genes are quite similar, but sequence divergence becomes gradually stronger further upstream. The 5′-flanking regions of the *MIP II* and *V* genes are also very similar, except for a few interspersed stretches of pronounced sequence divergence. By contrast, the 5′-flanking region of the *MIP III* gene has no sequence resemblance to those of other *MIP* genes. The upstream regions, the signal peptide, and the first amino acids of the B chain in the *MIP IV* and *VI* genes are very similar to each other. Also, the upstream regions do not resemble those of other *MIP* genes. In the *MIP* genes, differences in the DNA sequences upstream to transcription initiation may be important in the evolution of the differential, stimulus-inducible expression pattern of the *MIP* genes in the LGCs (see page 292). The *MIP VI* gene probably is a pseudogene, because an insertion of seven nucleotides in exon 2 causes a shift of the reading frame resulting in a stop codon at the end of exon 2.

Biosynthesis and Structure of the MIPs and Their Precursors

The MIP precursors encoded by the completely characterized *MIP I, II, III* and *V* genes represent preproinsulin-related proteins containing a signal sequence, A and B chains and a connecting C peptide, as well as dibasic amino acid processing sites for the generation of MIPs and C peptides (Figure 25). Pulse-label and pulse-chase analysis of newly synthesized proteins and peptides in the LGC system *in vitro* showed that putative MIP precursors were present in the LGC somata after a 20 min pulse with radioactive cysteine (Figure 26). The synthesis and subsequent conversion of the proMIPs to end-products probably is confined to the LGC somata (and perhaps the proximal parts of the LGC axons that were not studied in these experiments). The MIPs and C peptides were transported to the LGC axon terminals in the median lip nerves, where they appeared between 1.5 h and 6 h following the pulse period. Sequencing of the material purified from the median lip nerves showed that various MIPs were present as encoded on the genes. However, the A and B chains of MIPs I, II and V appeared to be N-terminally blocked (pyroglutamate). The B chain N-terminus of MIP III is two amino acids longer than predicted by the gene work. Moreover, the two C-terminal amino acids of all B chains are post-translationally removed (Figure 27) (K. W. Li, unpublished results). In conclusion, these data indicate that preproMIPs are processed to form mature 2-chain MIP molecules, that together with the various C peptides are stored in the LGC axon terminals. Comparison of MIPs I, II, III and V revealed that they are homologous with only about 45–75% of the amino-acid residues being identical among them throughout the A and B chains (Figure 27). However, all MIPs share the amino acids that

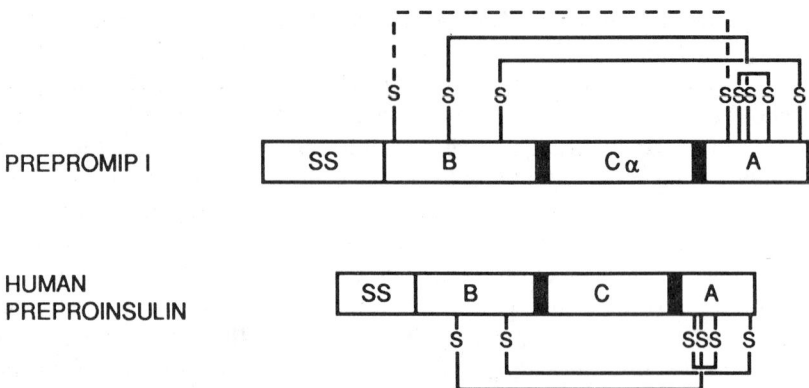

Figure 25 Schematic representation of the precursors of MIP I and human insulin. The precursors are aligned on the positions of the cysteine residues involved in the interchain disulphide bridges in the B chain domains. SS, signal sequence; B, B chain; A, A chain; Cα, Cα peptide; C, C peptide; S, position of cysteine residue. The extra putative disulphide bridge in MIP I is indicated by a dotted line, others by solid lines. Vertical black bars indicate proteolytic cleavage sites

LGC SOMATA   LGC AXON TERMINALS

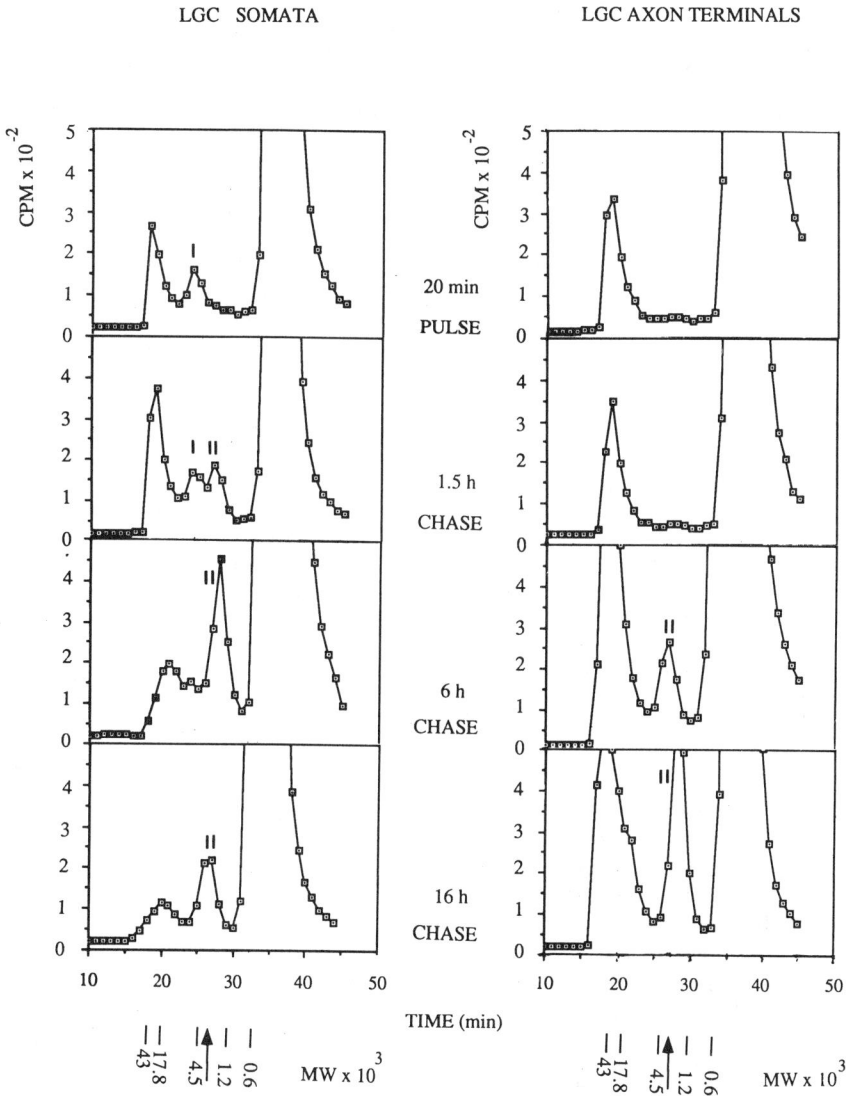

Figure 26 High-performance gel permeation radiograms of newly synthesized peptides in the LGC system of *L. stagnalis*. LGC systems (30 per time period) were pulse-labelled for 20 min in Ringer containing [^{35}S]cysteine and chased in Ringer containing non-radioactive cysteine. LGC somata and lip nerves were dissected separately. Peak I represents proMIPs and peak II the MIPs. Several molecular weight markers were run concurrently (in kD, indicated at the bottom of the figure). The elution of bovine insulin (molecular weight approximately 6.5 kD) is indicated by an arrow. Insulins, and for that matter MIPs, and their precursors, show a slightly aberrant elution profile, taking into consideration their molecular weight, and elute later, due to their globular structure. CPM, counts per minute

A Chains

		-4	-3	-2	-1	1	2	3	4	5	6	7	8	9	10	11	12	13	14	15	16	17	18	19	20	21	
Insulin(-related)																											
MIP I	Lymnaea	pQ	G	T	T	N	I	I	V	C	E	C	C	M	K	P	C	T	L	S	E	L	R	Q	Y	C	P
MIP II	Lymnaea	pQ	R	T	T	N	L	V	C	E	C	C	F	N	Y	C	T	P	D	V	V	R	K	Y	C	Y	
MIP III	Lymnaea	E	S	R	P	N	I	V	C	E	C	C	Y	N	Q	C	T	V	D	D	V	L	E	Y	C	I	
MIP V	Lymnaea	pQ	R	T	T	G	I	V	C	E	C	C	Y	N	V	C	T	V	D	V	L	A	E	Y	C	Y	
Bombyxin II	Bombyx	–	–	–	–	G	I	V	D	E	C	C	L	R	P	C	S	V	D	V	L	L	S	Y	C		
Insulin	Sponge	–	–	–	–	I	I	V	S	G	Q	C	T	S	G	I	C	R	G	S	L	Y	Q	C			
(-related)																											
IGF I	Human	–	–	–	G	I	V	D	E	C	C	F	R	S	C	D	L	R	R	L	E	M	Y	C	A	⋮	
IGF II	Human	–	–	–	G	I	V	E	E	C	C	F	R	S	C	D	L	A	L	L	E	T	Y	C	A	⋮	
Relaxin	Human	R	P	Y	V	A	L	F	E	K	C	C	L	I	G	C	I	R	K	D	I	A	R	L	C	–	
Relaxin	Whale	R	–	M	–	T	L	S	E	K	C	C	Q	V	G	C	I	R	K	D	I	A	R	–	–		
Insulin	Hagfish	–	–	–	G	I	V	E	Q	C	C	H	K	R	C	S	I	Y	N	L	Q	N	Y	C	N		
Insulin	Guinea pig	–	–	–	G	I	V	D	Q	C	C	T	G	I	C	T	R	H	Q	L	Q	S	Y	C	N		
Insulin	Rat I	–	–	–	G	I	V	D	Q	C	C	T	S	I	C	S	L	Y	Q	L	E	N	Y	C	N		
Insulin	Human	–	–	–	G	I	V	E	Q	C	C	T	S	I	C	S	L	Y	Q	L	E	N	Y	C	N		

B Chains

		-12	-11	-10	-9	-8	-7	-6	-5	-4	-3	-2	-1	1	2	3	4	5	6	7	8	9	10	11	12	13	14	15	16	17	18	19	20	21	22	23	24	25	26	27	28	29	30	31
Insulin(-related)																																												
MIP I	Lymnaea	pQ	F	S	–	H	T	C	C	N	I	D	R	R	H	P	R	G	V	L	C	G	S	A	L	A	D	L	V	D	F	A	–	C	S	S	N	Q	P	A	M	V	–	G
MIP II	Lymnaea	–	S	S	–	–	–	–	–	A	Y	L	S	P	H	P	R	G	I	L	C	G	S	N	L	L	A	V	D	F	V	V	C	G	S	N	T	S	S	M	V	–	–	S
MIP III	Lymnaea	Q	T	T	–	H	S	A	C	W	S	T	R	R	P	A	R	H	L	C	G	S	H	L	A	R	T	L	A	Q	W	I	–	C	S	T	Y	T	S	K	V	–	–	–
MIP V	Lymnaea	pQ	F	S	–	–	–	–	–	–	–	–	–	F	V	D	R	H	L	C	G	S	D	L	V	K	R	L	A	D	I	V	C	G	S	R	N	Q	P	A	M	V	–	–
Bombyxin II	Bombyx	–	–	–	–	–	–	–	–	–	–	–	–	Q	P	Q	A	V	H	T	Y	C	G	R	H	L	A	R	T	L	A	D	L	C	W	E	R	G	F	Y	T	M	S	–
Insulin	Sponge	–	–	–	–	–	–	–	–	–	–	–	–	F	V	N	V	H	L	C	G	S	H	L	V	E	A	L	Y	L	V	C	G	E	R	G	F	F	Y	T	P	M	S	–
(-related)																																												
IGF I	Human	–	–	–	–	–	–	–	–	–	–	–	–	G	P	E	T	L	C	G	A	E	L	V	D	A	L	Q	F	V	C	G	D	R	G	F	Y	F	N	K	P	T	G	–
IGF II	Human	–	–	–	–	–	–	–	–	–	–	–	–	A	Y	R	P	S	E	T	L	C	G	G	E	L	V	D	T	L	Q	F	V	C	G	D	R	G	F	Y	F	S	R	P
Relaxin	Human	–	–	–	–	–	A	Y	W	K	D	D	L	K	W	K	D	D	V	I	K	L	C	G	R	E	L	V	R	A	Q	I	A	I	C	G	M	S	T	W	S	K	R	S
Relaxin	Whale	–	–	–	–	–	–	–	–	K	W	S	T	N	D	L	K	K	R	E	L	V	R	A	A	I	D	L	T	A	I	L	V	C	G	V	S	W	G	R	T	A	L	–
Insulin	Hagfish	–	–	T	T	–	–	–	–	–	–	–	–	R	T	T	G	H	L	L	C	G	K	D	L	V	N	A	L	T	I	V	C	G	Q	V	G	F	F	Y	D	P	T	K
Insulin	Guinea pig	–	–	–	–	–	–	–	–	–	–	–	–	F	V	S	R	H	L	C	G	S	N	L	V	E	T	L	Y	S	V	C	Q	D	D	G	F	F	Y	I	P	K	D	–
Insulin	Rat I	–	–	–	–	–	–	–	–	–	–	–	–	F	V	K	Q	H	L	C	G	S	H	L	V	E	A	L	Y	L	V	C	G	E	R	G	F	F	Y	T	P	K	S	–
Insulin	Human	–	–	–	–	–	–	–	–	–	–	–	–	F	V	N	Q	H	L	C	G	S	H	L	V	E	A	L	Y	L	V	C	G	E	R	G	F	F	Y	T	P	K	T	–

are important in adopting the basic insulin configuration. This is apparent when MIPs are compared with other members of the insulin superfamily (Figure 27). In the A and B chains of the MIPs, cysteines are present at positions typical for the insulin superfamily, suggesting that the three characteristic disulphide bridges in the MIP molecules have been conserved. In addition, the important hydrophobic core residues of the globular insulin structure are either conserved as identical residues, or are replaced by residues with an equally hydrophobic character. The only exception is arginine at B15 in MIPs II and V. Also, α-helices, which are present in the A and B chains of vertebrate insulins, can be predicted for the MIPs.

Although the MIPs are two-chain peptides that will adopt the insulin core structure, they cannot be considered genuine insulin molecules. MIPs exhibit strong divergence of surface residues that are important in many functions of the vertebrate insulin molecules (Blundell and Wood, 1975), such as receptor binding, solubility of the molecule, processing of the precursor, and monomer and dimer interactions and hexamer formation. A striking example is the almost complete divergence of the amino acid residues involved in receptor binding, including residues at A1–A5, A8 and B23–26. Thus, it is unlikely that the MIP receptor is of the vertebrate type. Interestingly, these putative receptor binding residues are divergent among MIPs, which suggests either that each MIP binds a different receptor, or alternatively, that various MIPs bind the same receptor with different affinities. Thus, each MIP may fulfil a different function in the control of growth and associated processes in *Lymnaea*. In addition to these differences, MIPs possess features that classify them into a distinct group of the insulin superfamily. Both the A and B chains are N-terminally extended (Figure 27), and the B chain extension contains an extra cysteine at B − 6 that may form a third interchain disulphide bridge with an extra cysteine at A4. Due to these properties, the MIPs are the most complexely folded molecules of the insulin superfamily.

Figure 27 (*opposite*)   Amino acid sequence comparison of MIPs I, II, III and V with those of other insulin(-related) peptides based on both cDNA and peptide-sequencing data. The sequence similarity in the A and B chains of the MIPs ranges from 45% to 75%. The sequence similarity of the MIPs to bombyxin II, sponge insulin-related peptide, and vertebrate insulins, relaxins and IGFs is 20–40%. The sequence similarity among insulins and related peptides from vertebrates is 55–95%. In the MIP A and B chains cysteines are present at positions A6, A7, A11, A20, B7 and B19, an arrangement which is typical for members of the insulin superfamily. Two additional cysteines are present at positions A4 and B − 6. Like the insulins, MIPs have a glycine at B8, but lack glycines at B20 and B23, which are present in most insulins and introduce a sharp turn in the B chain. Most residues of the hydrophobic core of insulin are conserved as hydrophobic in the MIPs, namely A2, A11, A16, A20, B11, B15 and B19, except for Arg at B15 in MIPs II and V. Other hydrophobic residues are identical or conserved: A3, A19, B6, B12 and B18. Residues A1–A5, A8, and B23–B26, which interact with the insulin receptor, are diverged among MIPs. Note that the A and B chains of MIPs I, II and V are blocked N-terminally. The two C-terminal amino acids (which are indicated in the figure) of the B chains in all MIPs are in fact post-translationally removed. Number 1 designates the first residues of the A and B chains of human insulin

Stimulus-induced Differential Expression of *MIP* Genes in the LGCs

Expression of the *MIP I, II, III* and *V* genes in adult animals is entirely restricted to the LGCs, as could be assessed by various methods. Northern blotting experiments showed that MIP I, II, III and V transcripts are only present in the cerebral ganglia of the CNS. No MIP IV and VI transcripts could be identified. Because the *MIP VI* gene probably is a pseudogene, this is not surprising. For the same reason the MIP IV transcript may not have been found. Alternatively, however, *MIP IV* gene transcription may take place under hitherto unknown conditions. The MIP I, II and V specific transcripts each had a length of 650–700 nucleotides. Two MIP III specific transcripts of 800 and 1150 nucleotides were found that are probably generated by the use of two distinct termination signals in the 3'-region of the *MIP III* gene.

Hybridization histochemistry showed that the *MIP I, II, III* and *V* genes are expressed in the LGCs and in the canopy cells of the lateral lobes (Figure 28). No other cell type of the central nervous system showed a positive signal. Unexpectedly, MIP transcripts were also detected in LGC axons. The significance of this phenomenon is not well understood and further experiments addressing this question are in progress. The immunohistochemistry was in agreement with the *in situ* hybridization studies and showed immunostaining of only LGCs and canopy cells. Furthermore, it revealed a complex axonal topology of the LGCs and canopy cells that confirms the dye injections and the ultrastructural studies in all details (cf. Figure 22). To determine the intracellular localization of the (pro)MIPs more precisely, immunogold electron microscopy was performed (Figure 28). Immunogold labelling in the LGCs and canopy cells was observed above neurosecretory granules budding off from the Golgi apparatus, above mature granules in both cell bodies and axon terminals, and over exocytosis profiles in LGC axon terminals. This suggests that proMIPs are packaged into granules in the Golgi apparatus and transported to the axon endings, where the peptides derived from the precursors are released (see also page 295). There is endocrinological evidence that the lateral lobes are involved in the control of the synthesis and release activities of the LGCs and of female gonadotropic centres in the cerebral ganglia (Geraerts, 1976b). Therefore, the canopy cells probably are specialized LGCs that transmit regulatory stimuli to both the LGC clusters and the female gonadotropic centres (cf. Figure 22) of the cerebral ganglia.

Since each MIP may have a different function, we reasoned that physiological conditions with different effects on growth and associated processes in *L. stagnalis* (Geraerts *et al.*, 1988b; Joosse, 1988) might induce a differential pattern of expression of the *MIP* genes in the LGCs. We first investigated the effects of starvation on MIP transcript levels. During starvation growth is arrested and glycogen stores are considerably depleted. Northern blot analysis of MIP II and III transcripts in the LGCs showed that during starvation the MIP II transcript had disappeared completely, while the level

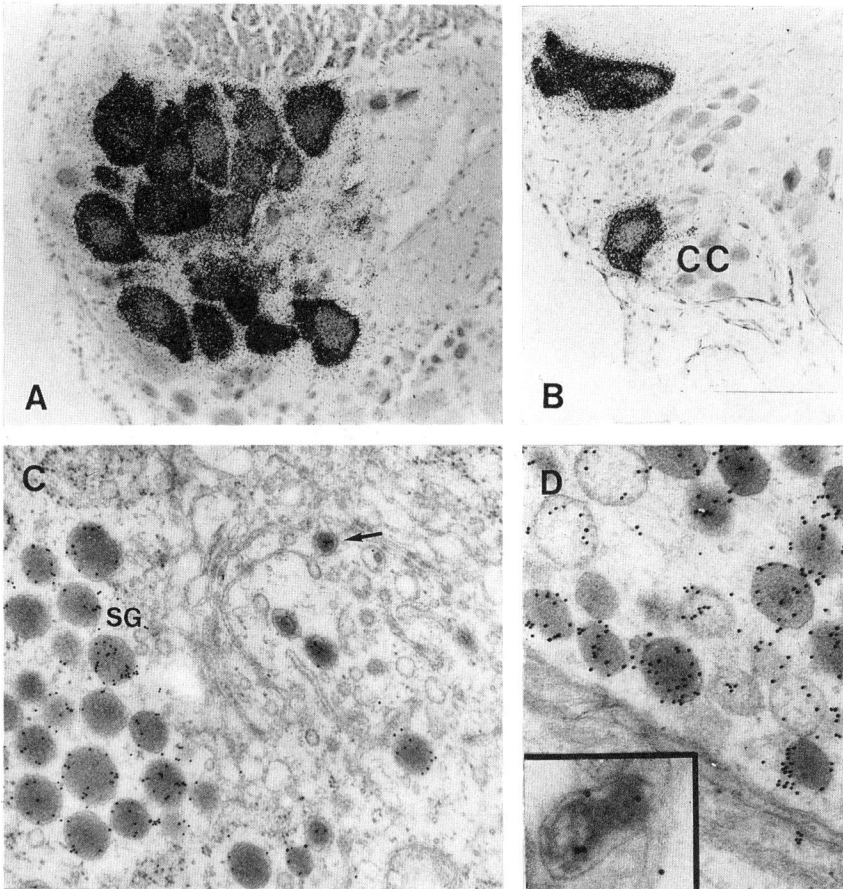

Figure 28 Localization of MIP I mRNA in the CNS of *L. stagnalis*. A: Localization in the LGCs. Shown is a section of the left cerebral ganglion with LGCs. All LGCs display a strong positive signal after hybridization to a MIP I cDNA. ×120. B: The canopy cell (CC) in the lateral lobes shows a strong positive signal by *in situ* hybridization using MIP I cDNA. In the upper part of the figure a positive LGC is seen. ×300. C: Immunogold labelling of the soma of a LGC with antiMIP Cα peptide. A secretory granule associated with a Golgi saccule shows immunoreactivity for antiMIP Cα (arrow). Mature secretory granules (SG) are also positive. ×44 000. D: Immunogold labelling with antiMIP Cα of secretory granules in neurohaemal axon terminals of the LGCs in the median lip nerve. ×57 000. Inset: immunogold labelling of an exocytosis profile of an axon terminal of the LGCs in the periphery of the median lip nerve. Electron-dense granule content released by exocytosis is immunoreactive for antiMIP Cα. ×63 000. Courtesy Drs van Minnen and van Heumen

of the MIP III transcript was severely reduced (Figure 29a). Also, the length of the MIP III transcript was reduced in starved animals, indicating changes in mRNA stability and/or translation efficiency. In a second series of experiments, the effects of extirpation of the lateral lobes, a treatment which causes giant growth and a depletion of glycogen stores, and the effects of a

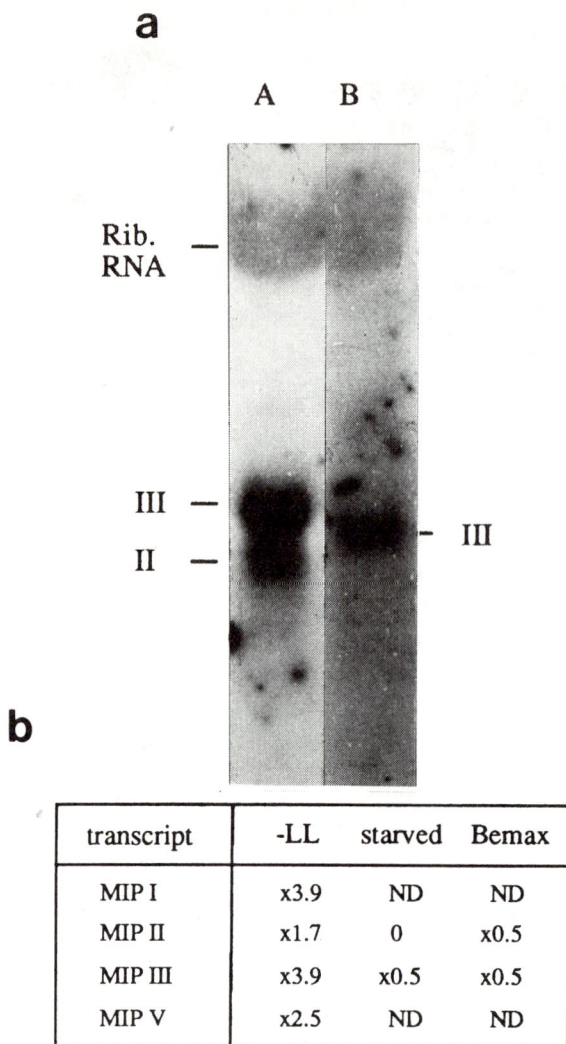

transcript	-LL	starved	Bemax
MIP I	x3.9	ND	ND
MIP II	x1.7	0	x0.5
MIP III	x3.9	x0.5	x0.5
MIP V	x2.5	ND	ND

Figure 29 Stimulus-dependent differential expression of the *MIP I, II, III* and *V* genes. A: Northern blot analysis of MIP II and III transcripts in the LGCs of starved (21 days) animals (lane B) and lettuce-fed controls (lane A). Oligonucleotide probes specific to MIP II and III mRNAs were used. II, MIP II transcript; III, MIP III transcript. Notice the total disappearance of the MIP II transcript and the reduction in length of the MIP III transcript in the starved animals. b: Summary of differential *MIP* gene expression, as determined by quantification of hybridization signals using MIP-specific oligonucleotides on Northern blots. The values indicate times the control level of MIP transcripts. Control animals were fed lettuce *ad libitum*. The hybridization signals were quantified by multiple scanning with an LKB Ultrascan XL densitometer. Animals were treated as indicated. −LL, animals deprived of the lateral lobes. Bemax, animals fed the carbohydrate-rich wheat product Bemax. ND, not determined

carbohydrate-rich diet, which results in an arrest of growth and enormously increased glycogen stores, were studied. The results, which are summarized in Figure 29b, suggest a stimulus-dependent differential pattern of expression of the *MIP* genes in the LGCs.

Electrical Activity and Release of MIPs

Data concerning the electrophysiological characteristics of the LGC system are restricted to *in vitro* experiments on LGCs in the isolated CNS or on dissociated LGCs in primary culture. These *in vitro* studies have shown that the LGC system can act as a site of integration of diverse information. Among the first messengers involved in the regulation of LGC activities are several peptides and amino acids, as well as dopamine and glucose. Only dopamine and glucose responses are studied in some detail. The LGCs of *Lymnaea* display a complicated response to dopamine (de Vlieger *et al.*, 1987). Initially, the LGCs are rendered inexcitable. This is caused by a hyperpolarization, due to the opening of K channels, and by a concomittant reduction of the voltage dependent Ca current. The effect on the K channels is mediated via a D2-like receptor. This initial phase of the response lasts from one to a few minutes and is followed by a slow rise in excitability, during which the cells gradually depolarize. This effect is mediated through a D1-like receptor. Because no effects of dopamine application on intracellular cAMP levels of the LGCs were found, it is unlikely that the responses are mediated through inhibition or stimulation of adenylate cyclase activity, as is the case in the classical vertebrate D2 and D1 receptors. However, an increase in the intracellular levels of cAMP using non-hydrolysable analogues, such as

5 mM

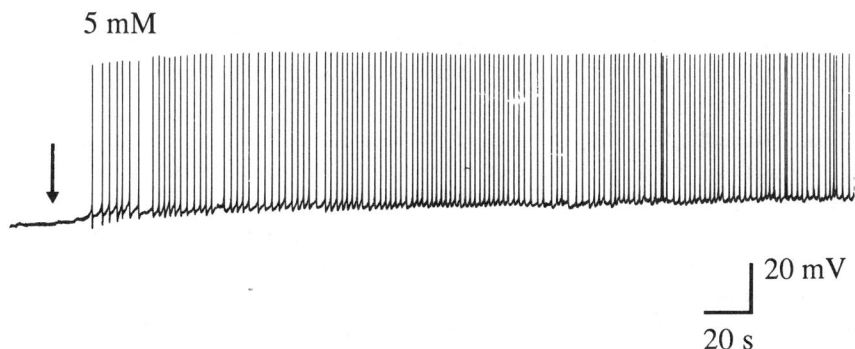

Figure 30 Excitatory effects of glucose on LGCs. D(+)-glucose directly evokes long-lasting spiking activity in the LGCs of cerebral ganglia *in vitro*. Glucose was applied at the arrow. The threshold is 5 mM glucose. The effect is not seen with L-glucose or with other monosaccharides such as galactose, fructose, etc. Courtesy Dr Kits

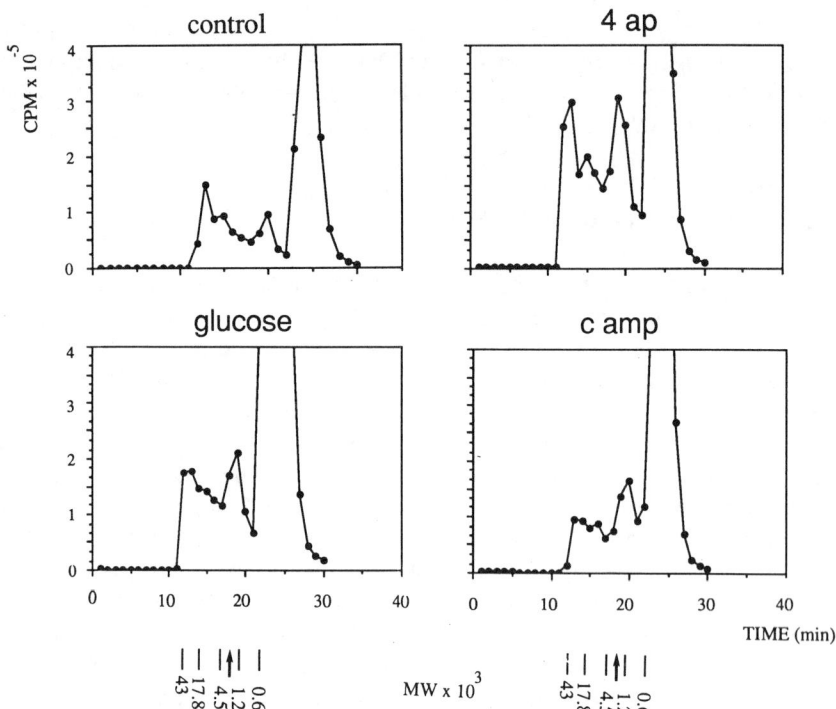

Figure 31 *In vitro* release of MIPs during electrical activity of the LGC systems of *L. stagnalis*. LGC systems were prelabelled overnight in Ringer containing [^{35}S]cysteine, washed with several rinses of Ringer and placed in a small dish with fresh Ringer. Electrical activity and release of the LGC system was induced by several compounds as indicated. After 1 h, releasates were analysed by high-performance gel permeation chromatography. Glucose was D(+)-glucose (2 mM); 4 ap, 4-aminopyridine (0.5 mM); c amp, 8-CPT-cAMP (0.25 mM). For further details, see Figure 26 and text

8-CPT-cAMP, prevented the inhibitory response and mimicked the stimulatory one. Therefore, the role of cAMP in the regulation of the responses to dopamine remains as yet unresolved.

An interesting finding is that physiological concentrations of glucose (0.1–10 mM) applied *in vitro* can induce long-lasting discharges of action potentials in the LGCs (Figure 30). Thus, blood glucose may play an important role as an excitatory first messenger. This creates an interesting parallel with the regulation of the electrical activities of the β-cells in the pancreas of vertebrates (Petersen *et al.*, 1986). There is strong evidence that the regulation of LGC excitability involves cAMP acting on Ca-channels (Kits and Lodder, 1988). When the level of cAMP is experimentally increased, inexcitable cells turn into excitable ones and cells that already displayed enhanced excitability initiate a long-lasting spiking activity. Application of 8-CPT-cAMP, IBMX and forskolin cause enhancement of the Ca current, which can be mimicked by intracellular application of the catalytic subunit of cAMP-dependent kinase. This suggests that the effect is brought about by phosphorylation of Ca channels or associated proteins. Therefore, it is thought that an increase in the intracellular levels of cAMP and calcium is necessary for release of MIPs from the LGCs. This is entirely corroborated by the results of *in vitro* experiments employing LGC systems, prelabelled with radioactive cysteine and treated with cAMP. Application of cAMP clearly stimulates release of MIPs above background levels (Figure 31). Other compounds that induce spiking activity in the LGCs, such as glucose and 4-aminopyridine are also capable of stimulating the release of MIPs (Figure 31).

Evolutionary Perspective

The insulin superfamily of regulatory peptides signals essential steps in growth, development, reproduction and metabolism in both vertebrates and invertebrates. The members belonging to the insulin superfamily are quite divergent structurally and functionally. In vertebrates the two-chain insulins are released by the pancreas and function as metabolic hormones, whereas the single-chain IGFs and the two-chain relaxins are produced by different tissues, bind different receptors and serve other functions. IGFs are important growth regulators, and relaxins have a role in reproduction (Froesch *et al.*, 1985; Steiner *et al.*, 1985; Girbau *et al.*, 1987). In invertebrates bombyxins are found in insects, where they might be involved in the control of moulting (Kawakami *et al.*, 1989), and MIPs are involved in growth and associated metabolic processes in molluscs (Geraerts *et al.*, 1988b; Joosse, 1988). The function of sponge insulin-related peptide is still unknown (Robitzki *et al.*, 1989). The members of the insulin superfamily can be subdivided into distinct groups of related peptides, and their phylogenetic relationships can be tentatively proposed as shown in Figure 32. The functional and structural diversity of the members of the insulin superfamily raises many important questions and urges the development of new concepts concerning the evolution, phylogenetic distribution and function of the peptides belonging to the insulin superfamily. Some of these issues will be discussed below.

All members of the insulin superfamily share the basic insulin globular configuration, indicating that an early genesis of this information-rich structure has been an important step in the evolution of the insulin superfamily (Steiner and Chan, 1988). Because this basic insulin motif is found in vertebrates, insects and molluscs, it must have been present in the common ancestors, the Archaemetazoa, which date back as far as 6×10^8 years ago. Insulin-related peptide of sponges exhibits very high amino-acid sequence similarity with the vertebrate insulins (cf. Figure 27). However, the intrachain disulphide bridge in the A chain is absent. Moreover, the positions of the other cysteine residues are atypical, due to a deletion in the A chain and an insertion in the B chain. These modifications may have important conse-

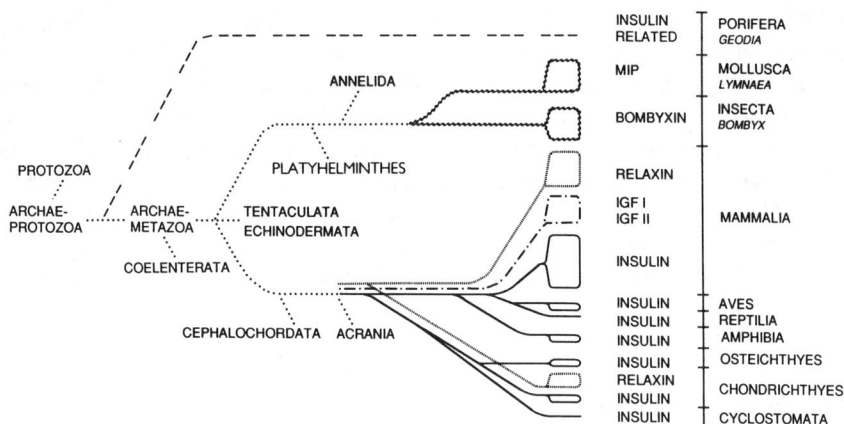

Figure 32   Tentative scheme of the phylogenetic relationships of the animal phyla and the known members of the insulin superfamily. Dotted lines, hypothetic phylogeny. Dashed line, insulin-related peptide of sponges. Wavy lines, insulin-related peptides of insects and molluscs. Cross-hatched lines, relaxins of vertebrates. Dashed/dotted lines, IGFs of vertebrates. Solid lines, insulins of vertebrates

quences for the three-dimensional structure. The absence of the intrachain bridge in sponge insulin-related peptide may perhaps indicate that a simpler ancestor molecule, probably possessing only two disulphide bridges, has been present in the Archaeprotozoa, from which both sponges and Archaemetazoa have arisen. The occurrence of a fourth disulphide bridge in the MIPs represents very likely a relatively recent development towards a more complex insulin core structure. The studies on the *MIP* genes for the first time make it likely that the ancestral insulin-related peptides of the Archaemetazoa were encoded by genes that already possessed the structural organization of the *insulin* gene. They furthermore suggest that these ancestral peptides were proteolytically cleaved from a prohormone in much the same way as the insulins and MIPs. Thus, the *IGF* genes, which have a modified intron–exon organization (Daughaday and Rotwein, 1989) and code for single-chained peptides, and the *bombyxin* genes, which lack introns altogether (Kawakami *et al.*, 1989), represent probably more recently evolved modifications of the ancestral *insulin* genes.

Interestingly, in the molluscs and insects the insulin-related peptides are produced by neuroendocrine cells in the CNS. The claim that insulin is produced by neurons in the CNS of vertebrates is controversial; however, in view of the growing evidence that pancreatic islet cells share a number of features with neuroendocrine cells (Petersen *et al.*, 1986; Alpert *et al.*, 1988), it seems possible that in the Archaematazoa the evolution of the insulin superfamily may have been within primitive neuroendocrine cells, probably associated with the digestive system (Steiner and Chan, 1988). In *Lymnaea* and other invertebrates there is evidence for the presence of immunoreactive

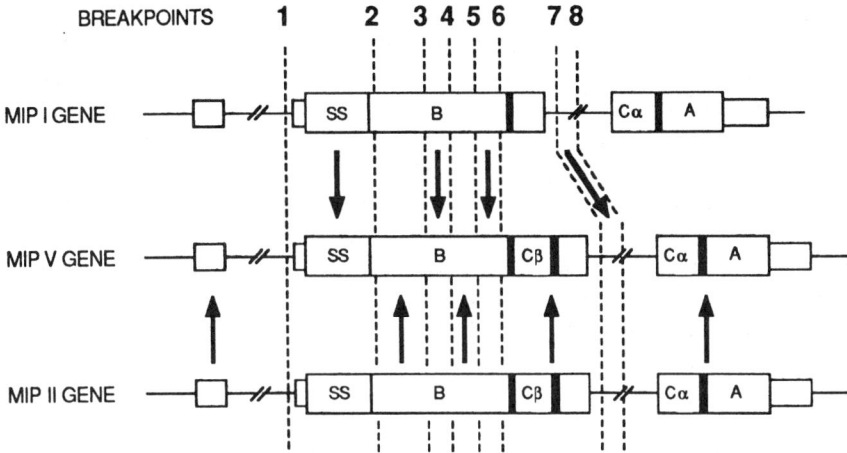

Figure 33 Schematic representation of the hybrid *MIP V* gene. The *MIP V* gene may have evolved by an exchange of large stretches of the parental *MIP I* and *II* genes, very likely by intergenic crossing-over. Breakpoints refer to putative DNA crossing-over sites, as indicated by the nucleotide sequence data. SS, signal sequence; A, A chain; B, B chain; Cα, Cα peptide; Cβ, Cβ peptide

insulin in the gut; however, structural data about intestinal insulins of invertebrates are as yet not available.

An intriguing aspect of the evolution of the insulin superfamily concerns the striking difference in the degree of conservation of its members. The vertebrate insulins and the highly similar sponge insulin-related peptide and to a lesser extent also the bombyxins are conserved, suggesting a low acceptance of mutational change. By contrast, the MIPs, like the relaxins, are widely divergent among themselves, indicating a high degree of acceptance of mutational change. Could different mechanisms account for these uneven rates of evolution in the insulin superfamily? Blundell and Wood (1975) have previously pointed out that in insulins most amino acid replacements are deleterious, due to a critical interdependence of the various residues in the molecule and their strict relationship to the three-dimensional structure and the role of this structure in the physiology of (pro)insulin—e.g. synthesis, cleavage, packaging, transport and receptor interaction. All these aspects could act as restraints during the evolution of insulin, resulting in a highly selective fixation of random amino acid replacements. This model, however, does not hold for the extensive molecular differences of MIPs and relaxins.

The *MIP* genes possess structural patterns that are reminiscent of important macroscale events that have taken place during evolution. The A and B chain domains of the *MIP* genes code for highly different peptides, while other parts, for example, those encoding C peptides, are rigorously conserved. Also, in the introns, conserved and diverged regions alternate. These phenomena can be explained by macroscale events, such as (un)equal crossing-over and/or gene conversion. A convincing example is the *MIP V* gene, which is clearly organized as a complex mosaic pattern of nucleotide sequences derived from the *MIP I* and *II* genes. Here, crossing-over events have created MIP diversity, which is especially clear in the B-chain domain of the *MIP V* gene (Figure 33). The duplication of an ancestor *MIP* gene very likely has been an initial step towards MIP diversity. This early event released the constraint on mutational divergence, and subsequent exchanges of large parts of the *MIP* genes significantly enhanced the rate of successful sequence variations. Whether this molecular mechanism is at the basis of the relaxin sequence diversity remains an intriguing question. The macroscale evolutionary events as described for the *MIP* genes may have a wider significance—i.e. in the generation of complex proteins in general.

4.   *Concluding Remarks and Future Trends*

From the studies on the molluscan peptidergic model systems several interesting conclusions can be drawn. As we have seen, the mechanism responsible for the control of such complex behaviours as egg-laying in *Lymnaea* and *Aplysia* involves the synthesis of large prohormones containing multifunctional sets of different peptides that are essential in mediating the full physiological and behavioural array associated with egg-laying. These peptides are released during long-lasting bursts of electrical activity of the peptidergic systems in order to act as neuromodulators, local hormones (non-synaptic release or paracrine actions), or circulatory hormones on targets in the CNS and the reproductive tract. Several peptides act as autotransmitters and initiate discharge activity in all cells of the peptidergic network. In addition, the electrotonic coupling among the cells probably is a means for the synchronization of the activities of the constituent neurons. These features provide the means for the sudden release of large amounts of bioactive peptides. Other peptide-secreting systems displaying episodic release in, e.g. the hypothalamus and pituitary of vertebrates, may have similar properties. The peptides derived from the egg-laying peptide precursors are packaged in distinct vesicle classes that have unique subcellular localizations. The peptides are not recovered in stoichiometries defined by the prohormones, which suggests that cellular trafficking, not precursor structure, defines the levels and sites of release of the various bioactive peptides. This separation of synthesis, packaging, transport and release expands the information content of a prohormone by generating various vesicle classes containing different combinations of bioactive peptides.

The neuropeptide gene families controlling egg-laying and growth in molluscs code for different though related (sets of) bioactive peptides. This has several interesting consequences. First, the diversity and complexity of physiological and behavioural processes that can be controlled by a gene family coding for different though related sets of neuropeptides is greatly expanded. Thus, neuropeptide gene families coding for different peptides are extremely well suited for the regulation of vital and often long-lasting life processes. Second, the expression of the members of neuropeptide gene families may be controlled in a tissue-specific way. The CDCH and ELH genes are expressed in neurons of the CNS and of the peripheral nervous system and in secretory cells of the reproductive tract. It seems likely that the peptides generated in these tissues have a role in the co-ordination of some (behavioural) aspect related to egg-laying. Thus, tissue-specific expression of neuropeptide gene families is a means to control local processes that are part of a larger physiological or behavioural programme. Third, a large number of or even all members of a neuropeptide gene family may be expressed in one type of neuron. In *Lymnaea* several genes of the *MIP* gene family are expressed in a stimulus-dependent way in the LGCs. A neuron's ability to express alternative peptides indicates that it has available a greater number of codes for communication with its targets; therefore, this type of differential expression and release of different neuropeptides endows the peptidergic neuron with a considerably increased adaptive function for information-handling.

Acknowledgements

The authors wish to thank Prof. Joosse and Dr Kits for a critical reading of the manuscript.

References

Alpert, S., Hanahan, D. and Tertelman, G. (1988). Hybrid insulin genes reveal a developmental lineage for pancreatic endocrine cells and imply a relationship with neurons. *Cell*, **53**, 295–308

Benjamin, P. R., Swindale, N. V. and Slade, C. T. (1976). Electrophysiology of identified neurosecretory neurons in the pond snail *Lymnaea stagnalis* (L.). In *Neurobiology of Invertebrates. Gastropoda Brain* (ed. J. Salanki). Akademiai Kiado, Budapest, pp. 85–100

Blundell, T. L. and Humbel, R. E. (1980). Hormone families: pancreatic hormones and homologous growth factors. *Nature*, **287**, 781–787

Blundell, T. L. and Wood, S. P. (1975). Is the evolution of insulin Darwinian or due to selectively neutral mutation? *Nature*, **257**, 197–203

Boer, H. H., Groot, C., de Jong-Brink, M. and Cornelisse, C. J. (1977). Polyploidy in the freshwater snail *Lymnaea stagnalis* (Gastropoda, Pulmonata). A cytophotometric analysis of the DNA in neurons and some other cell types. *Neth. J. Zool.*, **27**, 245–252

Brownell, P. H. (1983). Neuroendocrine mechanisms of visceromotor behavior in *Aplysia*. In *Molluscan Neuro-Endocrinology* (ed. J. Lever and H. H. Boer). North-Holland, Amsterdam, pp. 78–81

Brussaard, A. B., Ebberink, R. H. M., Schluter, N. C. M., Kits, K. S. and Ter Maat, A. (1990). Discharge induction in molluscan peptidergic cells requires a specific set of four autoexcitatory neuropeptides. *Neuroscience* (in press)

Brussaard, A. B., Kits, K. S., Ter Maat, A., van Minnen, J. and Moed, P. J. (1988). Dual inhibitory action of FMRFamide on peptidergic neurons controlling egg laying behavior in the pond snail. *Brain Res.*, **447**, 35–51

Buma, P., Roubos, E. W. and Pieters, F. A. L. (1983). Significance of calcium and cAMP for the control of neurohormone release by the neuroendocrine caudo-dorsal cells of the freshwater snail *Lymnaea stagnalis.* In *Molluscan Neuro-Endocrinology* (ed. J. Lever and H. H. Boer). North-Holland, Amsterdam, pp. 74–77

Chiu, A. Y., Hunkapiller, M. W., Heller, E., Stuart, D. K., Hood, L. E. and Strumwasser, F. (1979). Purification and primary structure of the neuropeptide egg-laying hormone of *Aplysia californica. Proc. Natl Acad. Sci. USA*, **76**, 6656–6660

Coggeshall, R. E. (1967). A light and electron microscope study of the abdominal ganglion of *Aplysia californica. J. Neurophysiol.*, **30**, 1263–1287

Coggeshall, R. E., Yakstra, B. A. and Schwartz, F. J. (1970). A cytophotomeric analysis of DNA in the nucleus of the giant cell, R-2, in *Aplysia. Chromosoma*, **32**, 205–212

Daughaday, W. H. and Rotwein, P. (1989). Insulin-like growth factors I and II. Peptide, messenger ribonucleic acid and gene structures, serum, and tissue concentrations. *Endocr. Rev.*, **10**, 68–91

Dictus, W. J. A. G., de Jong-Brink, M. de and Boer, H. H. (1987). A neuropeptide (calfluxin) is involved in the influx of calcium into mitochondria of the albumen gland of the freshwater snail *Lymnaea stagnalis. Gen. Comp. Endocrinol.*, **65**, 439–450

Ebberink, R. H. M., van Loenhout, H., Geraerts, W. P. M. and Joosse, J. (1985). Purification and amino acid sequence of the ovulation hormone of *Lymnaea stagnalis. Proc. Natl Acad. Sci. USA*, **82**, 7767–7771

Fisher, J. M., Sossin, W., Newcomb, R. and Scheller, R. H. (1988). Multiple neuropeptides derived from a common precursor are differentially packaged and transported. *Cell*, **54**, 813–822

Froesch, E. R., Schmidt, C., Schwander, J. and Zapf, J. A. (1985). Actions of insulin-like growth factors. *Ann. Rev. Physiol.*, **47**, 443–467

Geraerts, W. P. M. (1976a). Control of growth by the neurosecretory hormone of the light green cells in the freshwater snail *Lymnaea stagnalis. Gen. Comp. Endocrinol.*, **29**, 61–67

Geraerts, W. P. M. (1976b). The role of the lateral lobes in the control of growth and reproduction in the hermaphrodite freshwater snail *Lymnaea stagnalis. Gen. Comp. Endocrinol.*, **29**, 97–108

Geraerts, W. P. M. and Bohlken, S. (1976). The control of ovulation in the hermaphrodite freshwater snail *Lymnaea stagnalis* by the neurohormone of the caudodorsal cells. *Gen. Comp. Endocrinol.*, **28**, 350–357

Geraerts, W. P. M. and Hogenes, Th. M. (1985). Heterogeneity of peptides released by electrically active neuroendocrine caudodorsal cells of *Lymnaea stagnalis. Brain Res.*, **331**, 51–61

Geraerts, W. P. M., Ter Maat, A. and Hogenes, Th. M. (1984). Studies on release activities of the neurosecretory caudo-dorsal cells of *Lymnaea stagnalis.* In *Biosynthesis, Metabolism and Mode of Action of Invertebrate Hormones* (ed. J. Hoffmann and M. Porchet). Springer-Verlag, Berlin, pp. 44–50

Geraerts, W. P. M., Ter Maat, A. and Vreugdenhil, E. (1988a). The peptidergic neuroendocrine control of egg-laying behavior in *Aplysia* and *Lymnaea.* In *Endocrinology of Selected Invertebrate Types* (ed. H. Laufer and G. H. Downer). Alan R. Liss, New York, pp. 141–231

Geraerts, W. P. M., Vreugdenhil, E. and Ebberink, R. H. M. (1988b). Bioactive peptides in molluscs. In *Invertebrate Peptide Hormones* (ed. M. C. Thorndyke and G. Goldsworthy). Cambridge University Press, Cambridge, pp. 377–468

Girbau, M., Gomez, J. A., Lesniak, M. A. and de Pablo, F. (1987). Insulin and insulin-like growth factor I both stimulate metabolism, growth and differentiation in the postneurula chick embryo. *Endocrinology*, **121**, 1477–1482

Jansen, R. F. and Bos, N. P. A. (1984). An identified neuron modulating the activity of the ovulation hormone producing caudo-dorsal cells of the pond snail *Lymnaea stagnalis. J. Neurobiol.*, **15**, 161–167

Jansen, R. F. and Ter Maat, A. (1985). Ring neuron control of columellar motor neurons during egg-laying behaviour in the pond snail. *J. Neurobiol.*, **16**, 1–14

Joosse, J. (1964). Dorsal bodies and dorsal neurosecretory cells of the cerebral ganglia of *Lymnaea stagnalis* L. *Arch. Neerl. Zool.*, **15**, 1–103

Joosse, J. (1988). The hormones of molluscs. In *Endocrinology of Selected Invertebrate Types* (ed. H. Laufer and G. H. Downer). Alan R. Liss, New York, pp. 89–140

Kaczmarek, L. K., Finbow, M., Revel, J.-P. and Strumwasser, F. (1979). The morphology and coupling of *Aplysia* bag cells within the abdominal ganglion and in cell culture. *J. Neurobiol.*, **10**, 535–550

Kawakami, A., Iwami, M., Nagasawa, H., Suzuki, A. and Ishizaki, H. (1989). Structure and organization of four clustered genes that encode bombyxin, an insulin-related brain secretory peptide of the silkmoth *Bombyx mori*. *Proc. Natl Acad. Sci. USA*, **84**, 6843–6847

Kandel, E. R. (1979). *Behavioral Biology of* Aplysia. W. H. Freeman, San Francisco

Kauer, J. A., Fisher, T. E. and Kaczmarek, L. K. (1987). Alpha bag cell peptide directly modulates the excitability of the neurons that release it. *J. Neurosci.*, **7**, 3623–3632

Kits, K. S. (1980). States of excitability in ovulation hormone producing neuroendocrine cells of *Lymnaea stagnalis* (Gastropoda) and their relation to the egg-laying cycle. *J. Neurobiol.*, **11**, 397–410

Kits, K. S. and Lodder, J. C. (1988). cAMP increases excitability in growth hormone producing neurones by enhancement of Ca-current. In *Neurobiology of Invertebrates; Transmitters, Modulators and Receptors. Symp.Biol. Hung.*, **36**, 655–667

Kupfermann, I. (1967). Stimulation of egg laying: possible neuroendocrine functions of bag cells of abdominal ganglion of *Aplysia*. *J. Neurophysiol.*, **33**, 877–881

Mahon, A. C., Nambu, J. R., Taussig, R., Shyamala, M., Roach, A. and Scheller, R. H. (1985). Structure and expression of the egg-laying hormone gene family in *Aplysia*. *J. Neurosci.*, **5**, 1872–1880

Mayeri, E., Brownell, P. H. and Branton, W. D. (1979a). Multiple, prolonged actions of neuroendocrine bag cells on neurons in *Aplysia*. II. Effects on beating pacemaker and silent neurons. *J. Neurophysiol.*, **42**, 1184–1197

Mayeri, E., Brownell, P. H., Branton, W. D. and Simon, S. B. (1979b). Multiple, prolonged actions of neuroendocrine bag cells on neurons in *Aplysia*. I. Effects on bursting pacemaker neurons. *J. Neurophysiol.*, **42**, 1165–1184

van Minnen, J., Dirks, R. W., Vreugdenhil, E. and van Diepen, J. (1989). Expression of the egg-laying hormone genes in peripheral neurons and exocrine cells in the reproductive tract of the mollusc *Lymnaea stagnalis*. *Neuroscience*, **33**, 35–46

van Minnen, J., van der Haar, Ch., Raap, A. K. and Vreugdenhil, E. (1988). Localization of ovulation hormone-like neuropeptide in the central nervous system of the snail *Lymnaea stagnalis* by means of immunocytochemistry and *in situ* hybridization. *Cell Tiss. Res.*, **251**, 477–484

van Minnen, J., Reichelt, D. and Lodder, J. C. (1980). An ultrastructural study of the neurosecretory Canopy Cell of the pond snail *Lymnaea stagnalis* (L.), with the use of the horseradish peroxidase tracer technique. *Cell Tiss. Res.*, **214**, 453–462

Nagle, G. T., Painter, S. D. and Blankenship, J. E. (1989). Post-translational processing in model neuroendocrine systems: precursors and products that coordinate reproductive activity in *Aplysia* and *Lymnaea*. *J. Neurosci. Res.*, **23**, 359–370

Nagle, G. T., Painter, S. D., Blankenship, J. E. and Kurosky, A. (1988). Proteolytic processing of egg-laying hormone-related precursors in *Aplysia*. Identification of peptide regions critical for biological activity. *J. Biol. Chem.*, **263**, 9223–9237

Nahon, J. L., Presse, F., Bittencourt, J. C., Sawchenko, P. E. and Vale, W. (1989). The rat melanin-concentrating hormone messenger ribonucleic acid encodes multiple putative neuropeptides coexpressed in the dorsolateral hypothalamus. *Endocrinology*, **125**, 2056–2065

Nambu, J. R. and Scheller, R. H. (1986). Egg-laying hormone genes of *Aplysia*: evolution of the ELH gene family. *Neuroscience*, **6**, 2026–2036

Newcomb, R., Fisher, J. M. and Scheller, R. H. (1988). Processing of the egg-laying hormone precursor in the bag cell neurons of *Aplysia*. *J. Biol. Chem.*, **263**, 12514–12521

Newcomb, R. and Scheller, R. H. (1987). Proteolytic processing of the *Aplysia* egg-laying hormone and R3–14 neuropeptide precursors. *J. Neurosci*, **7**, 854–863

Petersen, O. H., Findlay, I., Suzuki, K. and Dunne, M. J. (1986). Messenger-mediated control of potassium channels in secretory cells. *J. Exp. Biol.*, **124**, 33–52

Robitzki, A., Schroder, H. C., Ugarkovic, D., Pfeifer, K., Uhlenbruck, G. and Muller W. E. G. (1989). Demonstration of an endocrine circuit for insulin in the sponge *Geodia cydonium*. *EMBO Jl*, **8**, 2905–2909

Rothman, B. S., Mayeri, E., Brown, R. O., Yuan, P.-M. and Shively, J. E. (1983). Primary structure and neuronal effects of α-bag cell peptide, a second candidate neurotransmitter encoded by a single gene in bag cell neurons of *Aplysia*. *Proc. Natl Acad. Sci. USA*, **80**, 5753–5757

Roubos, E. W. (1984). Cytobiology of the ovulation neurohormone producing caudo-dorsal cells of the snail *Lymnaea stagnalis*. *Int. Rev. Cytol.*, **89**, 295–346

Roubos, E. W., van Leeuwen, J. P. T. M. and Maijers, A. (1985). Ultrastructure of gap junctions in the central nervous system of *Lymnaea stagnalis*, with particular reference to electrotonic coupling between the neuroendocrine caudo-dorsal cells. *Neuroscience*, **14**, 711–722

Scheller, R. H., Jackson, J. F., McAllister, L. B., Schwartz, J. H., Kandel, E. R. and Axel, R. (1982). A family of genes that codes for ELH, a neuropeptide eliciting a stereotyped pattern of behavior in *Aplysia. Cell.*, **28**, 707–719

Schmidt, E. D. and Roubos, E. W. (1987). Morphological basis for nonsynaptic communication within the central nervous system by exocytotic release of secretory material from the egg-laying stimulating neuroendocrine caudo-dorsal cells of *Lymnaea stagnalis. Neuroscience*, **20**, 247–257

Smit, A. B., Vreugdenhil, E., Ebberink, R. H. M., Geraerts, W. P. M., Klootwijk, J. and Joosse, J. (1988). Growth-controlling molluscan neurons produce the precursor of an insulin-related peptide. *Nature*, **331**, 535–538

Steiner, D. F. and Chan, S. J. (1988). Perspective: An overview of insulin evolution. *Horm. Metab. Res.*, **20**, 443–444

Steiner, D. F., Chan, S. J., Welsh, J. M. and Kwok, S. C. M. (1985). Structure and evolution of the insulin gene. *Ann. Rev. Genet.*, **19**, 463–468

Stuart, D., Chiu, A. and Strumwasser, F. (1980). Neurosecretion of egg-laying hormone and other peptides from electrically active bag cell neurons of *Aplysia. J. Neurophysiol.*, **43**, 488–490

Shyamala, M., Nambu, J. R. and Scheller, R. H. (1986). Expression of the egg-laying hormone gene family in the head ganglia of *Aplysia. Brain Res.*, **371**, 49–57

Ter Maat, A., Dijcks, F. A. and Bos, N. P. A. (1986). *In vivo* recordings of neuroendocrine cells (caudo-dorsal cells) in the pond snail. *J. Comp. Physiol.*, **158A**, 853–859

Ter Maat, A., Geraerts, W. P. M., Jansen, R. F. and Bos, N. P. A. (1987). Chemically mediated positive feedback generates long-lasting afterdischarge in a molluscan neuroendocrine system. *Brain Res.*, **438**, 77–82

Ter Maat, A., Lodder, J. C. and Wilbrink, M. (1983a). Induction of egg laying in the pond snail *Lymnaea stagnalis* by environmental stimulation of the release of ovulation hormone from the caudo-dorsal cells. *Int. J. Invert. Reprod.*, **6**, 239–247

Ter Maat, A., Roubos, E. W., Lodder, J. C. and Buma, P. (1983b). Integration of biphasic synaptic input by electrotonically coupled neuroendocrine caudo-dorsal cells in the pond snail. *J. Neurophysiol.*, **49**, 1392–1409

de Vlieger, T. A., Kits, K. S., Ter Maat, A. and Lodder, J. C. (1980). Morphology and electrophysiology of the ovulation hormone producing neuro-endocrine cells of the freshwater snail *Lymnaea stagnalis* (L.). *J. Expl. Biol.*, **84**, 259–271

de Vlieger, T. A., Lodder, J. C., Werkman, T. R. and Stoof, J. C. (1987). Change in excitability in growth hormone producing cells of *Lymnaea stagnalis* induced by dopamine receptor stimulation. In *Neurobiology: Molluscan Models* (ed. H. H. Boer, W. P. M. Geraerts and J. Joosse). North-Holland, Amsterdam, pp. 172–178

Vreugdenhil, E., Jackson, J. F., Bouwmeester, T., Smit, A. B., van Minnen, J., van Heerikhuizen, H., Klootwijk, J. and Joosse, J. (1988). Isolation, characterization, and evolutionary aspects of a cDNA clone encoding multiple neuropeptides involved in the stereotyped egg-laying behavior of the freshwater snail *Lymnaea stagnalis. J. Neurosci.*, **8**, 4184–4191

Wendelaar Bonga, S. E. (1970). Ultrastructure and histochemistry of neurosecretory cells and neurohaemal areas in the pond snail *Lymnaea stagnalis* (L.). *Z. Zellforsch.*, **108**, 190–224

Index

305